Hospital Administration

Hospital Administration

Third Edition

CM Francis
MBBS, PhD (Cambridge)
Consultant
Planning and Management
Community Health Cell, Bangalore, India

and

Mario C de Souza
MBBS, FIIMB
Medical Superintendent
The Royal Hospital
&
Advisor, Hospital Administration
Ministry of Health
Sultanate of Oman
Muscat

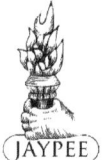

JAYPEE BROTHERS MEDICAL PUBLISHERS
The Health Sciences Publisher
New Delhi | London | Panama

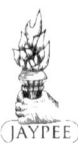 **Jaypee Brothers Medical Publishers (P) Ltd**

Headquarters
Jaypee Brothers Medical Publishers (P) Ltd
4838/24, Ansari Road, Daryaganj
New Delhi 110 002, India
Phone: +91-11-43574357
Fax: +91-11-43574314
Email: jaypee@jaypeebrothers.com

Overseas Offices

J.P. Medical Ltd
83 Victoria Street, London
SW1H 0HW (UK)
Phone: +44 20 3170 8910
Fax: +44 (0)20 3008 6180
Email: info@jpmedpub.com

Jaypee-Highlights Medical Publishers Inc
City of Knowledge, Bld. 235, 2nd Floor
Clayton, Panama City, Panama
Phone: +1 507-301-0496
Fax: +1 507-301-0499
Email: cservice@jphmedical.com

Jaypee Brothers Medical Publishers (P) Ltd
Bhotahity, Kathmandu, Nepal
Phone: +977-9741283608
Email: kathmandu@jaypeebrothers.com

Website: www.jaypeebrothers.com
Website: www.jaypeedigital.com

© 2000, CM Francis and Mario C de Souza

The views and opinions expressed in this book are solely those of the original contributor(s)/author(s) and do not necessarily represent those of editor(s) of the book.

All rights reserved. No part of this publication may be reproduced, stored or transmitted in any form or by any means, electronic, mechanical, photocopying, recording or otherwise, without the prior permission in writing of the publishers.

All brand names and product names used in this book are trade names, service marks, trademarks or registered trademarks of their respective owners. The publisher is not associated with any product or vendor mentioned in this book.

Medical knowledge and practice change constantly. This book is designed to provide accurate, authoritative information about the subject matter in question. However, readers are advised to check the most current information available on procedures included and check information from the manufacturer of each product to be administered, to verify the recommended dose, formula, method and duration of administration, adverse effects and contraindications. It is the responsibility of the practitioner to take all appropriate safety precautions. Neither the publisher nor the author(s)/editor(s) assume any liability for any injury and/or damage to persons or property arising from or related to use of material in this book.

This book is sold on the understanding that the publisher is not engaged in providing professional medical services. If such advice or services are required, the services of a competent medical professional should be sought.

Every effort has been made where necessary to contact holders of copyright to obtain permission to reproduce copyright material. If any have been inadvertently overlooked, the publisher will be pleased to make the necessary arrangements at the first opportunity. The **CD/DVD-ROM** (if any) provided in the sealed envelope with this book is complimentary and free of cost. **Not meant for sale.**

Inquiries for bulk sales may be solicited at: jaypee@jaypeebrothers.com

Hospital Administration

First Edition: 1991
Second Edition: 1995
Third Edition: 2000
  Reprint: 2004
  Reprint: **2019**
ISBN 978-81-7179-721-9

Preface to the Third Edition

Two major developments in recent times have had a profound effect on the working of hospitals the world over: (i) came the tenet that hospitals are obliged to guarantee an acceptable standard of care, and (ii) the insistence that the desired clinical outcome be assured at a reasonable or even predefined cost. Hospital trustees, patients, third-party payers and the public at large are no longer willing to tolerate lesser efficiency and productivity on the part of hospitals as compared to other industries. It is for this reason that professionalism in Hospital Administration and Hospital Management as a discipline, has grown tremendously in the last few decades.

In India too, more and more there is the conviction that hospitals must be run by trained professionals. Gone are the days when a doctor, just by virtue of seniority or social standing in clinical circles, could take on the reins of a hospital. Beyond exposure to basic clinical aspects and the general workings of hospitals, Hospital Administrators of today require knowledge and skills in various fields, including personnel management and labour relations, financial management, materials management, management engineering, hospital law, patient relations, etc. In response to this felt need, several hospital management courses have been established in India during the last 15 years. But extensive reading material on this subject, specific to the Indian context, is lacking. Thus, the need for this book, *Hospital Administration,* first published in 1991. It was extremely well received. A second edition was brought out in 1995.

The first two editions were focussed on the practical needs of the Hospital Administrator. Yet, the book was being prescribed for and used by students of Hospital Management in various universities and courses of study.

This edition is an attempt by the authors to significantly improve on the previous editions and also focus on the educational needs of students of Hospital Management without losing the practical approach. Several chapters have undergone major revision to include as much authentic and reference material as may be required by students and practicing professionals. These revised topics include: Hospital Administrator—Role and Responsibilities, Hospital Organization—Structure and Function, Hospital Committees, Medical Staff Organization, Nursing Service, Medical Records. There are also new chapters that have been added in this edition: Day Care, The Operating Department, Quality Management in Our Hospitals, Quality Management Programs: Techniques and Tools, Ethics, Laws Applicable to Hospitals, and Consumer Protection Act.

It is hoped that this revised and improved version will prove itself extremely useful to students, serve as a working guide to professionals in the field and help in the better administration of our hospitals.

CM Francis
Mario C de Souza

Preface to the First Edition

Hospitals represent a sizable investment of resources. There is increasing concern to improve the quality of administration in our hospitals to meet the rising expectations of people. There are new needs and new demands. New pressures require better responses from improved administration. These pressures include demands for the availability of newer diagnostic and treatment procedures, equity, accountability, and many others.

Many hospital administrators, facing the complex problems in administering hospitals had asked me to write a book, based on my experience. This book is the result. It is hoped that the book will help the hospital administrators to identify and solve many of the problems faced by them. As present problems are solved, new problems come to the fore; it is a continuous process. The administrator must not only solve problems as they arise but also anticipate them and prevent them.

A hospital is a service organisation. The problems and their solutions are different from a manufacturing concern. The objectives are different. The ways of tackling the problems are also different. There is often a feeling that the problems in the governmental and voluntary sectors of hospital administration are different. The similarities are far more than the differences. If we go to the roots of the problems, the causes are exactly the same.

The objective of any hospital is to help people attain and maintain health. The hospital provides service such that people can regain health and remain healthy, improving the quality of life. Compassion and competence should mark that service. In recent times, with the shift in emphasis to competence, compassion is being neglected. This is bringing hospitals into disrepute. The human aspect of care should never be lost sight of.

A hospital administrator must constantly make decisions. This is not easy. He must choose between alternatives which will have direct and indirect effects on individuals, families and the community served by the hospital.

The cost of providing hospital care is increasing with alarming speed. How is an administrator to hold the line on cost? There are pressures on administration by the professionals who want more and more sophisticated tests and procedures. The users want the cost to be reduced. With the present economic situation in the country most of the members of our society cannot (and most do not need to) afford the high cost technologies. Others demand them. Here is the dilemma.

A hospital has a diversity of people with different backgrounds, training and outlook. The administrator has to bring about harmony and ensure smooth, efficient and comprehensive working of the entire hospital to achieve its objectives. The people in the hospital have to be motivated to give the best possible care within the resources available.

The health care system needs change. The hospital administrator has a major role in bringing about the change. It is a challenge and an opportunity as well.

CM Francis

Contents

Section 1
Introduction

1. Introduction -- *1*

Section 2
Hospital Administrator

2. The Hospital Administrator – Role and Responsibilities --- *6*
3. Profile of an Effective Hospital Administrator --------------- *12*

Section 3
Managerial Skills

4. Planning -- *19*
5. Information System -- *24*
6. Communication --- *31*
7. Delegation --- *37*
8. Decision Making --- *41*
9. Monitoring and Evaluation -------------------------------------- *46*
10. Managing Time --- *52*
11. Meetings --- *58*
12. Negotiations -- *64*
13. Innovation --- *67*

Section 4
Hospital Organization

14. Hospital Organization—Structure and Function ----------- *75*
15. Hospital Committees -- *93*

Section 5
The Clinical Services

16. The Medical Staff Organization ----------------------------- *107*

Section 6
The Nursing Services

17. Nursing Service -- *124*

Section 7
Specialized Service Areas

18. Casualty Services -- *138*
19. Disaster: Be Prepared --------------------------------------- *150*
20. Outpatient Services --- *155*
21. Day Care --- *163*
22. The Operating Department ---------------------------------- *171*
23. Diagnostic Services -- *180*
24. Medical Records --- *185*
25. Pharmacy -- *204*

Section 8
Human Resources

26. Personnel -- *221*
27. Performance Appraisal System ------------------------------ *233*

Section 9
Materials Management

28. Materials Management -------------------------------------- *247*

Section 10
Finances

29. Finances --- *271*
30. Activity Based Costing in Hospitals ------------------------ *293*

Section 11
Quality Assurance

31. Quality Management in Our Hospitals --------------------- *305*
32. Quality Management Programs:
    Techniques and Tools -- *315*

Contents **xi**

Section 12
Infection Control

33. Control of Hospital Acquired Infection -------------------- *329*

Section 13
Ethics and Law

34. Ethics --- *341*
35. Laws Applicable to Hospitals -------------------------------- *355*
36. Consumer Protection Act, 1986 ----------------------------- *359*

Section 14
India's Health Policy

37. Hospitals in the Framework of
India's Health Policy -- *371*

Section 15
Summing Up

38. Summing Up -- *380*

Index -- *383*

Section 1: Introduction

CHAPTER

1

Introduction

---

*"but they shortly found out
That the Captain they
Trusted so well
Had only one notion for
Crossing the ocean
And that was to tingle his Bell".*

Lewis Carroll, in
The Hunting of the Snark

Managing a hospital to serve its purpose requires specialized knowledge and skills as also a proper frame of attitude. Gone are the days when a skilled clinician or a person trained in business administration could be expected to manage a hospital. Specialized courses are available today. They are run by the Universities and Management Institutions. Such courses of study help the student to specialize in this frontier area between Medicine and Management. Hopefully, students trained in these institutions, with continuing education and experience, will be able to manage the hospitals effectively and efficiently.

A Hospital Administrator is primarily a manager of resources. These resources are many and varied. They are also scarce. This is especially so in a country like India. The success of the hospital administrator depends on how well he or she organizes and utilizes the available resources. The resources may be:

- People—professionals, skilled and unskilled;
- Methods;
- Measurements;
- Materials;
- Machines and equipment;
- Money;
- Time (only resource which cannot be extended);
- Information (highly valuable and expanding fast).

A hospital administrator can be compared to a conductor of an orchestra, making optimum use of each resource.

In addition to being a manager of all types of resources, the hospital administrator is:
- Conceiver of goals,
- Policy formulator, strategy planner, and
- Initiator of changes.

QUITE COMPLEX

A hospital is a complex organization and has all the attributes of an organization. But there are many special features of management and administration which are not visible in many other organizations and systems.

A HOSPITAL

- Provides personalized and individualized care; each person (patient) is unique, even when there are many persons suffering from the same disease;
- Must be highly responsive to the expectations of the individual, the family and the community;
- must be involved in primary health care and community health, even when providing secondary and tertiary care;
- Must cope with emergency care; management of crisis (accidents and emergencies) is an integral part of management of a hospital;
- Cannot make mistakes, which may end up with loss of life, or life-long disability or chronic disease;
- Has teams of professionals who expect and demand freedom for decision-making and action;
- Has difficulty in providing individual rewards or punishments; and

- Finds it difficult to evaluate its functioning, with ill-defined objectives and outcomes.

But in spite of these drawbacks, the persons working in the hospital find satisfaction. There is a sense of commitment and fulfillment.

This book has a two-fold purpose. It gives the principles of Management and Administration. It also gives the practical ways avoiding problems and, should they arise, of handling them successfully. It deals with problem avoidance and problem solving.

Hospital administration is not easy; it is highly complex. But it need not produce anxiety neurosis, if properly handled. And this book gives you help to handle situations and problems that may arise. It aims at giving you the knowledge, skills and attitude to avoid problems from arising and to solve problems should they happen. Whatever your situation, problems big and small, are bound to crop up.

Administration is often tense; it is a process. Things happen in spite of the best rules. Problems do not respect rules and regulations, or procedures. You may win or lose, depending on how you handle people and problems. Insolvable-looking problems may melt away with surprising ease, like the shadows at dawn.

Problems which looked small and simple may snowball into extremely difficult issues. Be watchful.

Do not tell a problem is difficult. If it was not difficult, it will not be a problem.

This book will help you to cope up with problems. You will deal with the problems more efficiently and effectively.

Do not make premature assumptions. Be open to all suggestions and comments.

I have often heard administrators complaining of lack of authority. I have also heard of others complain that the administrator does not use his authority. He is reluctant to use it. He is afraid to use it—afraid of criticism, afraid of subsequent action by the higher authorities or by the employees.

There was a complaint that there were not enough medicines in the District Hospitals of a State. The Health Minister of the State wanted to help. In the month of March (towards the end of the financial year), some funds became available from another head of account. He placed Rs. 4 lakhs (a large amount at that time) at the disposal of each of the District Officer of Health (who was also the Medical Superintendent) with specific instructions to use the funds immediately (without lapsing) for the purpose of urgently required medicines. Only two out of the nine officers used the funds fully. With some prodding, four more used the funds partially. Three surrendered the funds wholly.

Hospital administrators often complain of increasing competition. There is competition all around. There is a sudden growth in the number of "corporate" hospitals. This brings on a commercial outlook and environment. They often bring in advanced, sophisticated technology as part of the "investment" to make more profit. While selective technological upgradation is good, not all of the newer, costly technology are necessary or even desirable. The cost is often so high, that it prices out most of the people. These 'corporate', NRI and similar hospitals offer more attractive pay packets and more perquisites. There is a fear that they may take away the best of the doctors, nurses and the technicians. Such assumptions are often wrong. Do not panic. The fact is that a well-run hospital will continue to attract the required professionals and technicians. Do not underestimate the qualities of your hospital or overestimate those of your competitors. There is place for all. The country needs more hospitals and a variety of hospitals, governmental and non governmental.

Failure

Failure is a part of the human experience. If failure is seen as a challenge, you will find that it is truly a step on the road to success and personal growth. "Failure is only the opportunity to begin again more intelligently", remarked Henry Ford.

George Clemenceau, the French statesman has said: "To fail is not unworthy, since it implies that one had attempted something".

Roger Bannister, a medical student, was expected to win the gold medal at the 1952 Helsinki Olympics. He did not. But it spurred him to try to run a mile in less than four minutes. And he broke the four minute barrier, two years after his failure at the Olympics. Bannister has said that, if he had won the Olympic gold medal, he may not have pursued the attempt to break the barrier.

Have you become miserable because you made a mistake? You did not have the right answer at a particular time or answered wrongly? Do not worry. It can happen to the best of administrators. Nobody is infallible; nobody is right all the time. You have a right to make mistakes. The only person who never makes a mistake is the man who does nothing. But you must learn from the mistakes. You must profit from the mistake. It is a learning experience. This book aims to reduce the mistakes.

Section 2: Hospital Administrator

CHAPTER 2

The Hospital Administrator—Role and Responsibilities

...*the man on the white horse*......
...*the kingpin in the entire organization*......

The Hospital Administrator is the key executive of the hospital—'the' executive that everyone looks up to for direction. It is he who sets the tone for performance and largely determines how efficiently and effectively the hospital will function. It is therefore, the Hospital Administrator who is to be finally held responsible for success or failure of the hospital.

In the past, in India and in most other countries, it was the general tendency for a hospital to be headed by a doctor. A clinician rose in stature to be ultimately appointed as the Director or Chief Executive of the hospital. But being relatively untrained in management, he was unable to cope with general administration, personnel laws and labour relations, finance, planning, materials management, etc. Consequently, *the hospital lost an excellent clinician but gained a poor administrator.* Further, such a clinician administrator was often supported by an untrained (not incompetent) non medical administrator: a bureaucrat in Government hospitals, a clergy

The Hospital Administrator—Role and Responsibilities 7

representative in the case of hospitals run by religious organizations, a confidante of the owners in the case of proprietary hospitals. With Hospital Management as an established discipline, it is now possible to have medical, nursing and non medical persons undergo hospital management training and be able to function effectively as Hospital Administrators.

Depending on one's background (medical or non medical), ownership of the hospital, and appointment of other top management executives, a Hospital Administrator—as chief executive—may be designated as: Chief Executive Officer (CEO), Director, Hospital Administrator, or Medical Director/Superintendent.

In medium and large hospitals, there is need for more than one Hospital Administrator, in which case the senior-most non medical administrator will function as the CEO/Director, while a Medical Superintendent—at times a practising clinician—may be appointed to look after medical administration. Alternatively, the CEO may be a Medical Director/Superintendent assisted by a non medical Hospital Administrator. In large hospitals, there may also be need for one or more Assistant Hospital Administrators, each overseeing a group of ancillary and support service departments.

The role and responsibilities of a Hospital Administrator, therefore vary depending on the job title, availability of other medical/ non medical administrators, and the specific duties assigned to him or her by the Management (Government / Governing Board / Trustees / Owners) of the hospital.

Duties of a Hospital Administrator

In general, the duties of a Hospital Administrator functioning in the capacity of a CEO/Director include the following:
- Being the **legal representative** of the Management, the CEO:
  — is responsible for compliance by the hospital of all Government rules, legal, ethical and statutory requirements;
  — under the principle of 'respondeat superior' (let the master answer), he is responsible for acts of all staff of the hospital: full-time, part-time, visiting.
- As the **executive arm** of the Governing Board:
  — has a general duty to oversee every activity taking place in the hospital;

- has ultimate responsibility to ensure that the mission/philosophy and objectives of the hospital permeate to its departments and staff;
- transmits, interprets and implements the Management decisions, and rules of the hospital;
- in keeping with the policies of the Management, he formulates major rules, regulations and procedures, and supervises their implementation;
- promotes effective utilization of hospital resources—human, money, materials, physical facilities and space;
- coordinates long term and annual plans for the hospital, and on approval of the Management, directs their implementation;
- submits to the Governing Body, on an annual basis, budgetary proposals, performance reports and audited statement of accounts;
- while a hospital is in the construction/equipping stage, liaises with the Management, architects and engineers on one side and with the medical/nursing professionals on the other in establishing the need for departments, facilities, equipment, furnishing and staffing;
- ensures financial viability of the organization by promoting proper marketing efforts, high turnover, and economy in use of resources.

- The CEO is also the **official link** between the Management and the employees and hence:
  - advises the Governing Board on the salary structure, service benefits, major staff grievances;
  - it is he who is ultimately responsible for healthy employer-employee relations and negotiations with employee union.

- As the **leader** of the organization:
  - creates a favourable organizational climate, resolves major organizational conflicts, promotes high employee morale and job satisfaction;
  - works closely with other key executives including the Medical Superintendent, Nursing Superintendent and Asst Hospital Administrators forming a cohesive management team to deal with day-to-day affairs;
  - selects other senior executives, department heads and senior staff, appropriately delegates duties and responsibilities to them, and makes them accountable;

The Hospital Administrator—Role and Responsibilities 9

— ensures that these executive and administrative staff function effectively and thereby run the hospital smoothly and efficiently;
— is responsible for effective communication within the hospital—between departments and sections, and between the hospital and its employees—and thus issues circulars and attends inter-departmental and departmental meetings, and reports to the Management on relevant activities of the hospital.
- As **employer**, the CEO has major responsibility for personnel management:
  — appoints staff as required and as recommended by the heads of the respective departments, and fixes their remuneration in accordance with their qualifications and experience, relative grade/level in the organization, approved salary scales and budgetary limits;
  — contracts out those services which can be more efficiently and economically performed by firms specialized in that activity;
  — is responsible for the personnel policies, adherence to service rules and staff discipline, and maintenance of accurate personnel records;
  —is the final disciplinary authority in the hospital.
- Being the **custodian** of hospital funds and property:
  — establishes a good system for the careful, economical and proper use of hospital finances, develops adequate financial controls, ensures proper upkeep of accurate financial records, and prevents misuse of hospital funds and property;
  — advises the Management on the fees/charges for various services;
  — oversees the acquisition of facilities and purchase of equipment and materials, and ensures their proper use;
  — takes action to prevent/cope with disasters, fire, theft;
  —ensures that medical records are properly maintained, and that written records of all business transactions, correspondence, and reports are properly safeguarded.
- Since the hospital exists primarily to provide care, even if not of medical background, the CEO has fundamental responsibility for the **quality of care** provided. Thus:
  — takes all necessary steps to ensure high standard of service—professional, technical and supportive.

- ensures that proper procedures are in place for the efficient admission, care and discharge of patients;
- monitors the performance of the hospital, its turnover, efficiency, effectiveness and quality of medical and nursing care provided;
- ensures that physical facilities and equipment are adequately available and functioning properly to support good and speedy patient care;
- implements a system to periodically review and improve the professional competence of staff through quality assurance, on-the-job training, and their continuing professional enrichment by involvement in continuing education, scientific activities and research.
- Being the official representative of the hospital, the CEO has responsibility for **external activities** too:
  - promotes a positive image of the hospital and develops good public relations with the Government, official agencies, vendors and the public at large;
  - maintains close contact with the Community served by the hospital;
  - liaises with Government and non-Government organizations in developing and implementing health policies and in solving health problems of the Community;
  - takes active interest in and encourages professional forums, publications, and educational activities.
- He/she carries out such other duties as may be reasonably called upon to discharge as the CEO of the hospital.

As it is not physically possible for the CEO to personally attend to all the above duties, some of them may be delegated to other key executives such as the Medical Superintendent, Hospital Administrator, Asst Hospital Administrator/s. However, the ultimate responsibility rests with the CEO/Director.

A Hospital Administrator with a designation of Medical Director/Superintendent has additionally direct responsibility for the following activities in medical administration:

- Heads the medical staff organization and is responsible for the effective functioning of clinical and ancillary services.
- Works closely with the heads of clinical and ancillary service department in developing and improving the quality and range of clinical services, diagnostic and treatment facilities, and protocols for efficient patient care.

The Hospital Administrator—Role and Responsibilities 11

- Works closely with the nursing service in developing proper procedures for good nursing and supportive care to patients.
- Assists in the appointment of technical faculty, and approves clinical privileges, which define their scope of work.
- Adopts systems to monitor and improve the quality of care, utilization of facilities, turnover, and performance of staff.
- Develops policies and procedures to safeguard staff and patients against iatrogenic injuries and nosocomial infection.
- Organizes committees for clinical audit, operation theatre, control of hospital infection, drugs and therapeutics, patient research.
- Ensures proper upkeep and confidentiality of medical records and patient documentation.
- Oversees the medico-legal, ethical and research issues concerned with patient care and coordinates with the respective clinicians in this regard.
- Promotes continuing professional education of medical, nursing and paramedical staff.

If the Medical Director/Superintendent is the CEO, many of the non medical activities—general administration, personnel, finance, materials management, maintenance of physical facilities—are more specifically delegated to a non medical Hospital Administrator.

CHAPTER

3

Profile of an Effective Hospital Administrator

...An Administrator who isn't "fired with enthusiasm" should be fired, with enthusiasm......

With the changed perspective of what hospitals are and how they should be run, the traditional role of a Hospital Administrator has undergone profound change. The Hospital Administrator is no longer merely an honest manager of resources concerned with the welfare of his hospital and its patients. The Hospital Administrator of today has to be the *conceiver of the mission of the hospital*, the *policy formulator*, the *strategy planner*. He has to be *creative* and *innovative*. He has to not only manage within the available resources but to *raise resources* to meet the challenges ahead. He has to run the hospital like an *efficient industry*, while at the same time not lose sight of the *humane touch*. He has to carve out a *unique niche* for the hospital, simultaneously keeping up with technology advances and social changes.

Abilities and Role Profile of a Hospital Administrator

- *Competence*, which comes from *knowledge*, *skills* and *experience*.
- *Sensitivity* to organizational problems, people's needs, unrealized potential of staff.
- Ability to *analyze, synthesize* and *integrate* diverse information.
- Ability to *see ahead* and *plan* accordingly: planning for the future while managing the present.
- Ability to imbibe new and creative ideas, being an *agent of change*.
- Willingness to *take risks* so as to get the new ideas accepted and implemented. The greatest failure is not to try!
- Ability to *coordinate*, bringing about harmony and collaboration; organizing, allocating resources and controlling.

- Ability to *delegate*, making effective use of his own time and that of others around him.
- Good personal *motivation* and ability to motivate and develop the people working in the hospital.
- Ability for *hard-work*. A little more determination, a little more pluck, a little more work—that's luck!
- Ability to *introspect* and *evaluate*, making adjustments as necessary.
- Sense of *equity, fairness* and *social justice* in all dealings within and outside the hospital.
- Ability to *manage stress* through patience, a sense of humour, a state of optimism, an ability to withstand unwarranted criticism. Like the Irish saying, "A man should be like his tea: his real strength appearing when he gets into hot water."

Prerequisities for Effectiveness

Understanding the Situation

You are in charge of the hospital. Find out the objectives of the institution. Each organization is unique, even though there will be many similarities. You have to understand the particular situation and the challenge. You might think that you know all about your hospital's objectives, having served in the same institution for a long time. You will be surprised!

The Hospital Mission Why was your institution established? What were the objectives then? Have the objectives been changed? Why? What are the changed objectives? Are they relevant today? Have they been achieved? If not, what have been the constraints? Can they be overcome? What are the strengths and weaknesses of your hospital? What opportunities lie ahead? Are all those working in the hospital aware of its objectives? How can these objectives be translated into concrete action plans?

The People You have to work with the people who are already there. Others may join. Some would have been selected by you; others may come on transfer or appointment by other persons or organizations. You will have to understand them, their motivations and aspirations. How best can their yearnings be channeled to serve the interests of the institution?

There will be professionals—medical, nursing and paramedical—and others. You have to knit them together as cohesive teams.

There may be power groups in the Management and among the staff in the hospital. There may be a union to work with. There will be groups of patients, employees, external organizations and the public with whom you have to interact.

Service Every hospital provides service through its resources—people, equipment, materials, others. Are these resources optimally utilized? Are certain resources in excess? Which service needs improvement? How can you amend the service with minimal increase in resources?

It is not enough if you know the situation prevailing in your hospital. Your hospital is not an island by itself. You have to look around. There are many other health care institutions to learn from. You have to work in collaboration and in healthy competition with other hospitals around. It is also important to know the situation in the country. What are the important elements of the national health policy? How does your hospital fit into the framework of this policy? What is happening in the world? What are the advances in health care—knowledge, skills, technology, attitudes.

Integrating/Coordinating

Being at the top of the organization you are able to see the hospital as a whole. Each department head visualizes the part he is chiefly concerned with. And each individual is overwhelmed only with what directly relates to him. There will be conflicts of interest and emphasis. But, you must have an integrated view of what is required. None of the departments are totally independent; they are inter-dependent. Whenever changes are suggested, you have to ask yourself—and others—the question: "what implication does this suggestion/demand have on the hospital as a whole?"

(For example: The Prosthetic and Orthotic Centre in Hospital M changed the working days in a week to five and a half days. There was immediately a demand from other departments to follow suit. The decision had to be reversed, as the hospital, as a whole, couldn't afford this.)

It is necessary to integrate with other hospitals and health care institutions—referrals, outreach centres, private practices. Whatever be the type of your hospital, you will not have all the necessary expertise. You will have to refer the patients to other institutions or call in their experts. Understand the capabilities of those institutions and maintain good relations with them. Your hospital can also function as a referral centre for other health care facilities. A referred patient should necessarily be back-referred, in the patient's interest, and if you want the relationship with the referring doctor / healthcare facility to grow. It is also necessary to integrate with the national programmes, for control of tuberculosis, malaria, immunization, leprosy, etc.

Leading

An effective Hospital Administrator provides the necessary leadership for the growth and development of the institution and overall improvement of the health of the people. A leader must have many qualities, important among them being:

- *Integrity* This is the most important attribute for long term leadership. A leader must not only be honest in his dealings, but he must also 'appear to be honest'. Only then will people trust and stand by you. Integrity is especially necessary in the field of health care. There must be respect for truth, confidentiality, impartiality, morality. Uphold high standards of conduct, honesty, ethics and demand the same of others.

- *Mastery over fear* A leader is prepared to take risks when indicated to bring about changes. Fear is the dungeon of the mind, into which it runs and seeks seclusion. Fear of failure can only result in failure. Every setback is a blessing in disguise for it teaches you a much-needed lesson. And you must profit from your mistakes so that you will not make the same mistake again. Do not be afraid of criticism or opposition. Remember, the kite rises against the wind!

- *Self-confidence* A leader trusts in his own ability to handle the ordinary as also new, future or extraordinary problems. Only if you believe in yourself will you demand of yourself persistent and continuous action to attain the objective. The more faith you have in your idea, the more will others accept it and comply.

- *Decision-making* It is the heart of all administrative and managerial function. Within the authority given to you, you must take decisions and act. Define the problem, analyze it, develop alternative solutions, ask the right questions and select the best option under the circumstances.

- *Constructive activity* An Administrator is always active, improving constantly the physical and other facilities. He is never idle. As Socrates said,
  > *"I call that man idle
  > who might be better employed."*

- *Initiative* It makes a person do what ought to be done. It looks out for opportunities, for new approaches, for improvements. A leader does not have to be told what is to be done. *A leader dreams things that never were and says why not!* Leadership is doing the right thing, in the right manner, at the right time, as a matter of right.

- *Enthusiasm* You must be enthusiastic about all that you do. And you must be able to transmit this enthusiasm to others, so that together you can reach your goal. Enthusiasm is contagious. Let everyone catch it!

- *Willingness to serve* There must be a genuine desire to be of service to as many as possible. This does call for sacrifice. Great achievements come with great service.

- *Singleness of purpose* Decide what you want to be done and follow it till it is accomplished. Concentrate on your objective.
  > *"Singleness of purpose is one of the
  > chief essentials for success in life."*
  > ... **John D. Rockefeller, Jr.**

- *Ability to cooperate with others* You have to work with people who have different perceptions. You must subordinate your personal objectives to the objectives of the institution and to the common good.

- *Sensitivity* You should have a mastery over what is happening in the hospital and in health care in general. You must have perceptual ability—to perceive events, problems, implications, and consequences.

Building a Team

Only a cooperative effort can produce the best results. Recognize the perceptions of the Governing Board, your colleagues and peers

Profile of An Effective Hospital Administrator 17

and your employees. Discourage power brokers and individualistic approaches. Encourage all working in the hospital to participate in planning out the various activities. This will automatically enlist their cooperation and support and ensure success of the activity. Understand the needs of others and be sensitive to day-to-day behaviour.

There are various teams working in the hospital: administrative, therapeutic, diagnostic, supportive. Build those teams and knit them together to provide *efficient, compassionate* and *competent* care.

Knowledge, Skills and Attitude

You must be knowledgeable in administrative practices and fully conversant with the rules and regulations of the Hospital. Keep abreast with the ever-changing Government rules related to personnel, labour relations, finance. Develop a means to stay up-to-date with new developments in medical technology, hospital practices, management techniques.

Knowledge of the processes, procedures, techniques and methods is useful. You cannot be an expert in everything. You do not have to. But you should know who are the experts in each area and be able to call upon their advice when needed. This is particularly necessary when taking crucial decisions regarding new projects, investment in new technology, purchase of expensive equipment, engineering and safety requirements, terminating staff.

The Hospital Administrator should keep himself up-to-date by continuing education. This will lead to professional growth, with a positive attitude, competence and confidence.

Be Creative

Creativity is necessary to improve the functioning of any hospital. You have to be creative because each situation varies from hospital to hospital and you know your hospital best. You will face new situations, new opportunities and new threats. You have to respond to them perhaps with measures not tried before. Break new ground.

The ability of the hospital to foster innovation and creativity often determines its success. Otherwise, it declines gradually, becomes moribund and even decays.

All of us have the quality of creativity, to a greater or lesser extent. But we tend to resist the unfamiliar. We want to play safe and conform. We are afraid to change the status quo.

Search for innovative ideas. Generate, recognize, support and implement new ideas. Brilliant solutions to problems may come from those ideas, which may initially appear ridiculous. Consider the ideas carefully, think over them, analyze their merits, verify their validity and then put them to use. *Ideas not acted upon are useless.*

Encourage people working with you to be creative. Listen to them, probe them, and if the ideas appear sound, try them out.

Section 3: Managerial Skills

CHAPTER

4

Planning

A major responsibility of the hospital administrator is that of planning. At a personal level we plan to some degree. We are constantly making decisions; what to do, how to do it, and when to do it, what we will do tomorrow through plans for next month, next year and coming years.

Planning is looking ahead, determining the goals, objectives, policies, procedures and methods; considering the various alternatives. Select the best alternative under the circumstances. Work out a time frame; fix a target date. While various people are to be consulted, planning cannot be delegated to someone else. Planning assures the best utilization of resources and economy of performance. Planning raises all the questions of what, why, where, when, who and how, as also how much and how many.

There are various stages in planning, starting with the conceptual stage of setting up the hospital. Planning is a continuous process, affecting improvements in the services and solving problems encountered or likely to be encountered. The administrator must be conversant with the process of planning. Constant efforts must be made to improve the quality of planning, which in turn improves implementation. Indians are said to be good in planning but poor in the implementation. Poor implementation is to a large extent due to poor planning.

Planning can be divided into two parts:
  i. Strategic, and
  ii. Operational.

Strategic planning tries to meet the long term objectives of the hospital. It defines and tries to achieve the goals set for the hospital. It gives answers to questions such as
   i. What is the purpose (mission; general objectives) of the hospital?
   ii. What kind of service is to be provided and to whom?
   iii. What are the alternatives available and how to choose the best course of action (consistent with the strategy and resources).

Operational planning helps in implementing the strategic plan. It determines what should be done and how it is done within a time frame and within the resources. The operational plan translates the strategic plan into practice.

Approaches

There are many approaches to planning. One of the best among them is the objective-oriented, problem-solving approach. It is based on the analysis of the problem, to identify the core problem and then the objectives to be achieved by solving the problem.

Problem Analysis

Analyze the main problem. The object of problem analysis is to solve or reduce the main problem. It must be done at the grass root level. Also determine the causes and effects of the problem.

Problem analysis is carried out by participation by different groups. All interested (and even uninterested but affected) persons and groups in the organization must participate. The interests may be:
- Positive (supportive)
- Negative (opposing)
- Neutral (could not care less!)

The groups participating are the beneficiaries and those affected adversely by the plan. Inclusion of all shades of views and opinions will lead to better analysis of the problem and the cause and effect. It will also lead to better cooperation when the plan is being implemented and therefore, to a better and quicker solution of the problem.

The discussion must be free and fair to bring out all viewpoints (including controversial ones) at the planning stage itself, of those affected positively and negatively. The participative analysis aims at addressing the question: What is the core problem? The members of the team identify the core problem.

Many suggestions regarding the problem may be put forward but these need not be the core problem. Often they are the causes or effects of the core problem—specific or general and immediate or remote. *Do not rest till the core problem is identified.*

The next step is the analysis of the causes of the core problem as also the effects. Many of these would have come up while trying to identify the core problem. There will be others. Identify them.

The members of a group identified a core problem: the hospital laundry is not able to meet the needs of the wards for clean linen. *The causes could be*
- Not enough machinery or equipment
- Lack of adequate skilled or semi-skilled staff
- Drying facilities not sufficient
- Insufficient management
- Improper co ordination
- Not enough linen.

The effects could be
- Machinery over-utilized/under-utilized/spoiled
- Staff dissatisfied
- Cleanliness in wards compromised
- Cross-infection and longer stay in the hospital
- Increased inventory and loss of money.

A network of causes and effects can be worked out. We can also construct a problem tree: trunk (main problem), roots (causes) and branches (effects).

Objective Analysis

The problems which are stated in negative terms are rephrased to become positive conditions to be achieved. In the problem with the laundry, the overall goal or main objective is "clean linen to meet the needs of all the wards provided". It is better to state the objective as achieved. It may not be reasonable to think of 100 percent achievement all the time. An acceptable one may be to "provide clean linen to meet the needs of the wards at least 95 percent of the time". This will be the main objective. It has to be achieved by various means, which will have to be worked out in relation to the resources. Among the means may be:

- Purchase/repair and commissioning of the right type of machinery
- Employment of skilled and semi-skilled staff of the right number and right training
- Enough drying facilities
- Improvement of management
- Coordination between the wards and laundry.

These means are then evaluated. Depending on the findings, allocate priorities. Make choices depending on the urgency, cost/benefit ratio, availability of personnel and funds and other factors.

Planning requires working out a project planning matrix. Various questions require answers:
- What is the overall goal and purpose?
- What are the desired results or outputs to be accomplished by the project?
- What are the indicators of achievement of results/outputs?
- How can they be verified?
- What are the activities necessary to achieve the desired results/outputs?

The project planning matrix looks carefully into the resources and inputs needed for the various activities: men, materials, money, time.

In the example of supply of clean linen, among the various alternatives, the means identified to achieve the objective was making available more and better washing machines. It was decided that if the machinery is installed and worked, the overall objectives will be achieved. This raised many questions:
- Are enough funds available?
- Is the machinery available?
- How much time will be taken to place orders, and to have the machinery in proper working condition?
- Will there be back-up service?
- How to train sufficient number of the staff to work the new machines?
- Can the existing staff be retrained? Who will train them? Is there need to get outside staff? What will be the impact on the existing staff?
- What is the time frame?
- What do we do with the old machinery?

A realistic rational planning requires certain steps. They are enumerated as under:
1. Situational analysis. What is the present situation? What is the problem to be solved? What is the opportunity?
2. Priority, goal and objective setting. What is to be achieved? What are the aims and targets? What is the feasibility?
3. Appraisal of the options, based on the problem/opportunity, cost-effectiveness and other barriers.
4. Selection of best possible alternative.
5. Programming the preferred alternative.
6. Implementation.
7. Evaluation.

CHAPTER 5

Information System

You require many managerial inputs to function as an effective administrator. The larger the hospital and the more complex the services provided, the greater is the need to pay attention to these requirements. Among them is the need for up-to-date, reliable information. All administrative and managerial processes depend on proper information. Hence, you require a comprehensive Information System.

"A girl jumped down from the second floor of the hospital and sustained multiple fractures and is in a critical condition".

"The intravenous fluid administered to Mahadevan in the post-operative ward produced severe adverse reaction".

"There is no pethidine available in the pharmacy".

"The blood bank refrigerator did not work in the night".

"The bed occupancy in the medical wards has fallen to below 60 percent".

"The bank balance has reached a critical level".

"The senior anesthetist has not come for work and the operations are delayed/postponed".

There are tremendous numbers of bits of information and data generated within the hospital. Do they come immediately to the concerned person, who will make the necessary decisions and take appropriate action?

Information is generated not only internally; it has to be gathered from outside also, to enable the Administrator to take appropriate measures. Information has to be gathered from other hospitals, whether governmental or nongovernmental. Information has to be obtained regarding health policies in the country. Information has to be obtained regarding new drugs, new procedures, new equipment (as also about old ones when they have to be discarded or modified).

All of them affect the day-to-day and long term functioning of the hospital. The amount and variety of the information that flow to the Administrator go on increasing at an explosive rate. The Administrator has to be enabled to cope up with the information. There is need for a system. There is need to collect, collate, process, filter, sort, retrieve and use the required type of information. Some of the information will be very important and even vital for the running of the hospital. Most of the information details are of no immediate use for the proper management of the hospital. But some of these may be useful in the near or distant future.

Too much information coming directly to the Administrator may be as bad as too little information. Too many reports, too many papers to be seen or so many persons to meet can result in the Administrator being submerged by the information. The information must be selective, relevant and useful; irrelevant data can only delay action. The Administrator must be able to digest and absorb the information, so that suitable action follows.

The information must be relevant and valid. It must be as accurate and complete as possible. Inaccurate and incomplete information may be misleading. At the same time, it may not be possible to get complete information. The system must be such that adequate information can be obtained, starting from the incomplete data or information.

It is essential that the information is obtained on time. Delayed information is useless. It may, at best, enable corrections.

It is not enough to get the raw information. The information must be collated, filtered and regrouped, such that the information is understood in its proper context. Information from one area of service or department may make it necessary to get information from other areas, which may be affected beneficially or adversely by the action contemplated.

A hospital information system must provide the needed information, without spending unnecessarily the scarce resources of men, money and time. The Administrator has to know enough for various functions:
  i. Administrative
 ii. Clinical (therapeutic, diagnostic and supportive) and
iii. Financial.

All the three are inter-related. Absence of information in any one area will have repercussions on the others.

Information helps the Administrator to match the resources with the needs, as best as possible. It helps to increase the efficiency in the delivery of services and avoid waste. It can help to plan and implement priorities so that quality of care is assured.
The system must be such that the network provides the needed information in all directions. It should respond to the urgent and critical needs, where no delay should occur. It must inform unusual incidents. It should, at the same time, be able to gather and disseminate information on a periodical basis: daily (e.g., cash balance), weekly, monthly (census of admissions and discharges), quarterly, half-yearly and annually (e.g., income and expenditure statement). Depending on the policy of the hospital, it may provide immediate information regarding admission as inpatients of staff working in the hospital or very important persons connected with the hospital, iatrogenic problems, medico-legal cases, etc.

The information system should provide periodical reports on the functioning of the clinical, laboratory, radiology, operations (major and minor), deliveries and pharmacy. There is need for periodical reports on the number of outpatients and inpatients, together with analysis of length of stay, total patient days and number of deaths. Reports on medical and nursing care are important.

Reports on the functioning of stores, dietary, linen and laundry, central sterile supply, maintenance and personnel should be obtained periodically; so also there is need for periodical reports with analysis of finance and accounts.

There are a host of other areas on which information is available and needed. So also there is need to know what is happening outside the hospital, whether it be own outreach programmes in the slums or the villages or other hospitals. A hospital administrator must be up-to-date with respect to the health policy of the state and the country as also programmes of health care.

Each hospital has (or should have) a philosophy and objectives of its own. There is need to know where the hospital stands with respect to its philosophy, goals and objectives. Only if the Administrator knows the strengths and weaknesses, corrective or remedial measures can be taken.

The value of the information system depends on:
 i. Availability on time,
 ii. Quality, complete, correct and adequate, and
 iii. Quantity; not too much; not too little.

Information System

Information is only a tool for better administration. Information by itself is of no use but, if properly used, it helps in better administration. Without correct and adequate information it is very unlikely that you will be able to administer effectively your hospital.

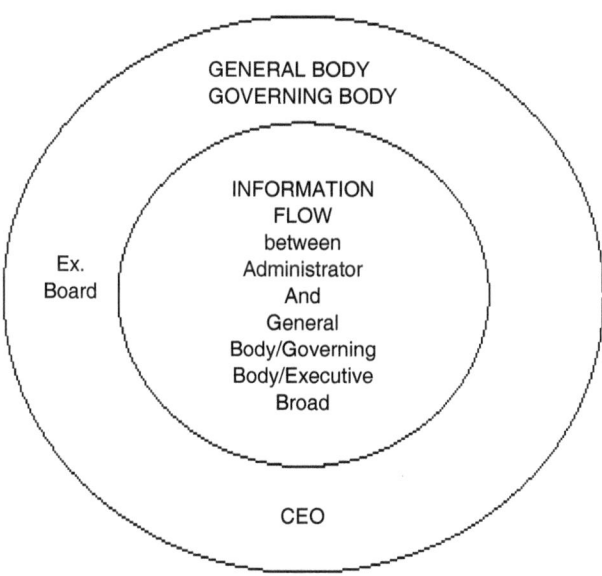

GB/EB to Administrator	Administrator to GB/EB	Between Administrator and GB/EB
Objectives	Reports	Meetings
Policies, strategies	Plans; projects	Conferences
Plans; projects	Suggestions	Reviews
Directives	Recommendations	Information
Appointments	Budget	
Feedback	Statement	

Hospital Administration

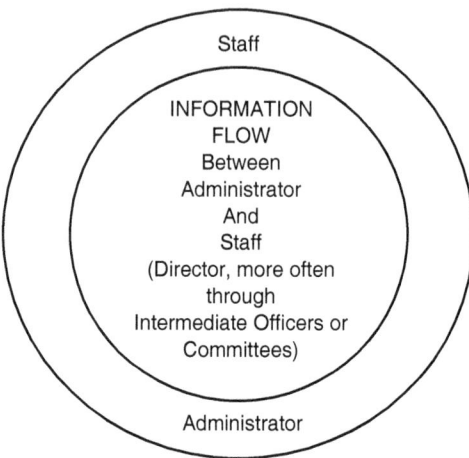

Administrator to Staff	Staff to Administrator	Between Administrator and staff
Objectives	Ideas and suggestions	Patient care
Policies and strategies	Information	Requirements
Plans; information	Reports of meetings	Meetings
Directives	Problems/grievances	Audit
Appointments	Exceptional/happenings	Social gatherings
Terms and conditions	Admission/Discharge	Newsletters
Rules and regulations	Deaths	Safety
Schedules	Accounts	Infection control
Performance appraisals	Budget proposals	
Reports	Achievements	
Education/training	Feedback	
Budget control		
Standards		
Commendations		

Information System 29

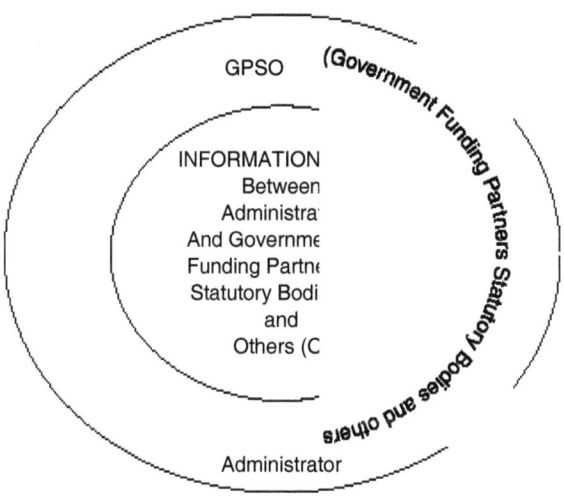

Administrator to GPSO	GPSO to Administrator	Between GPSO and Administrator
Reports	Rules and regulations	Suggestions
Suggestions	Reports (asked for)	Sharing information
Compliances	Inspections	Meetings

Fingle's law:

> The information you have is not
> What you want.
>
> The information you want is not
> What you need.
>
> The information you need is not
> What you can get.
>
> The information you can get costs
> More than what you want to pay.

30 Hospital Administration

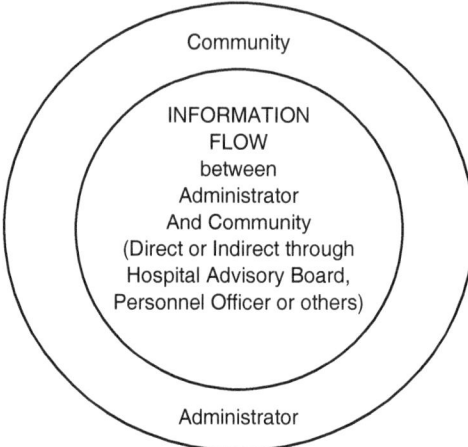

Administrator to Community	Community to Administrator	Between Community and Administrator
Objectives	Suggestions	Community health camps
Policies; plans	Requirements patients	Relatives and friends of
Seminars/workshop	Requests	Professional support
Community Health Information	Problems	

CHAPTER

6

Communication

A major part of your time as Administrator will be spent in receiving and sending information. Do you want to achieve your objectives? You have to do it through people. Communication is a two-way process, whether it be between individuals or between an individual and a group or between groups of persons. It is mutual. The people must share the idea before they can communicate with each other. All persons partaking in communication bring into the relationship their own thoughts, feelings, patterns of behaviour and points of view. Create a climate of good relationships through proper communication.

Communication is the means of imparting ideas and making oneself understood by others. Success of all administrative and managerial functions depends on effective communication. The Administrator must know what is happening in the hospital and be able to convey information to all those involved with the hospital—the employees, the patients and the public. Skills as a communicator help in the building up of morale in the hospital and confidence in the public.

What does communication involve? Communication implies that there is a *message* to be *transmitted*, that it is *received* and *understood*. Hopefully the message is accepted and, where action is indicated, the desired *action* is taken at the right time by the right people. There are many blocks to communication.
- The information does not get to the person who is to receive it.
- There is distortion by the sender, transmitter or recipient.
- There can be misinterpretation.

Ensure that the language is clear, concise and appropriate for the particular person or persons. One of the main barriers to good communication is lack of proficiency in the proper use of language. Try to be competent in the use of the local language. Verbal (spoken or written) communication is not the only means of communication. Others forms like touch and body language can be used effectively.

Even when all requirements are met, successful communication may not occur. "Still man hears what he wants to hear and disregards the rest". It is common observation that if we ask the persons who come out of meetings as to what was said by the different speakers, we get different answers. Each one focuses his or her attention on particular aspects. There can be a lack of attention; even if heard, it is not understood. There may be information overload; if too many things are said, most of it may not be retained.

People have preconceived ideas and personalized meanings. When a person speaks, he may be understood differently by the listener because of his own thinking.

Hospital M wanted to start a Cancer Detection Centre. A meeting of the Medical Staff was called. It became clear after a few minutes that there were two groups with different understanding. One group understood it in the way it was meant to be—detection of signs and symptoms in an *apparently asymptomatic person* while the other group understood it as a Cancer Diagnostic Centre, to diagnose cancer in a person with symptoms pointing to the *possible presence of malignancy*. The matter was clarified and thereafter the discussions focussed on Cancer Detection Centre.

To communicate effectively, whether in writing or by speaking, certain guidelines may be followed:

1. *Think* well what you want to communicate.
2. *Get the facts* If you wish to inform, to convince and to persuade the staff and others, mastery of facts is essential.
3. *Organize the facts* The facts should be arranged, so that they form a logical sequence, one leading to the other. Too many facts presented in a jumble form produce confusion.
4. *Outline w*hat you want to write or say before writing or speaking. Write down the points you want to make. Arrange them according to sequence and importance.
5. Have a good *introduction* It must have an impact. It must focus on the subject.
6. While writing, have *headings* and *subheadings*. In long reports, use numbering of paragraphs.
7. *Eliminate unnecessary details* Avoid facts that people can not see or use. While you must know as much detail as possible, too many details in your presentation can produce difficulties in understanding.

8. *Make one point* Every executive message should have only one main point; that point must be made quickly.
9. *Put yourself in the position of the recipient* Think how you would like to be told. Also consider his level of comprehension. Consider how the message will sound to the recipient. Who are the target people? Who will be listening to you or reading what you are writing. Keep your audience or readership in mind always.
10. Do not assume that what is known to you is known to everyone else. Most often, it is not so.
11. *Use precise, simple, ordinary language* The language must be such as is easily understood. Avoid jargon and technical language as much as possible. When you write, use short words (not more than 150 syllables to 100 words), short sentences (not more than 15 words) short paragraphs (not more than 5 sentences).
12. *Be concise* Shortening and condensing often make the matter more clear and easier to understand. Cut out unnecessary words.
13. *Be relevant* Is what you are saying or writing relevant to the topic? If not, leave it out.
14. *Maintain eye contact* If you are speaking to a person or a group of persons, maintain eye contact. There will be much greater attention paid as also more confidence in you.
15. *Be enthusiastic* Enthusiasm is contagious. Those who are to implement the plans, policies and programmes must catch it.

Often we use communication as an outlet for our emotions, for self-expression. This can be so to a limited extent. Do not overuse it. There must be a will to communicate, to explain your thought, your wish and instructions.

Communication is easier when there is mutual trust. That trust has to be earned over a long period of time. People must come to realize that the Administrator is one who keeps to his word, that he is a person of integrity.

Open Lines of Communication

There must be upward, downward, horizontal and diagonal or tangential communication within the hospital. There must also be lines of communications with other health care institutions, organizations (government and non governmental) and with the community. Build up a communication network. Effective communication, whatever be the form or medium, is an essential catalyst for good performance.

Both formal and informal channels of communication are important. One type of informal communication is the "grape vine". Do not overuse it. At the same time, do not completely avoid it. The information obtained via the grape vine path is most often inaccurate, half-truths, rumours, wishful thinking, suspicion or distorted information. Yet one should constantly watch for such information. It often reflects the mood of the people working with you. Where indicated, either directly or through the departmental heads or during conversation or talks the misinformation must be corrected.

James Callaghan, the British Prime Minister said: "A lie can be half round the world before the truth has got its boots on".

Hospital H terminated the services of an employee on probation. A rumor spread through the hospital that 13 employees in the dietary department were being retrenched, including regular employees. The incident precipitated a strike. Possibly, if the employees had been told of the exact situation, the strike could have been avoided. But the Administrator and the Personnel Officer thought it best to keep quiet.

Corrective information is very useful and should be given quickly. Unchallenged rumour often gets by as fact.

Communication serves different purposes. It can be social. It can *be imparting information*. It can be *therapeutic. Patient education* requires good communication. *Health education* needs effective communication.

Communication must often lead to appropriate action. The right information and direction must reach the right people at the right time. This is what once did not happen in JJ Hospital, Bombay, with tragic results. In the report of the Commission of Inquiry on what is popularly known as "Glycerol Deaths", Justice Lentin has this to say: "The Dean and the Medical Superintendent were negligent and guilty of dereliction in the discharge of their duties in not taking any action after receiving information of adverse drug reaction in the JJ Hospital". They should have communicated with all the users in the hospital to stop the use of the suspected drug. They should have ensured that the culprit drug was withdrawn.

Effective and quick dissemination of vital information is a must. If neglected, there can be disastrous consequences. The communication must be quick—avoid delay. It must be effective — the step taken must ensure the action desired.

When talking to the staff, call him or her by name. Every person craves for attention and to be recognized. It makes a tremendous difference when the Administrator recognizes him or her and calls him or her by name. The sound of his or her name is sweet and most important single word for that person.

If we agree that communication is a two-way process, the Administrator must listen and observe. Listening is not easy but you can and should cultivate the art of good listening.

i. Concentrate on what the other person is saying. Listen critically. The tone and emphasis can convey meanings which would be lost if you are not attentive enough. How the person said something may be more important than what he said. The unspoken words and subconscious thoughts of the person could often be understood, if you are alert.
ii. Be open to receive fresh ideas and information. Our mind is like a parachute. It does not function till it is open.
iii. Avoid distraction.
iv. Look at the person who is speaking to you. Observe the whole person. Watch for gestures, postures, facial expressions and actions.
v. Try to see things from the speaker's point of view. Tune in to his feelings. He/she will then talk freely. He/she may himself/herself find solutions to some of his problems or learn to live more peacefully with them.
vi. Encourage him to talk. Ask simple questions. Obtain clarifications. Obtain specific information.
vii. Be responsive. Show your responsiveness by your total behaviour. Show that you are interested in what he is saying. He will then communicate more freely.

"Give us grace to listen well".

Some Administrators are afraid to communicate, to inform. Information is a source of power. The Administrator might withhold information, thinking that the staff might use it in their negotiations. Negotiations must be based on facts. The staff give of their best when they understand their role and function and know what is happening. There is a very strong relationship between job satisfaction and good information. The well-informed staff perform better. They will also be more realistic in wage negotiations, especially in relation to ability of the hospital to meet the claims for increase in emoluments.

The doctors in hospital R wanted an almost 100 percent increase in emoluments. The Administrator showed them the audited statement of accounts and how the hospital was having deficit because of the care being given to the poor. The doctors settled for a smaller raise.

What are the major benefits of improved communication? Among the benefits are:

   i. Better understanding of the objectives of hospital. There is more likelihood of the achievement of the objective,
  ii. Better employer-employee relationships,
 iii. Better image of the hospital. This leads to improved quality in the recruitment of personnel, and
  iv. Better general public support, useful always, but more so in times of crisis.

CHAPTER

7

Delegation

A hospital administrator cannot do everything by himself/herself. Good management is also to get things done through others. It is therefore necessary to delegate (entrust) to others certain tasks. The hospital administrative team members often pass the buck above, to the Administrator, who may be flattered to agree and "I will do it". This tendency must be resisted. Delegate tasks. You will end up being more successful in your administration. Through effective delegation, the administrator's time can be released to perform the important jobs.

How to Delegate?

List all the jobs which have to be got done. Mark those jobs which can be got done (perhaps even better than by you) through others. Delegate these jobs. While entrusting the job, make sure that the job is spelt out in detail. Provide sufficient authority. *Delegation can be effective only if the person is given authority along with the responsibility.* Fix a deadline (time frame) for completion and make it clear to the person. Extract an obligation from the subordinate to perform effectively. Remember that the ultimate responsibility still rests on you. Monitor progress through periodic progress reports. You cannot get away saying : I entrusted the job to Keshav and he did not do it.

To Whom to Delegate?

The choice of the person is important. Delegation develops people second in command. "When a man realizes he can call others in to help him do a job better than he can do alone, he has taken a big step in his life", points out Andrew Carnegie. Assess the subordinate and then delegate. The person to whom responsibility and commensurate authority are delegated must have attitudes, abilities, knowledge and skills to carry out the delegated responsibility, utilizing the given authority.

What to Delegate?

The administrator cannot delegate his own function. The purpose of delegation is to enable the Administrator to concentrate on his own job. Delegation cannot be indiscriminate. The work to be carried out by the person to whom the responsibility is delegated has to be chosen carefully. Determine which job is to be done by you and which can be done by others. What are the jobs which
- You must do yourself;
- You must do with someone else's help;
- You could do but others also can do;
- Others should do with your help; and
- Others must do.

When delegating tasks, it is also necessary to give sufficient authority to match the requirements of the tasks. If authority is not delegated, the person to whom the task is delegated will not be able to perform the task. He or she will be considered a failure, for no fault of theirs. Delegation without authority is not delegation.

Why do Administrators not Delegate More Often?

There can be many reasons:
- The administrator thinks that he can do the job better and faster by himself. Even if this is true, the administrator must delegate. He develops a subordinate who can then be entrusted the task with confidence. At the same time, the administrator is free to do other important jobs with greater attention.
- The administrator may feel that none in his group or team is competent enough to carry out the job efficiently. There can be fear of the other person making mistakes. Take the risk. You will find that the fear was unwarranted in the majority of instances.
- The administrator may not want to delegate. There can be a feeling of job insecurity. Will the other person take over? Will the management find me superfluous?
- The administrator may not be willing to let go of his power. By delegating you will actually become more powerful.

- The administrator may not know how to delegate.

Why do Team Members not Like to Take up the Job?

Sometimes even when the Administrator is keen on delegating, the team members may not be willing to take up the responsibility (and the authority). It is always much easier to make someone else do it, especially if there is great responsibility attached to it. The member is also not sure of his/her authority. He / She may not be sure of support from the Administrator and others in the hospital. Very often, the member does not think that the extra work (with extra responsibility) will help him in his career. "Why should I take up added responsibility when there are no monetary or material benefits"?

Other reasons are fear of criticism for mistakes, lack of needed information to do the job well and lack of self-confidence. The most important factor is psychological, especially fear of making mistakes. But taking that responsibility, with the superior there to guide and correct, will certainly help in the development of the subordinate.

How to Motivate?

It is essential to motivate the subordinates to take up the extra responsibility. Put yourself in the shoes of the subordinate. Reflect on the relationships. Trust the subordinate and discuss the job with him. Assure the sub-ordinate of all necessary help in the performance of the job. Provide all necessary information and inputs.

When There is to be Delegation?

Delegation involves decision-making and implementation of decisions. There are various ways of decision-making and implementing decisions. Depending on these, there may be delegation, participation, consultation or none of them:
1. The administrator decides independently using information available or obtaining the necessary information from the subordinate. The administrator may or may not explain the reasons underlying the decision. — No delegation; no participation

2. The administrator
    i. Makes tentative decisions, discusses the problem and tentative decisions with the subordinate and then decides himself.
    ii. Presents the problems to the subordinate, gets ideas and suggestions and then decides himself.

    Consultation; no delegation.

3. The administrator and subordinate discuss the problem, develop and evaluate alternative solutions and make the decision:
    i. Administrator plays major role
    ii. Both play equal role
    iii. Subordinate plays major role.

    Participation; partial delegation.

4. The subordinate makes the decision
    i. Subject to approval by the administrator
    ii. And informs the administrator
    iii. Without informing the administrator.

    Delegation

Good management calls for delegation of what can be delegated. It is a major duty of the administrator to develop the subordinates. The administrator must guide and help the subordinate in carrying out the task entrusted, when such guidance is required but should not interfere unnecessarily. The administrator should foster an atmosphere of trust. The subordinate must be enabled to carry out the task independently but free to approach for guidance should he or she feel the necessity for it.

CHAPTER

8

Decision Making

Decision-making is the heart of all administrative and managerial functions. Within the authority given to you, you must take decisions. It is your duty to tackle problems as and when they arise in the hospital and make decisions. Ensure that the responsibilities you undertake are within the limits of your capacity. Do not accept more than you can carry out without neglect to the field to which your position is related. Others working with you might like to thrust on you the responsibility for decision making (passing the buck) because of fear of criticism or lack of interest or other reasons. Departmental problems should be tackled by the departmental heads, except when the departmental head seeks your help or it is essential that you should get involved in the problems immediately.

Decision may be *positive* or *negative*. Positive decisions may be to do something or not to do it, to cease action or to prevent action. Negative decisions are decisions not to decide and are as important as positive decisions. The decision not to decide may be taken because:
- The question is not pertinent,
- The question is pertinent but there are not enough data to take a final decision,
- The question is pertinent but the decision is to be taken by someone else (e.g., governing body), and
- You do not consider yourself competent enough to take the decision.

Decision making and problem solving are not the same. The decision may or may not lead to solution of the problem at that time.

Ramesh, an employee, was dismissed after due enquiry. The Union wanted him to be reinstated. The management decided not to reinstate him.

The decision did not solve the problem. All the same, it was a decision.

A decision may be made in various ways. It may be based on previous experience or on intuition or hunch. Decision may be taken on the basis of precedences. In the administration of the hospital, decision making must be rational. It cannot be arbitrary. There is need for scientific approach to decision-making.

For most day-to-day, common, repetitive problems, we have ready-made solutions. They are dealt with by the rules and regulations, standing orders and well-recognized procedures. When new problems arise, covering unfamiliar situations, recourse must be taken to a decision-making process.

There may be limitations to your making the decisions:
- Superiors (instructions from the Secretary to Government, Governing Body).
- Subordinates : the decision has to be implemented through the Staff working under you. One important principle is that orders will not be issued that cannot, or ordinarily will not, be obeyed. Otherwise, it can destroy authority, discipline and morale.
- Governmental regulations : Local, State and National. There may be restrictive legislation and interpretation of the legislation by the Courts, e.g., the Drugs and Cosmetics Acts, the Minimum Wages Act, the Industrial Disputes Act.
- Agreements entered into with other organizations may restrict the freedom to decide independently.
- Agreements with Union may stipulate certain kinds of action.
- General social order determined by custom, tradition, etc.

Steps in Decision Making

 i. Define the problem—Dig deep to locate the real problem. Find out the root cause. Find out what is the cause of the cause.
 ii. Analyse the problem—There will be many components to any problem. To analyse the problem we must try to get as much of the facts as possible but remember that we will not get all the facts all the time. This should not be an excuse for delay in decision making.

Case Studies

1. There are two administrative heads of departments who are in mutual conflict often. It was thought to be due to personality

differences. But on probing deeper, it was seen that the functions and duties had never been really defined. There were overlapping responsibility and authority. Each head of the department was asked to write down their perceptions of their duties and responsibilities. Based on their response, a decision was taken, after consultation, assigning specific duties.
2. The department of Physiotherapy in a hospital had a large turnover of physiotherapists. It was thought that the large turnover was because of the low pay. The head of the department suggested a higher pay but this was not acceptable to the management: it would create demands for higher pay in other departments for personnel of similar qualifications, and experience and the salary compared favourably with what was being offered in other similar institutions. The matter was looked into further. It was found that the Chief Physiotherapist, while capable and enthusiastic in her work, was unable to handle the juniors. She was sent for a course in middle management and things settled down.
3. Develop alternative solutions –ask the right questions. You have every right to put off decisions, if you need more information, more facts and more time to consult others and sort out the issues. Do not allow yourself to be stampeded to a decision. But there is no point in deferring decisions unnecessarily, in hope that the problem will solve by itself.

Once the problem has been defined and analyzed, we must search for alternative solutions. Some alternatives may be provided by your colleagues and subordinates. You must consider them and also conceive of more and better alternatives. Test each alternative, as if it has already been put into effect. Consider the probable impact and consequences. Remember, each decision has an effect on the entire hospital system.
4. Decide on the best solution under the existing circumstances.
Risk/Benefit Ratio: Every solution has some risks and some benefits. Select the one with least risks and most benefits. Doctors are aware of the risk/benefit ratio in choosing therapeutic procedures or drugs.

Economy of Effort and Expenditure Where there are similar solutions, with risk/benefit ratio more or less equal, the

alternative which calls for less effort and less expenditure of resources (men, money, materials, time) will be selected.
Acceptability The solution must be acceptable to those concerned. There is no use of a solution which is not acceptable. At the same time, it must be remembered that most solutions may not be accepted fully by everyone.
5. Implement the decision and follow it up.

Sharing Decision-Making

It may be a good idea to share the decision making with others directly affected by the decision. Decision making involves the selection of one alternative from among two or more alternatives. We must:
 i. Be aware of the alternatives,
 ii. Define each of these alternatives and the consequences of the selection of each of them, and
 iii. Exercise a choice.

The staff working with us can be involved in the decision making, especially the first two and even the third. But in this case, though the choice may be made by the whole group, unanimously or by consensus, the responsibility remains with the Administrator. He can and should overrule the majority opinion if he is convinced that the risks involved in the choice are proportionately more than the possible benefits. But in the large majority of instances, it should be possible to go along with the group's decision.

The purchase of a blood gas analyzer by Hospital M was discussed by a group of doctors and nurses involved. They considered the parameters to be analyzed and, thereby, the choice fell in certain categories of equipment. The manufacturers meeting the specifications were requested to quote and invited for discussions with the group. Considering the quality, meeting the requirement and the cost, selection was made.

The advantages of sharing decision-making are:
 i. To make possible better quality of product, meeting the particular requirements of the hospital,
 ii. Readiness of all those involved to ensure greater success in the working of the equipment, and
 iii. Satisfaction of the members in having participated in the decision making, which can bring about greater cohesion.

Muddling Through

Often, administrators are reluctant to take a rational, comprehensive decision. They would rather go slow and tackle the problems by small changes as the problems arise. This has its own advantages. It maximizes security in making change. Changes are limited. Such a policy may work out in certain circumstances.

 i. The present policies are in the main satisfactory; only marginal changes are sufficient for achieving an acceptable improvement.
 ii. There is high degree of continuity of the nature of the problem and in the available means for dealing with the problem.

Some solutions may work out in some instances for some time. But a more scientific way of solving the problems will be called for in course of time.

CHAPTER

9

Monitoring and Evaluation

Monitoring and evaluation are integral parts of the planning cycle. They have to be achievement and person oriented, focussing on both quantity and quality. Monitoring deals with ongoing assessment of programmes and activities to make appropriate corrections in the inputs; evaluation is more concerned with terminal, midterm or other long period assessment.

MONITORING

An administrator must always know what is happening in the hospital. Are you really aware of what is happening? Do you know how the hospital services—medical, nursing, pharmacy, laboratory, radiology and supportive—are being run? Are they functioning in a way they should to achieve the objectives?

A hospital organization is complex. You cannot be involved directly in everything. But you need to know what is happening in the critical areas and be able to get the information when needed.

If your hospital is well-organized, the activities will go on smoothly. If you have delegated the responsibilities to competent persons and given them commensurate authority as well, the services can be expected to be carried out without any hitch and according to the objectives of the hospital. Even then there will be exceptions which will need your intervention. There may be unforeseen problems or unexpected opportunities. Circumstances may have changed. You may have to reassess the situation, taking a comprehensive and long term perspective.

Monitoring is knowing what is going on. Closely associated with it is the function of controlling—making changes to keep the activities on course. Monitoring and controlling are mainly concerned with day-to-day activities. Evaluation is concerned with longer term assessment.

Why Monitoring?

Monitoring observes critically the activities during their implementation. It measures outputs against inputs, in achieving the objectives. The inputs may be manpower, money, materials, time and other resources. Outputs may be numbers of outpatients and inpatients, operations done, medicines dispensed, health education conducted and so on. Are the budgets being overspent or underspent by the departments and sections? Are the staff sufficient to carry out the duties? Is there under-utilization of the staff? Are there drug shortages? The questions are many and varied.

Monitoring brings out the unusual and unexpected. The Administrator can then concentrate on such happenings, whether positive or negative.

Monitoring also helps the staff to perform better. They know there is someone interested in their work, appreciates their achievements, listens to their problems and tries to solve them. Too rigid a monitoring can have an adverse effect. It has to be done judiciously. An effective administrator is always alert and on the look-out for warnings of unusual occurrences, irregularities and opportunities.

Monitoring provides feedback which could help in revision and fine tuning activities to enhance their quality and effectiveness.

Indicators for Monitoring

To monitor effectively, we need to develop appropriate indicators. Both quantitative and qualitative indicators are important.

Quantitative

- Simple counts of events or activities (numbers).
- Rates, measuring the frequency at which the events occur per day, per week or per month.
- Ratios, proportions, percentages of the work accomplished to the total.

Qualitative

In hospital qualitative indicators are particularly important. These must be developed specifically for each activity.

For an administrator, management indicators are important. Among them are processes of evolving policy, review of policy and decision-making, knowledge, skill and attitude of personnel, turnover of staff and employees, periodical review of work responsibilities and performance assessment.

An important part of monitoring will be satisfaction of the patients, their families and relatives and the community.

Financial management review is both quantitative and qualitative. It includes financial achievements, regularly of financial reports, maintenance of records and comparison of actual financial performance to budget (proportionate).

Steps for Monitoring

 i. Specify the objectives of monitoring
 ii. Decide on the scope of monitoring
 iii. Select indicators or Standards
 iv. Choose sources of information
 v. Develop methods of data collection
    a. Collect data
    b. Analyze data
    c. Take appropriate action.

How to Monitor?

Many methods are available for monitoring

Observation

Visits to wards, departments and sections. It is essential that the administrator gets about and has a very good first-hand knowledge of what is going on in the hospital. See what is happening. Spend time with the staff and discuss their problems.

Reports

These may be verbal or written. Both are equally important. The written reports may be at fixed intervals as also when they are considered necessary. The reports must be short and to the point. They must let the administrator know how the work is going on and what are the difficulties. Give feed backs on the reports.

Checklists

These can help in reviewing the activities in the hospital. If these are carried forward, they could help in having continued information.

Meetings

They help to review the objectives and targets. These meetings may be at fixed periodical intervals or can be on an adhoc basis.

Opinions

There may be complaints or appreciation. They may be made by patients, relatives, neighbourhood community, press and others. Complaints must always be investigated, even if they are anonymous and action taken. Appreciation must be fed back to the people involved. Encourage constructive criticism. It would help in improving the services.

Monitoring should be done tactfully in a hospital. Doctors and other health professionals often resent over monitoring. They guard their rights to decide what should be done for any given patient.

Peer review and medical audit are systems by means of which doctors of similar status can monitor the work and achievement of each other.

Monitoring systems have to be reviewed periodically in the light of experience.

An important requirement provides prompt feedback to the personnel concerned.

EVALUATION

Evaluation is the process of collecting data and using the data to form judgements. It often helps to reach decisions about the activity being evaluated. There is overall appraisal of direction, efficiency, costs and outcome of the programme.

Evaluation is an integral part of planning. It may be:

- *Formative* carried out while the activity is still going on. It is part of continuous monitoring. It helps to identify features where improvements are possible.

- *Summative* carried out on completion of the project or activity. It is terminal. It enables judgement on what has been done.

Purpose of Evaluation

1. Was the activity worth doing? In the case of formative evaluation, it helps to determine whether the activity should be continued or abandoned, or modified.
2. Has the activity accomplished/is likely to accomplish the objectives? It can also help to decide whether the activity should be extended.
3. If the activity did not achieve its purpose, why was it not achieved?
   Failures may be due to deficits in:

- *Inputs or resources* Were they sufficient? Were they applied on time and in the best possible manner?

- *Outputs or services* Are the services provided appropriate, relevant and adequate, both in quantity and quality? Are the services efficient? Are they acceptable to the community and utilized by the people.

- *Outcome* What was intended to be achieved? Are any health improvements the direct result of the activity? Did the activity produce any other effect, positive or negative?

Methodology

The design of evaluation must be kept simple, commensurate with getting the answers sought after. Evaluation should include the plan (goals and priorities), the process (the way in which the plan was implemented) and the outcome (product).

There are four stages in evaluation methodology:

Setting Out the Questions

Setting out the questions that the evaluation is expected to answer. We need to have:
- Baseline information describing the situation before commencing the activity and the statements about policies, priorities and programmes;
- Input information the resources used in the programme; and
- process information, describing the situation after the activity or during the activity (changes or achievement in the service period).

Sources of Information

- Hospital statistics: All relevant data must be available and used judiciously.
- Surveys, which include attitudes of communities and users of services. The surveys may be quantifiable or qualitative.
- Feedback from the staff and management of the hospital.

How to Obtain the Information?

It is essential to decide how to get relevant and reliable information.

How and by whom the Information will be assessed?

It is necessary to determine who carries out the evaluation. The persons selected must be knowledgeable and have the appropriate skills and attitude.

Who Carries Out the Evaluation?

Different groups of persons may be selected to carry out the evaluation.

Outsiders with skills These are the experts who have been involved in similar activities. They are usually objective. There must be relationship of trust and cooperation between external evaluators and those whose activities are being evaluated.

Service providers These are the people who administer the services. They are interested in the evaluation but could be biased in favour of the outcome.

Users These are the beneficiaries of the services. They are likely to be critical.

A judicious mix of all three groups (or getting information from representatives of the groups) could bring about a more accurate evaluation. Evaluation is best as a cooperative process.

CHAPTER 10

Managing Time

One of the greatest resources is time. Do not squander it. Time cannot be increased unlike other resources. But you can improve the use of the available time.

> You have 24 hours a day
> 168 hours a week
> 8760 hours a year

It is the same amount of time for all. Some achieve a lot with that amount of time; some only a little. In practical terms, the time available is much less; may be 8-10 hours a day and about 300 days a year.

How can you use this limited time to the best advantage? You can do so, if you plan and organise your work.

The demands for time are many. It is not possible to give time to all the demands. You have to choose.

Have you thought of how much time is wasted? Time is perishable. It does not return. Listen to what Sir Walter Scott says:

> *"Does thou love life, then do not squander time,*
> *For that is the stuff that life is made of".*

There are many ways of wasting time:
 i. Inappropriate work habits;
 ii. Not setting goals and priorities;
 iii. Afraid to take decisions;
 iv. Doing things less important;
 v. Allowing others to waste your time; and
 vi. Doing work which ought to be done by others.

Case Study

Dr MS is the Medical Superintendent of H Hospital. Below is how he used his time on Monday.

Managing Time 53

Dr MS had been to a late party on Sunday. Woke up late on Monday, with a headache. Had some coffee and a tablet of aspirin. Got ready fast; had a hurried breakfast. Drove to the hospital. Was late for the staff meeting arranged for 9 am that day. Could not concentrate on the issues. Adjourned the meeting. It was his admission day. Went to OPD. Was angry at the large number of patients making a chaos. Shouted at the nurse on duty for poor management of the crowd. Saw a few patients and asked the junior to look after the rest. Went to the ward for the rounds. Phone call from the Secretary to Government. He had wanted some information about the hospital. The Finance Manager had offered to get the information but Dr MS had brushed aside the offer. Had thought of getting the information ready first thing on Monday morning but it escaped his memory in the hurry. Apologized to the Secretary and promised to have the information ready by 2 pm Coming out, there was a person with a complaint of negligence by a specialist in the hospital. Told him that he had no time to look into the matter at that time. Asked him to meet him (Dr MS) at 4 pm There was a heated exchange of arguments. The person ultimately left angry saying that they will meet in the Consumer Court. Rushed back to the ward. The patients took longer than expected, in spite of hurrying. Prescribed the medicines. One patient's relative was an old friend. He had waited to meet the doctor for a serious discussion on the prognosis of his relative. Dr MS, being in hurry, had no time for the relative. Told him to meet him next day. Went back to the office to work on the details to be furnished to the Secretary. The Finance Manager had left a note that he will not be coming in the afternoon. No one else knew about the required information. Skipped lunch to work on the data. Had no time to recheck. Gave the information to the Secretary, who said that the figures given earlier and now did not tally. Went back to work on the figures. Call from the Anaesthetist saying that the oxygen in the theatre had run out and the store did not have full cylinders. All cylinders had been exhausted during the weekend when there were a number of unexpected emergencies. Phoned up the Reliable Oxygen Supplies. They said that the supply can be made only the next day. Passed on the information to the Anaesthetist who said that he cannot be held responsible if something untoward happened for want of oxygen. Went back to work on the figures. Unable to set it right. Remembered that he was expected at an important meeting at 4 pm It was already 4.30 pm Found that the meeting had already started. Some of the decisions were not the right ones, according to him. There was heated exchange of views. All left angry at the end of the inconclusive meeting. Arrived home at 6.30 pm Wife had been waiting to go shopping which was cancelled. Had some snacks, one more aspirin and retired to bed exhausted.

How did Dr MS use his time? How did he cope with his work?

Being Busy

Some people are perpetually busy; it does not mean that they are making optimum use of their time.

There are two kinds of being busy:
- Chaotic, disorganized
- Calm, effective

Become a skilful user of time.

How Should You Plan Your Time?

Have a clear idea of how you want to use your time. Think what you want to do when, to achieve your goals and objectives.
- Consider your responsibilities. Strike a balance between various aspects of your job.
- What can I do?
- What can I do better than others?
- What must I do?
- What can I delegate?
- What can I train others to do?
- Prioritize each element of your job. Translate the priorities into action. Do you stop to think whether you are using your time effectively? If you wish to make better use of your time, stop. Look at how you are currently using your time, yesterday, during the past week, during the past month. Did you waste your time? Did your spend time on relatively unimportant matters? Did you spend your time on routine tasks which one of your subordinates could have done, may be even better.
- Were you able to recall what you did last week/last month? If you are keeping a diary, it would help. It is an important management tool. It helps you to plan ahead; to fix and keep appointments; to look back how you spent your time.

- Analyse what you did during the past one week/one month. Your activities fall into three categories:
   i. Tasks which had to be done by you (key responsibilities and obligations).
   ii. Tasks which other people expect, persuade or pressurize into doing.
   iii. Tasks you do because you want to (your own choice).

Activities can be classified into:
- Urgent and important;
- Urgent but not important;
- Not urgent but important;
- Not urgent, not important.

—**Stephen R. Covey**

Review your schedule every morning. Arrange them into:
Must,
Should,
Might
Be done today.

Earmark some time for an emergency or unexpected event. A hospital administrator must be ready to meet the unexpected.

How to Organize your Time?

Have a day plan and a "to do" list. Additionally, have a week plan, monthly plan and annual plan. May be you can have even a five year plan. You must plan for new opportunities, new careers, refresher courses and continuing education, leading to advancement in your career or better performance.

Stick to the plans as far as possible. No plan is worth it, if you do not stick to it but do not be too rigid. New opportunities might call for changes.

How to Prepare a "To Do" list?

i. Make a list of all the things you have to do or want to do that day.
ii. Think what you want to achieve by the end of the day.
iii. Think what you want to achieve on long term basis; set aside some time for it. It will help you to do what is important but may not be so pressing.

iv. Go through the list; decide on your priorities. Classify them into high priority, medium priority and low priority.
v. Concentrate on your high and medium priorities.

When Should you Prepare the List?

Spend the first 15 minutes in the morning before you start your work or you can review your day's activities at the end of the day and plan what you want to do the next day.
- Work closely with your secretary. Get a suitable person as secretary; induct him/her on to the job; give on-the-job training.
- Build a relationship of trust; share information and confidentiality. Actively seek ideas from the secretary as to how to improve your work. Let your secretary know your priorities and movements. Have a daily session with your secretary to deal with mail, routine matters and dictation. Train your secretary to deal with minor matters. Get your secretary to deal with telephone calls in your absence. Involve your secretary in meetings. Back up your secretary's decisions; sort out problems or difficulties that occur. Do not let your secretary take over.

A Diary

Always carry with you a pocket diary. Keep it up-to-date. Encourage your colleagues to keep a diary. Obtain diaries for your colleagues.
- Make fixed appointments for important meetings and visits. Try to stick to the timings. Try to make others also stick to the times. Avoid delayed commencement of meetings because some come late. It wastes the time of all others.
- Take your diary to meetings; future meetings can be fixed then and there, while the participants are present.
- Update your diary regularly; review your diary from time to time. See how you have used your time. Ensure that you plan the use of your time better, if there had been any waste.
- Build spare time into your schedules for some unforeseen events. They will crop up and should not upset other schedules.
- An annual planner is useful. Get your team to use it.

Positive Attitude to Time

Cultivate a positive attitude to good use of time. It will lead to better use of human resources, facilities, transport, etc.
- Do not put things off into the indefinite future. Do it at the earliest. Do not waste time on non essentials. Use your time for tackling important matters.
- Always give time to *key people*. It helps in achieving your goals and objectives. But they also should not waste your time. A President of a prestigious University in USA once told me "I do not give more than 15 minutes to anyone to explain matters; if the matter cannot be explained satisfactorily in that time, it needs further detailed study. I ask the person to reduce it in writing". It saves time and clarifies matters better.
- Learn to say 'No' graciously. An administrator will be requested to attend many social functions. Do so, if you can spare the time. But it should not be at the expense of important duties or committed responsibilities.
- Control your time; let not others control your time. I have seen a poster. "If you have nothing to do, do not do it here"; a very wise prescription. Do not allow others, who have nothing better to do, waste your precious time.
- Make full use of other people. Do not do yourself what someone else can do better. Delegate responsibilities and tasks. Give commensurate authority to enable the person to perform the tasks.
- Foster team spirit. Do not waste time in unnecessary arguments. Even if you win the argument, you lose in goodwill.
- Do not brood over past failures and mistakes. It is a time waster. But learn from past mistakes.
- Set time frames and deadlines for important tasks; stick to them. A strong point in the slogan "Health for All by 2000 AD" is the fixing on the time frame.
Let time serve you. Let it not be your master but your servant.

CHAPTER 11

Meetings

A large part of the time is taken up by meetings. These meetings can be very useful. Meetings help in the *meeting of minds*. The usefulness of meetings depends on the quality of the meeting and the seriousness with which the members participate. Success depends greatly on the preparation which has gone into the organization of the meeting. Plan well ahead:
- Preparation of the agenda
- Clarity of objectives
- Background papers and their distribution
- Leadership
- Effective participation.

Who are to be Invited?

Determine carefully who should be invited to the meetings. At least in the initial stages, it is necessary that all persons affected positively or negatively must be invited. There may also be neutral persons but who will be able to contribute effectively to the deliberations. Invite the right people. It is also necessary to decide the number to be invited. Large groups have advantages and disadvantages.

Advantages

i. There is more knowledge and abilities available.
ii. More people interact.
iii. Greater representation for differing view points.

Disadvantages

i. There is more likelihood of conflict.
ii. Subgroups might form.
iii. Contribution from each member is reduced.
   Have an optimum number, considering the matter for discussion.

Arrangements

Seating in a circle is the best; it gives equality and equal eye-contact. The chairs should be comfortable. It is better to have them all of the same type, size and height. The room should be well-lit and ventilated, with least disturbance. The recording is done through a recording secretary, unless tape recording is desired; this would need transcription later. Interruptions must be avoided, as far as possible. Have a chalk board or flip chart available to focus attention and to make problems visible.

Duration

Meetings of about 90 minutes' duration may be optimal. If the meeting is likely to last longer, break it up into more sessions.

Purpose

Every meeting must have a purpose or goal. This must be clear from the beginning. Meetings have different purposes and goals:
- Informative
- Consultative
- Executive
- Combinations of the above.

Informative Meeting

The purpose is to pass on information, e.g., blood transfusion and AIDS, passing on the information received from Government and other agencies. Action may or may not arise out of such information.

Consultative Meeting

You would like to get new ideas and suggestions, e.g., how to get more voluntary blood donors? With people of different background participating, it is quite likely that many suggestions will be made.

Executive Meeting

These meetings help to make decisions and to get them executed effectively, e.g., a hospital decides not to have blood bought from commercial blood banks. The decision is taken together and therefore, implementation will have the cooperation of the participants.

Agenda

Meetings must have an agenda. The agenda should preferably be detailed. This enables the participants to prepare in advance and come with information, data, etc. Sometimes, the agenda is general to explore the views of the participants. The agenda should specify the time available. Enough time must be provided for useful exchange of ideas.

Starting

Start on time, even if it mean that a few persons may come later. A delay of, say, 10 minutes may be allowed. There is no justification in keeping people waiting too long for the late comers. Once you have established a name for punctuality, the participants will start coming on time. In a hospital, some can be expected to be late because the members may be involved in unforeseen emergency patient care.

Opening Statement

Determine beforehand the message you want to convey. Say what you have to say in precise, concise terms. The message must be clear. Highlight the points for discussion and decision. Let the group know its exact role to react, to recommend or to decide.

Discussion

Give every person a chance to speak. There will be a tendency to wander away from the agenda. The speaker must be gently prodded to stick to the item on the agenda. Make discussions as pleasant as possible.

Effective Participation

Make your remarks as concise as possible, stating your position, giving the reasons and examples, if relevant. Listen attentively and learn to disagree agreeably.

How Decisions Are Made?

Every member of the group influences the group for good or bad. Even if a member does not speak, he/she is still influencing the group by his/her attitude. Sometimes one individual dominates and makes the decision, when the other participants are passive or silent or timid. At other times, a small vociferous or articulate minority in the group makes the decision, even though the wish of the majority might be different. The group leader must draw out the views from as many people as possible. The decision then will be the decision of the group. Sometimes, votes are taken; this is better avoided as voting breaks the group into winners and losers. Most often, decisions are made by consensus. This is usually the next best to a unanimous decision.

Disagreement

Disagreements can be of immense value. They must be constructive. They often bring about better analysis of the problems, provided we make use of the differences of opinion wisely to:
  i. Gather more information,
 ii. Clarify issues, and
iii. Seek better alternatives.

But no one should persist in disagreement and obstruct decision-making, provided he/she has been given full opportunities to present his/her reasons and others have understood him/her.

Group Behavior

Groups Exhibit Different Behaviors.

Functional behavior helps the group towards its tasks or pulls the group together. This is often done by the leader by initiating, seeking and giving information and by coordinating and summarizing periodically. He/she encourages people to present their views and sees that everyone has a chance to speak. He/she summarizes to express the group feeling.

Dysfunctional behavior attacks other views and disagrees beyond reason. Such a person may dominate or withdraw sullenly.

Discussion Leader

You have to play the role of leader, expediter, observer and decision-maker but not of a lecturer. You have to protect the expression of minority opinions. Keep looking around to see who wishes to make a contribution. Guide the meeting along constructive channels. Keep the atmosphere open for discussion. Cut off tactfully if a speaker continues to talk for too long. Be ready to seek whether the group is ready for a decision. Take time to summarize and to decide what needs to be done next.

Buzz Group

When discussions have gone on for sometime, it may be useful to break into small units of 3-5 people to discuss the issue. The purpose of these buzz groups is to:
- Clarify a point
- Consolidate views
- Aid problem solving
- Provide feedback, and
- Ease tension.

The buzz group session should last only 10-15 minutes, when the larger group will be reconvened.

Brain Storming

A very useful procedure is to have a brain storming session. This is especially useful when the group is faced with a particularly difficult problem or when priorities are to be fixed. The members contribute ideas at random, without discussion, comments or criticism, until all ideas have been aired and recorded. The group then proceeds to use those which seem to be appropriate for the task. Some of the ideas will automatically be thrown out because of nonfeasibility or for other reasons, narrowing down the choice.

Minutes

Once the meeting is over, prepare the minutes promptly. The format must be consistent. When the names of some of the contributors to the discussion are given, give the names of all who contributed significantly. People like to see their names and feel offended when their name is omitted but others are given. The minutes must reflect faithfully the proceedings and contain all the salient points. Circulate the minutes as early as possible, when the memory is still fresh in the minds of the participants.

Meeting Individuals

Care must be taken when we meet individuals. Here again seating arrangements are important. Seats must be comfortable and equal. People may sit in different positions. This itself can give some idea. Normally it is face to face; this would indicate a desire for an honest discussion and put forward the views. It can also be competing. An informal seating corner to corner or corner to end is not a desirable way of seating. When people are invited to sit side by side, it indicates a desire to cooperate. If the person tends to sit far away (distant opposite end to end or end to corner or corner to corner), it may indicate independence. It would be a good idea to invite him to come closer.

CHAPTER 12

Negotiations

As an administrator, one has to negotiate with various people, directly or indirectly. One has to negotiate with:
  i. Unions within the hospital. They may put up charter of demands for revision of wages, better facilities and many other issues.
  ii. Suppliers, when one wants to purchase equipment, drugs, imaging films, furniture and other items.
  iii. Government and other organizations and firms, when they want some activity to be carried out by the hospital.

Negotiations should always lead to satisfaction for both parties. Is the union always happy, if the employees get large increases in wages? Is the management always happy, if the management gets away with a very small increase? Not necessarily. An important aspect in negotiation is satisfaction. Satisfaction often depends on the process—how that rise was got or was given; how that facility was agreed to or denied. Each party must come from the negotiating table feeling that they got something out of the negotiations. If the management gave in easily, the Union is likely to think that they might have got even more, if they had pressed for more. In a way, they might feel cheated. The members of the Union might feel that the office-bearers were not smart enough to demand more. Their positions become insecure. Next time, they will pitch much higher and expect much more.

The management also needs satisfaction. They may feel that the administrator could have held on longer and got away with less concessions and benefits. Next time, they may be more tough.

Often, during negotiations, it is necessary to say 'no' one more time before saying 'yes'. We do not say 'absolutely no' and break off. Time must be given for both parties to consider and deliberate on the demand. Time must be taken to go over the figures and study the implications of the proposals.

How much time should be taken? That depends on the situation. The Union should feel that they had to work at least to some extent to get what they wanted. And they certainly will be much more happy about it.

Remember that each negotiation affects the succeeding one. If the present one was satisfying, the next one has a greater likelihood of being satisfying.

The administrator's job should be to make the Union happy, feeling good about the final deal struck. At the same time, one has to safeguard the interests of the institution. There is a long-term relationship between the hospital management and employees. That should be kept in mind; then all will be happy.

Making Concessions

When negotiating, one has to make concessions. How to make these concessions are often more important than what concessions are actually made. It is wise to concede in small increases; give in slowly. Let it be a considered response. One might have to consider the impact of the concessions being asked for or one might think that one has all the answers. In either case, take time. Ask for time to think and work out the implications. Similarly, one has to give time to the Union also, should they need more time.

Have patience. "He who can have patience can have what he will".

Always think and work out the total impact of the concessions being given.

The Union of Hospital C had a charter of demands. One of them was a weightage of Rs. 3/- p.m. for every year of service. The management had offered another formula of weightage. Rs. 10/- p.m. for 5-10 years of service, Rs. 20/- for 11-15 years and Rs. 30/- for 16 years and above. On the face of it Rs. 3/- appeared to be attractive. But the impact depends on the hospital and the duration of service of the employees. Hospital C was an old one with most of the employees having long years of service. Always take time to work out the implications.

Striking Work

A voluntary, not-for-profit hospital, started as a leprosy asylum with 200 beds. With multi-drug therapy, the number of patients with leprosy got reduced. The hospital was restructured as a general hospital with 90 beds for leprosy patients, mainly for reconstructive surgery and 120 beds as an acute care general hospital. Most of the workers are those cured of leprosy. They were given jobs as part of rehabilitation. A management study showed that the number was in excess of the real need of the hospital.

The salary is reasonable, being higher than the minimum wages prescribed for the categories of staff but less than the government scales. The workers demanded parity with government employees.

The income of the hospital has decreased as the donor agency provides grant only for the leprosy affected patients. Income from the other (general) patients is low because most of them are poor or belong to the lower middle class.

The Union has given notice of strike. You are the administrator. How will you tackle the situation?

Negotiating for purchases is important. Very often there is a large margin of profit in health care equipment. By careful negotiations, the price can be brought down. The savings can be significant. Be careful that nothing significant is left out of the offer. At the same time, there may be options which are not useful or necessary. All the accessories and spare parts required for good working conditions should be included. Take the advice of others knowledgeable in the working of the equipment. Ask for details of the hospitals where such equipment has been installed. Refer to them. If you are then satisfied, start the negotiations.

Hospital H wanted an ultrasound machine. Eight firms were asked to quote. From a preliminary review, four were selected. They were given the exact requirements of the hospital and asked to present the features of the item quoted by them and to give the lowest quotation. Each firm was given one hour. Based on the presentation and the final quotations, two were selected for further negotiations, and ultimately one was selected. There was a saving of over Rupees one lakh.

When negotiating for purchase of equipment, it is essential to ensure that the firm or their agents will be able to service the equipment promptly and supply spare parts as may be required in a reasonable future period of time. The down time must be reduced to the absolute minimum. Necessary clauses should be incorporated in the order/agreement.

CHAPTER 13

Innovation

The only constant feature in this world is *change*. While all the change may not lead to progress, there can be no progress without change. This is true for the individual, institution, organization or the country. Civilization owes its existence to change. The success or even survival of an institution or organization depends on making necessary changes.

To innovate means to introduce something new; to be *creative*. An administrator must be innovative: an agent of change. Changes are imperative in the swiftly moving economy, political scene, science and technology, and expectations of the people. If there is no change, the organization/institution/country stagnates and goes down. Innovation is a *social value* of immense proportions.

Innovation is brought about by a series of processes. It starts with *thought*. Imagination is the workshop of the mind. It is the act of constructive thinking, grouping knowledge, skills and attitude into *new, original* and *rational ideas*. Old ideas and established facts are reassembled into new combinations and put to new uses. Imagination is both *interpretative* and *creative*. It can receive impressions and form new combinations and build them into ideas. These ideas are then translated into *plans* and then into *activities*. Our activities and achievements grow out of organized plans, first created in our imagination. Creative thinking requires that we keep our minds open and in a state of *expectancy* to achieve our objectives. Our minds are compared to parachutes; they function only when they are open.

We often do not attempt innovation because we are:
- *Afraid*: of failures; of opposition; of the unknown;
- Lacking adequate and correct *information*;
- Reluctant to *experiment*;
- Bound by *custom* and *tradition*; and
- Unaware of our *strengths* for achievement.

When a person proposes a change, there will be many who will resist. Discouraging remarks will be heard:
- "We tried that years ago; it did not work".
- "Nothing will ever change around here".
- "This requires extensive and thorough analysis".
- "There is need for change but the climate is not right just now".
- "I have never stood in the way of progress, but....".
- "Things are fine now; why risk a change?".
- "It will not work".

The excuses are many. A large number of reasons will be given why a thing cannot be done. But *those who think they can and dare, get new things done.*

To be innovative, one has to be something of a *dreamer* and a *doer*. Even if one does not possess these qualities, one can introduce innovations. One can support and encourage a dreamer and a doer.

A successful innovator or change agent:
- Identifies opportunities for improvement or overcoming major problems;
- Has a readiness to accept change;
- Creates a climate for innovation;
- Supports and sustains the change effort;
- Evaluates, reviews and modifies activities appropriately for effective change; and
- Continues the effort till the desired goal is achieved.

Innovation could lead to a new product or a new service. It may involve a new method or process. It can be a new mode of management. Innovation covers everything from the inception of a new idea to the use of the new product or service. The change may be a minor one or it may be radical. Radical changes are relatively rare. Usually, there are small changes, punctuated by occasional major changes. Innovation may make obsolete the existing equipment and machinery, materials and components, skills and managerial expertise.

It is similar to what happens in the drug industry. Occasionally a new drug is developed, based on a new concept. But, most often, the new drugs produced are as a result of minor changes in the molecule.

To bring about innovation, there is need for:
  i. *A definite purpose*. If you wish to succeed, you must have a definite aim and purpose. Anticipate the needs of your

organization. Anticipate the needs of the future. Work out the general and specific objectives. The objective must be clear.
ii. *Initiative* It is the pass-key that opens the door to opportunity.
iii. *Knowledge of facts* Get as much information as possible. Without accurate information, one cannot produce the desired change.
iv. *Self-confidence* Most often, the only limitation to one's trying out the new is lack of confidence in one's-self and in the organization. If one thinks one can, one will succeed most of the times.
v. *Persistent effort* One does not succeed because one gives up at the least difficulty or resistance. One has to be persistent and put up even greater efforts when faced with resistance. Many examples can be given of the successful application of these principles. Take the discovery of the electric bulb by Thomas A Edison. He had a definite purpose: produce light using electricity. He took the initiative and developed the idea. He had the facts with him: light could be produced by heating a thin wire with electricity. He had immense self-confidence. He knew he could do it. Edison tried heating thousands of wires of different metals. Light was produced but the intense heat also burnt the wire. He did not give up. He persisted.

Edison combined another known fact: there can be no combustion without oxygen. Solution to the problem: shut off all oxygen by placing the wire inside a glass globe (vacuum or inert gas). The incandescent electric bulb was born. Edison had a definite purpose, took the initiative, knew the facts, had ample self-confidence and persisted in his efforts.

Or, take the example of the discovery of insulin. Dr Banting had a definite purpose: to discover the active principle in the pancreas, which would reduce the level of blood sugar. He took the initiative of experimenting with animals. He knew the facts. Pancreas contained the active principle. This principle is destroyed by the proteolytic enzymes produced by the pancreas. If we ligate the pancreatic duct, the enzyme producing cells will be destroyed. He had immense self-confidence. Even though discouraged, he persisted. Success crowned his efforts.

Factors leading to change

a. *Dissatisfaction with status quo* The dissatisfaction may arise from our desire to do better, to bring about improvement over

the existing situation. More often, it may be forced upon us by outside influence: other organizations are doing better or we cannot survive if we continue the same way. The external and internal environment of the organization changes. The changes may be in
   i. Client needs (for product or service),
   ii. Technology, or
   iii. Competition.

Major changes are being forced upon the medical profession and health care institutions by the application of Consumer Protection Act. Large damages are being awarded for medical negligence. Greater care is being exercised. Doctors and institutions are getting themselves covered by insurance.

b. **Opportunities** Newer developments in science, technology, financing, management, etc. may provide opportunities for improvement.

c. **A shared vision** There must be a critical mass of persons within the organization for the change. Shared vision gives drive and encouragement.

d. **Knowledge of first steps** The first steps are important to get acceptance of the idea by others in the organization. Many persons or groups of persons do not know how to take the first step. It requires knowledge, skills and attitude to take acceptable first steps.

Change has high costs: *psychological* and *organizational*. Throughout the change process, the old systems have to continue along with the new ones. It produces a dilemma in the organization. While introducing innovation, there is need to guarantee efficiency (product or service); a proper balance has to be maintained.

Organizational change can be helped by a number of factors:
   i. A common, shared sense of purpose.
   ii. Improved quality and reliability of information.
   iii. Commitment and sense of responsibility
   iv. Flexible and informal systems, procedures and practices.
   v. Encouragement and support to initiatives and experimentation.
   vi. Teamwork, coordination and good communication.
   vii. Delegation of responsibility and authority.

viii. Open style of managing differences and conflicts.
ix. Willingness to tackle problems and persistence.
x. Active learning environment.
xi. Valuing individuals and individuality.

An important requirement for innovation is learning from experience. The administrator encounters a situation where something is happening which was not expected to happen or was not wanted. The administrator thinks:
    What is the problem?
    Is it the result of inadequate personal competence?
    Technology and process?
    Organization and procedures?
    Motivation and control?
    Monitoring and evaluation? Singly or in combination?

The administrator then starts to analyze the problem, its cause and results. All persons who may be affected (and even those not affected but can contribute to the analysis and even solution of the problem) are called together, pooling the resources. After analyzing the problem, objectives are set, looking into the means and ends, again involving all the persons and winning their consent. The administrator then directs, instructs, persuades, negotiates, monitors and evaluates. The entire organization learns from the experience—success or failure.

While trying to introduce innovation, it is necessary to have an effective change plan:
i. Define the goals and the time frame.
ii. Link the activities to the goals.
iii. Be specific and be integrated; think of the effect on the entire organization.
iv. Sequence the plan; it must be taken through logically, step by step with series of stages or phases.
v. Be adaptable and acceptable to the people.

How to Manage Change?

Management of change involves many factors:
    i. **Technology** Technology is changing fast all the time. It is necessary to choose appropriate technology. Every new technology need not be suitable. Improved, suitable technology must be adopted/adapted, considering efficiency and cost-

benefit ratio. The cost includes not only the cost of the machinery and know-how but also of retraining personnel and gaining acceptance of the change.

There was a time when we used to give antibiotics, pectin and kaolin and other substances in the treatment of diarrhoea. Today we know that the major killer is dehydration and the answer is the salt-sugar solution.

 ii. *Political* There are problems of allocation of resources. Who gets what? How is the organization used? Will the proposed change bring about a change in the power equation within the organization?

Changes in legislation can affect the function of the organization. The management must respond to these changes adequately and in time.

 iii. *Cultural* People hold beliefs. It is difficult to change custom and tradition. The values held by various groups of people in the organization affect acceptance of change.

Organizations vary in their characteristics with respect to bringing about innovation. An innovative organization
- Accepts uncertainties and risks,
- Is willing to face temporary instability,
- Allocates sufficient resources for research and development,
- Delegates responsibility and authority,
- Has dynamic structure to be able to adapt to the changes in function and is flexible,
- Uses scientific and technological advances optimally, and
- Encourages creative thinking.

Transition

While effecting change, it is important to ask some questions.
Why do we want to change? (Objective).
Where are we? (present state).
Where do we want to reach? (future state).
How best can we reach there? (the process).
Who will carry out the change? (the people).
When do we want to complete the change? (time frame).
How do we monitor progress (indicators).

Present State

a. Identifying the system
   Environmental mapping
   Structures—formal and informal
   Cultural norms
   Behavior, skills and beliefs
   Resources—men, money, materials, methods, time
   Interaction of all the above.
b. Demands and needs.
c. Responses.

Future State

a. What types of changes are needed?
   Objectives
   Technology
   Attitudes and behavior
   Policies and practices.
b. Which systems are involved? Which part(s) of the organization?
c. Are the systems ready for change? What are the forces for and against change?
d. Are the changes suggested realistic?
e. What are the resources available for change?
f. What is your motivation?
g. Why should other people want change?
h. What is the capability and willingness of others to effect the change?
i. What is the linkage with other systems? Can we have a domino effect in removing blocks to change?

Readiness to Change

Some individuals and organizations are more ready to effect changes than others. This depends often on the degree of felt security. In turn, it depends on the knowledge, skills and attitude, self-confidence, tolerance to stress and motivation of the individuals. It also depends on the culture and climate for innovation, tolerance to ambiguity, the possibility of success or failure and the desire to learn. If there is optimal feeling of security, the individuals and organization respond to changes. If the feeling of security is too high or too low, the response to change will not be present.

Creating Lasting Change

Three factors are useful to create lasting change

Change Yourself

Determine what you want to do. The great leaders decided what they wanted to achieve. Inspiring examples are Gandhiji and Abraham Lincoln. We can be inspired by the examples of the great leaders and follow their paths.

Change Your Limiting Beliefs

Often tied down by beliefs. We have to remove those shackles. We must believe that we can meet the new standards set by us. Gandhiji believed in the power of ahimsa (non-violence) and he achieved what he wanted.

Change Your Strategy

Decide on the strategy which is likely to help us achieve what we want. Change the approach till we reach the goal. Have firm belief that we can change the circumstances.

"Man is not the creature of circumstances;
Circumstances are the creatures of man".

-Benjamin Disrachi

Change is crucial. Change is a must for progress.

Section 4: Hospital Organization

CHAPTER

14

Hospital Organization—Structure and Function

...Even in the present age, most hospitals function on the lines of the bureaucratic organizational model propounded by the great German sociologist Max Weber almost a century ago......

Organizational structure is the bureaucratic set-up of an institution by which its staff, facilities and other resources are organized in such a manner as to be most effective in accomplishing the purpose/s for which the organization was established. The nature of the hospital and its organizational set-up thus depend primarily on its objectives. While certain objectives are similar to most hospitals, others may be different. Even when similar, the emphasis may vary. This diverse mix of objectives determines the nature of the hospital, its organizational hierarchy, the scope and volume of activities, the number and size of departments, staffing pattern, etc.

This chapter discusses the objectives of a hospital, the types of hospitals, uniqueness of a hospital organization, general organizational principles, hospital organizational structure, and the role of the management and various key executives.

OBJECTIVES OF A HOSPITAL

In hospitals, *patient care* comes first. In larger hospitals, particularly those attached to medical colleges, there will be emphasis also on *training*. The more specialized centres will additionally have elements of *research*. More and more hospitals are getting involved in *community health* and *outreach programmes*. The various objectives of a hospital include:

Principal Objectives

- Central goal: Cure
  — diagnostic and treatment procedures
  — medication
- Supportive goal: Care
  — nursing care
  — provide an atmosphere for rest, quietness and comfort and thereby facilitate healing
  — reassure the patient
- Extended goals:
  — alleviate health problems of the community
  — teaching
  — research

Secondary Objectives

- Financial viability
- Staff satisfaction, motivation, productivity
- Quality service:
  — efficiency
  — effectiveness
  — economy

Depending on the emphasis that the Management wishes to give to achievement of some or all of the objectives/activities enumerated above, each hospital should develop and proclaim its **mission statement** or philosophy. This prioritized write-up of the list of objectives should be clearly understood by all the staff of the hospital and should be translated into concrete action plans to be pursued by all the departments and staff.

(For example: The Mission Statement of The Royal Hospital, Sultanate of Oman is as below:
- To provide state-of-the-art tertiary care services.

- To serve as the apex referral centre for Ministry of Health institutions.
- To strive for:
  — high quality care to be rendered with maximum efficiency, effectiveness, and economy;
  — high level of patient satisfaction;
  — minimum patient waiting time;
  — appropriate interaction and cooperation with Ministry of Health institutions in order to respond effectively to the healthcare needs of the country;
  —high staff morale, job satisfaction and employee commitment to the goals of the organization.
- As a teaching hospital, to:
  — provide excellent teaching facilities to Omani under-graduate and post-graduate medical and nursing trainees and to students of allied healthcare disciplines with a view to attaining Omanization and local self-sufficiency in the medical field;
  — promote clinical research and thereby contribute to further development of medical services in the Sultanate.)

The mission statement serves as a guideline to the management and senior executives in formulating long-term plans for the hospital and in focussing its activities in the short run. It gives meaning to the purpose of the hospital and tells an employee what the institution expects in terms of his contribution. The hospital philosophy and mission statement should therefore, be publicized widely and be internalized by staff and all those intimately involved in the affairs of the hospital.

Types of Hospitals

The objectives of the hospital determine its nature or characteristics, which in turn have a bearing on its organizational structure. The salient criteria often used to classify and describe the type of hospital include the following:
- Nature of **ownership**:
  — government/Public (e.g.: Central or State Government Hospital, District or Regional Hospital, Municipality, ESI Corporation)
  — non-government/Private Not-for-profit/Voluntary/Charitable (e.g.: hospitals run by philanthropic and charitable organizations like religious groups, Rotary/Lions clubs, trusts)
  — corporate/Proprietary/Investor-owned For-profit

- Nature of **specialization**:
  — general
  — specialist (e.g.: Tuberculosis, Leprosy, Infectious Diseases, Psychiatric, Industrial, Trauma, Cancer, Women's/Children's or Geriatric Hospital)
  —Super-specialist (e.g.: Cardiac or Neuro Centre, Eye Hospital)
- **Bed strength:**
  — small (less than 100 beds)
  — medium sized (100-300 beds)
  — large (over 300 beds)
- **Length of stay:**
  — acute-care / short-term stay (with mean length of stay 7-30 days)
  — long-term stay (average length of stay over 30 days)
- **Training of under- or post-graduate doctors:**
  — teaching
  — non- teaching
- **Level of expertise:**
  — primary-care
  — secondary-care
  — tertiary-care.

Uniqueness of the Hospital Organization

Although basic management principles apply to all organizations whatever the nature of activity, each institution has its own peculiarities, which in turn influence its organizational set-up. A hospital organization differs from other organizations in certain distinctive ways:

- In contrast to the production industry, a hospital is a **'service'** organization. And as with other service organizations, there is no clear conceptualization of output. It is thus not possible to quantify the level of output, except through the use of surrogates (e.g.: outpatient load, number admitted per year, number of various procedures performed, occupancy, mortality rate, etc.) which in fact do not correctly express productivity and quality of the service.
- A hospital renders mostly **personalized** service specific to each individual patient's needs. What is in the patient's interest is, therefore, the foremost guiding principle in deciding what care should be extended in each case. Humanitarian, social and

professional values assume prominence. Thus, though treatment/activity protocols are often laid down to ensure a particular standard of care, the application of these standing rules many a time require interpretation and modification depending on the unique circumstances prevailing. There is hence no hard and fast rule of what should be done, when and how, except by going by the guideline of what a professional with a similar level of competence would reasonably be expected to do in a similar situation.
- Hospitals work within the framework of accepted **ethical** norms. There is a moral obligation to extend emergency care, whatever the cost, irrespective of the patient's ability to pay. The relative usefulness of alternative procedures vis-à-vis improvement in the quality of life, and the constant dilemma of continuing or stopping treatment are of daily concern to professionals. Care cannot be withdrawn from one patient just because there is another patient who is more important, deserving or with better prognosis. Emergency care cannot be denied to a patient just because his infectious/contagious disease (HIV positive, Hepatitis positive, rabies, viral haemorrhagic fever, etc.) poses a risk to the staff involved.
- A certain **code of behavior** is expected of all staff. Patient confidentiality should be preserved at all times. Professional decisions should be rational and without emotion. There is no room for indiscipline or non cooperation.
- Notwithstanding an individual hospital's objectives, hospitals are becoming increasingly responsive to the health needs of the surrounding **community**. This factor should, therefore, be taken into account in defining the mission of the hospital and in planning its activities.
- Hospitals have certain **work constraints** not applicable to most other industries. Hospital operations cannot be shut down but must be assured on a 24-hour 365-day year-after-year basis, irrespective of nonavailability of personnel, employee strikes, environmental disasters, lack of budget, etc. Procedures cannot be interrupted or be left half-done even if there is a change of shift. Much of the work is of an urgent nature, and emergencies specially cannot be postponed to more convenient timings.
- There are several **grey areas** that cannot be categorized as purely administrative or clinical. Technical staff, even if subordinate

in the organization to certain administrative staff, must have the freedom to exercise their scientific discretion. And senior administrators should realize the boundaries of their authority and resist the tendency to influence technical decisions. Medical, nursing and technical professionals should not be faced with the dilemma of having to abide by administrative directives which conflict with the patient's/clinical interest.

HOSPITAL ORGANIZATIONAL PRINCIPLES

It is important to take note of the various organizational principles, which if not adhered to result in inefficient organizations and organizational conflicts:

Pyramidal Organizational Hierarchy

Employees are arranged in a pyramid of superiors and subordinates. This vertical chain of command, or scalar principle, ensures that each individual staff in the pyramid is in a specific authority relationship to a superior whose authority can be traced from the next level of authority, on up to the top level. Unity of command further guarantees that each individual will report to one, and only one, superior. This traditional organizational structure assures clear flow of authority and responsibility which is required for proper delegation of work, accountability, discipline. Thus we have:

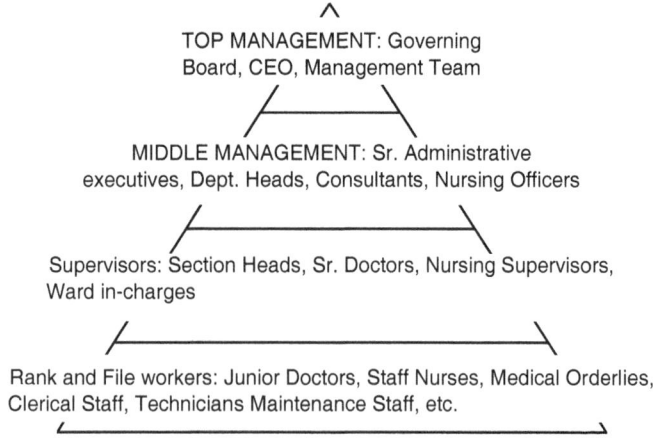

Tall or Flat Pyramid

This is determined by the number of levels between the top management and the workers. What factors influence the number of levels?
— size of the organization;
— complexity of the nature of functions and services;
— management style and attitude to authority;
— amount of delegation;
— span of control.

Flat structures have few levels of authority and are appropriate for small hospitals. They have short chains of command and broad span of control.

Tall structures have more levels of authority and are more formal. There is more specialization and standardization. There is less span of control and less delegation. This model is applicable for large specialist hospitals.

Matrix Structure

In contrast to Max Weber's vertical pyramid, where an employee works only within his superior's realm of activity, some of the more advanced hospitals use a horizontal approach. Here multidisciplinary teams are formed to accomplish specific tasks/goals/projects, and there is a lateral relationship between various categories of staff, all of whom work under the direction of a project manager and not their respective departmental heads. (For example, a nurse in-charge of a day care or managed care facility may co-ordinate doctors, nurses, technicians, clerks and other supportive staff. Again, in a large hospital, there may be various teams—patient care team, investigative team, support service team—to more effectively coordinate the care of patients in a ward.) Matrix structures are generally more efficient and effective since, with the team approach, individuals participate in the decision making process and therefore, feel more motivated and committed to the goals to be achieved.

Product-line Structure

This is a combination of the pyramid and matrix structure and has been widely adopted in the UK where it is also referred to as the cogwheel system. The hospital is organized on the basis of its major product lines (e.g.: Medical / Surgical / Child Health / Obstetrics and Gynaecology specialities and their associated sub/super-specialities), each of which is termed a Clinical Division/Directorate. A directorate has fair degree of administrative autonomy and looks after all categories of its staff including doctors, nurses, technicians and support staff. The role of the Hospital Administration in this model is more to monitor the individual performance of each directorate, to ensure harmonious relationship between the various directorates, and to provide ancillary and support services based on need.

Span of Control

There is a limit to the number of individuals who can be effectively supervised by a single superior. Higher up the organizational pyramid, direct control is best limited to 4-5, though at lower levels it is possible for a supervisor to efficiently supervise even double that number. (For example, with such broad range of responsibilities, it is possible for the CEO to have the Medical Superintendent, Nursing Superintendent, Asst Administrator, Finance Manager and Personnel Manager report personally to him. But to have many more, like the Hospital Engineer, Chief Pharmacist, Stores Manager and individual Clinical Heads report directly to him may be inviting trouble. In contrast, at a lower level, it may be possible for a Ward in-charge to effectively supervise even 20 Staff Nurses, Nursing Aides and Cleaners.)

Line Versus Staff Relationship

A line manager is part of the chain of command and hence has direct authority and responsibility for the work of his unit and for his subordinates. As against this, staff assistants provide only advice and technical support to line managers and should exercise their authority only through the respective line staff. (Example: Although the In-service Education Nursing Officer is a senior staff responsible for on-the-job training of all nurses, he can organize, his programmes only through the Nursing Administration and in coordination with the various Unit Nursing Officers. This also applies to other staff type positions like the Quality Assurance Officer, Personnel Department, etc.) An executive in staff position draws his authority from a line manager to whom he reports to and so should channel his advice/directives accordingly. Department heads should also remember that though they are line managers, when dealing with employees who are not within their jurisdiction, they are in a staff position and so cannot directly enforce discipline on staff of other departments except through their respective department heads.

Delegation

A subordinate's participation in decision making guarantees his commitment to the task/s to be accomplished. Delegation also economises on the superior's time leaving him free for more important tasks. It is, therefore vital to delegate decision making, especially of tasks of a routine nature, to employees who will actually perform the task. Delegation is of extreme importance in a personalized service industry such as health care, as it is one of the best ways to ensure commitment to a high standard of care. It must, however, be remembered that even if a decision or task is delegated, the ultimate responsibility is retained. Thus, the hospital management is responsible for the actions of its staff, and consultants are responsible for the quality of care provided by junior doctors and nurses.

Division of Labour

For a hospital to function effectively, there must be proper division of labour. The hospital is, therefore divided into departments on the basis of functions. This brings about specialization. Within a department, various levels of staff are assigned or authorized to perform specific tasks on the basis of their qualifications and competence. This is achieved through written job descriptions for various categories of staff and clinical privileges for doctors. Job descriptions help to:
 — select the right person for the job,
 — analyze and clarify what is involved in a particular job,
 — allocate responsibility and authority,

— review the effectiveness of the work done,
— determine the need for training to do the job more effectively, and
— evaluate performance by the person.

Rules and Regulations

To ensure an acceptable code of behavior amongst its employees, all formal organizations including hospitals, establish rules and regulations to be complied with by all staff. These specify the conditions for employment, work timings, holidays, discipline, etc.

Policies and Procedures

The larger an organization, more the need to have clear guidelines on the way in which work should be performed. This is particularly important in a hospital where the manner of performing a task cannot be left to the whim of individuals but is based on scientific teachings, accepted practices and standard norms. To ensure compliance by all staff, especially those trained under different schools of thought, each hospital should have its own written policies and procedures for common activities performed by large numbers of staff. These include: various treatment protocols, manual of nursing procedures, admission policies and procedures, ICU admission and management protocol, policies and procedures for coronary pulmonary resuscitation, disaster plan, infection control procedures, procedures for disposal of infectious waste, procedures for fire safety and prevention, purchase and stores procedures, etc.

Hospital Organizational Functions

There are two basic sets of functions that hospitals perform:
- Provision of medical care or the technical component:
  — diagnostic and treatment procedures
  — nursing care
  — technical/ancillary services (investigations, medications, rehabilitation, medical records and patient documentation, etc.)
- Provision of hotel-type services or the hotel component:
  — place to rest (bed, room)
  — physical amenities (food, water, linen, lighting, toilet, comfort)

Hospital Organization—Structure and Function 85

— hygiene (cleanliness, pest control, infection control)
— security (personal, of belongings)
— administration (front office management, efficiency, a fair charge, value for money).

The type of hospital and its objectives, and the various organizational principles and functions highlighted above determine a hospital's organizational structure. A typical **organizational chart** is displayed in the appendix to this chapter. However, this model may vary depending on:
— the nature of the hospital,
— whether the CEO has a medical or nonmedical background,
— the presence and job description of senior management executives,
— convictions/beliefs of the top management,
— examples of other similar (especially successful) hospitals,
— local/regional trends, custom and practice.

Functionally, the organizational structure of a hospital provides for the following **distinct groups of services**:

- Clinical and Diagnostic services (Anaesthesia, Internal Medicine, Cardiology, Clinical Haematology, Dermatology, Endocrinology, Gastroenterology, Nephrology, Neurology, Oncology, Respiratory Medicine, General Surgery, Cardiothoracic Surgery, Dental Surgery, Neuro-Surgery, Ophthalmology, Orthopaedics, Otorhinolaryngology or ENT Surgery, Paediatric Surgery, Plastic Surgery, Urology or Genitourinary Surgery, General Paediatrics and associated super-specialities, Neonatology, Obstetrics and Gynaecology and associated super-specialities, Blood Bank, Clinical Biochemistry or Chemical Pathology, Haematology, Histopathology, Microbiology, Immunology, Radiology, Nuclear Medicine, Radiotherapy, Staff Health, Community Health, etc.)
- Ancillary services (Physiotherapy, Occupational Therapy, Prosthetics and Orthotics, Respiratory Therapy, Pharmacy and Medical Stores, Infection Control, Medical Records and Computerized Clinical Information System, Medico-Social Work, Medical Library, etc.) In some hospitals, Radiology, Clinical Laboratory and Anaesthesia are grouped with the Ancillary services, but since these departments include doctors, it is preferred to group them with the clinical and diagnostic services.
- Nursing and Specialized service areas (Casualty or Accident and Emergency department, Outpatient department, Wards,

Operation Theatres, Intensive Care Unit, Coronary Care Unit, Daycare Unit, Dialysis Unit, Central Sterile Supply Department, etc.)
- Support services (Reception and Telephone, Dietary and Catering, Housekeeping and Environment, Linen and Laundry, Security, Engineering and Maintenance, Ambulance and Transport, etc.)
- Business and fiscal services (Administration, Admission, Finance, Billing and Cash, Human Resources or Personnel and Industrial Relations, General and Medical Purchase, General Stores, Internal Audit, Computers and Hospital Information System, Patient and Public Relations, etc.)
- Teaching/training services (In-service Education, attached Medical College, Nursing School/College, Institute of Paramedical Studies, etc.)

Organization and Functions of the Governing Body

Except for Government and proprietor hospitals, hospitals are owned and managed by Societies or Trusts. The Society is a legal entity registered under the Societies Registration Act. Any surplus generated from the activities of the Society does not accrue to any individual but is ploughed back to further its objectives. This non-profit status exempts the hospital from income tax and enables it to obtain grants and donations. In accordance with the rules of the Society, the members of the General Body:
- Guide, influence and formulate the philosophy and long term objectives of the Society.
- Elect competent persons to serve on its Governing Board to manage and control the affairs of the Society.
- Delegate decision making power to the Governing Body which is legally and morally responsible for operation of the Society.
- Retain the authority to restrict or curtail any action of the Board that is not in conformity with the philosophy and objectives of the Society.
- Exercise its power through annual and periodic review of activity reports of the Society.

The Governing Body is the highest management body of the hospital. It is a large forum that meets infrequently (usually once a year). Consequently it executes its functions through a Governing

Board, which is entrusted with the responsibility for governing the hospital and controlling its destiny.

The bylaws of the Society stipulate the size of the Governing Board (generally 8-15 members) and criteria for its membership—by nomination, election, ex-officio appointment. Nominated members could include the principal promoters of the hospital or their representatives, eminent persons who can contribute significantly to establishment and growth of the hospital (e.g.: prominent members of the community, persons of influence or affluence, hospital management experts, doctors, educationists, legal luminaries, Government officials, architects, etc.), and perhaps 1-2 senior staff of the hospital. Elected members could include a few of the Society elected for a fixed tenure. Ex-officio members include certain office-bearers of the Society, the Hospital Chief Executive Officer, and sometimes a few key executives of the hospital (e.g.: Dean of the Medical College, Medical Superintendent, Finance Director, Principal of the Nursing College, etc.) The Board generally meets 4-6 times a year and reports to the Governing Body.

The functions and activities of the Governing Body—more specifically carried out by its executive arm, the Governing Board - include the following:

Legal Representative

- It is the legal representative of the hospital.
- It is the highest management body responsible for all activities and lapses of the hospital.
- It ensures that the hospital complies with all relevant rules and directives laid down by the Government, Court, Health authorities and other statutory and regulatory bodies.

Mission and Goals

- It develops the mission and goals of the hospital with inputs from the general body, hospital administration, staff and others.
- It ensures a mechanism for communicating the institutional philosophy and goals to all the staff, patients and the community.
- It approves strategic plans for services and programmes intended to pursue these objectives.
- It approves department-wise objectives consistent with the institutional objectives.

- It receives regular reports from the administration on activities performed and goals achieved.
- It evolves a mechanism to monitor achievements and failures.
- It reviews the mission statement and makes changes on a periodical basis.

Organization and Direction

- It approves the organizational set-up of the hospital.
- It considers proposals for new services and departments.
- It selects and appoints the Chief Executive Officer, fixes his compensation, delegates to him duties and responsibilities, and defines the limits of his authority.
- It assists in the selection and approves appointment of key management and medical personnel, department heads and other senior staff, and approves their job description.
- It approves the staff budget including the grades and number of staff of each grade, salary scale, general and special perquisites;
- It appraises periodically the management of the institution and the performance of the CEO and other key personnel.

Policies, Rules and Regulations

- It lays down major policies, rules and regulations consistent with the objectives of the hospital, legal requirements, responsibility for patient care, code of conduct, discipline, efficiency of operations, safety of the institution, staff and public.
- It defines major policies for administrative action, financial transactions and record keeping, hospital admissions, co-operation with other organizations.
- It periodically revises the policies, rules and regulations in response to changed circumstances, advice from the administration, representations from staff.
- It ensures that there are written policies and procedures for resolution of apparent or potential conflicts and for redress of grievances.

Resources

- It is responsible for the provision of human, physical and financial resources required to fulfil the mission and goals of the institution;

- It approves the long term capital development plan for the hospital and plans for the forthcoming year/s.
- It develops, approves and assists in plans for raising resources required for additional projects.
- It approves merger, acquisition, sale of property.
- It approves the annual capital and recurring budget relating to revenue and expenditure.
- It approves purchase/disposal of major assets.
- It approves major contracts.
- It appoints a chartered accountant as the external auditor.
- It reviews the audited statement of accounts of the past year.
- It ensures that there is administrative follow-up on the recommendations made in the annual audit report, and seeks feedback from the administration on action taken.
- It ensures that there is a human resources plan for staff consistent with the hospital strategic plans.

Quality Assurance

- It is accountable for the provision of quality patient care.
- It adopts a policy for institution-wide quality assurance.
- It establishes a mechanism for receiving periodical reports on the quality assurance programmes in force at the hospital.

Utilization

- It receives and reviews utilization reports, work turnover and productivity.
- It appraises the CEO and other key executives on the effective and efficient management of resources.

Health and Safety

- It approves a programme for the health and safety of patients, staff and visitors.
- It ensures that the institution has taken measures to prevent fire and internal disasters.
- It reviews institutional preparedness to deal with internal and external disasters.

Senior Management Executives

In so far as the hospital is concerned, the Chief Executive Officer is the executive arm of the Governing Board and is responsible for implementation of its policies, rules and directives. The CEO is assisted in this task by the following senior management executives who oversee and manage the day-to-day affairs of the various functional areas of the hospital:
- Medical Superintendent / Hospital Administrator
- Nursing Superintendent
- Assistant Administrator/s
- Dean of the Medical College
- Principal of the Nursing College
- Finance Manager,
- Personnel Manager.

The role and responsibilities of each of the above executives will be discussed in the chapters dealing with the respective services.

Many hospitals find it convenient to appoint Hospital Administration Residents or Nurse Administrators as **Duty Directors**. During normal working hours, a Duty Director generally holds charge of the Patient Relations Department and, in which capacity he will:

— attend to patient complaints,
— assist VIP patients,
— supervise the registration and front office,
— manage queues,
— receive official guests,
— report to the concerned executive or department head any untoward incident noticed/reported.

During the evening and night shifts and on weekends, the Director on shift duty will attend to the aforesaid activities and also be administratively responsible for the hospital. In this latter capacity, he:

— represents the Hospital Administration,
— supervises the general working of the hospital during off-duty hours,
— is to be immediately notified of any major critical incident which occurs in the hospital,
— carries out rounds to inspect the uninterrupted functioning of facilities and nonavailability of staff,

- liaises with the Police and external agencies with regard to relevant urgent matters,
- provides on-the-spot cover for the CEO, Medical Superintendent and Hospital Administrator,
- filters matters and decides when the senior administrative executives ought to be contacted/summoned for major problems,
- submits a written report to the Hospital Administration on salient events that have transpired during that shift, and his observations regarding inadequate functioning of facilities and staff.

The Department Heads

Organizationally, reporting to the CEO and the senior management executives, are the various Heads of Departments. Each Department Head is responsible for all the activities that fall within the purview of that department and should ensure that the departmental objectives and activities are in line with the hospital's mission and objectives. In general, the job description of a Head of Department:
- He is overall responsible for quantity and quality of work performed by the department, proper utilization of its facilities, and adherence to its work protocols and procedures.
- He is responsible for staff posted under him. He should supervise their work, attendance, punctuality, discipline and performance.
- He is the primary authority to recommend leave applications of staff posted under him. He should maintain a leave roster and ensure that not too many staffs of the department are simultaneously on leave, or away from the hospital, such that their absence disrupts functioning or causes inconvenience to patient care. He is the authority to confirm attendance of his staff on their return from leave. He should notify the administration in case of unauthorized absence of any of his staff.
- He is responsible for materials and equipment made available for use by his department and staff posted under his charge. He is responsible for placing indents for drugs, consumables and equipment directly related to his department and its activities.
- He is responsible for records pertaining to patients treated by the department and activities carried out by staff of his department. He should ensure that such records are up-to-date, legible,

factual and bear the entries and name of the concerned staff. He should ensure proper upkeep and safe-custody of these records in accordance with the hospital records' retention policy.
- He should provide leadership in training and research activities and stimulate staff of his department to carry out similar activities.
- He should conduct periodical departmental meetings with his staff to review performance, conduct audits, address existing problems, ensure professionalism amongst staff, and promote productivity and efficiency of the department. Minutes of such departmental meetings should be forwarded to the concerned senior management executive/s.
- He reports to his immediate superior and thus should submit through proper channel his requests concerning staff, materials, equipment and any correspondence addressed to higher authorities. He should keep his immediate superior informed of all major issues concerning the department.
- He should promote the interests of the hospital in general and his department in particular, simultaneously ensuring that his department and its staff work in close cooperation with other departments.
- He should carry out such other tasks and functions as delegated to him by the appropriate hospital authority.

CHAPTER 15

Hospital Committees

*"Sitting on a committee is like sitting on a commode.
You make a lot of noise and finally
drop the whole matter."...*
　　　　　　　　Sir Winston Churchill

*"A group of men who individually can do nothing,
but as a group decide that nothing can be done."*
　　　　　　　　... Fred Allen

*"A group of the unfit, appointed by the unwilling,
to do the unnecessary."*
　　　　　　　　... Stewart Harrol.

The above quotes, made in lighter vein, express the frustration that many people experience with Committees: lack of direction, long winded discussions, indecisiveness, impotent recommendations, an executive's excuse to escape from prompt decision making, shirking of responsibility, a coffee club, a status symbol, a forum to settle scores, etc.

But despite these assertions of resentment, Committees are so essential to the present day mode of functioning that they have become institutionalized in the structure of most organizations. Committees, in fact, have the following merits:

- They foster shared decision making and participative style of management, which are vital for employee motivation, commitment and achievement of objectives.
- Committees facilitate better communication, team building, and inter-departmental cooperation.
- Committees bring out the combined wisdom of knowledgeable people, in that a problem is invariably viewed from various angles and finally a consensus emerges, which, hopefully is the best alternative. The final decision is thus likely to be more rational and objective.

- Committees which include members with varied expertise are useful in problem solving and project management.
- Many an executive dreads taking a very sensitive decision which has not been endorsed by a Committee. Since a Committee is a relatively anonymous entity, it is easier to ascribe the responsibility for the unpleasant decision to it rather than to have an individual executive handle the 'hot potato'. This is especially true if confidentiality is maintained, and the opinions of specific committee members are not divulged.
- Certain committees (e.g.: Purchase Committee, Appointments Committee, etc.) are set up as statutory bodies to prevent centralization of power, autocracy, corruption.
- Standing committees which meet at regular intervals (e.g.: Mortality Committee, Utilization Review Committee, Blood Utilization Committee, Infection Control Committee, etc.) set out clear time periods for review of certain topics and compel monitoring of progress on a periodical basis.

In large hospital set-ups, there are various committees that can be of great benefit if put to proper use. The Chief Executive Officer and the senior management executives (Hospital Administrator, Medical Superintendent, Nursing Superintendent, Quality Assurance Officer) are **ex-officio members** of all hospital committees. They should be notified of meetings, attend when possible/indicated, and minutes of meetings should be endorsed to them for information and needful action.

The various **standing committees** that generally exist in large hospitals, their **membership** and **terms of reference** are as follows:

MANAGEMENT/ADMINISTRATIVE COMMITTEE:

An executive ought to take decisions only within the limits of his area of authority. Any matter that concerns more than one area warrants prior joint consultation between the concerned executives. This is especially true at the senior management level where major issues generally do not fall into 'watertight compartments' but have 'grey areas' with implications on medical, nursing, financial and administrative services. The best forum to discuss such matters of common concern is the Management/Administrative Committee.

This committee includes the following senior management executives who work closely with the Chief Executive Officer to oversee and manage the day-to-day affairs of the hospital:

- CEO / Hospital Director *(Convener)*

- Hospital Administrator
- Medical Superintendent
- Nursing Superintendent
- Assistant Administrator/s
- Dean of the Medical College
- Principal of the Nursing College
- Finance Manager, and
- Personnel Manager.

The Management Committee should preferably meet on a weekly basis at a set day of the week and time.

Since this is a quasi-formal group, the meetings may or may not be minuted, though there needs to be a clear understanding of who will take action.

The terms of reference of the Management Committee are:
- To assist the CEO in the smooth and efficient running of the hospital.
- To foster a closely-knit team of senior executives who will work cohesively and present a united leadership front for the hospital.
- To provide a forum for executives to consult each other on issues that could have immediate or long-term implications on other functional areas.
- To apprise other executives of major issues and incidents peculiar to each area.
- To review utilization of resources and consider major changes in hospital procedures, rules and regulations that affect the hospital operations, staff and patient care in general.
- To advise the CEO on policies which require approval by the Governing Board.
- To help in preparation of the annual hospital report, capital and recurring budget, and long and short-term plans for the hospital.

MEDICAL COMMITTEE

The Medical Committee is the highest technical body in the hospital responsible for laying down its code of medical practice. It is the chief forum to approve general policies and procedures related to the safe and efficient delivery of patient care services.

The members of the Medical Committee include the following:
- Medical Director / Medical Superintendent / Chief of Medical Services *(Chairman)*

- Hospital Administrator *(Secretary)*
- Dean of the Medical College
- Principal of the Nursing College
- Nursing Superintendent
- Quality Assurance Officer
- Heads of Divisions of Medicine, Surgery, Pediatrics, Obstetrics and Gynecology, Laboratory
- Heads of Departments of Radiology, Anesthesia and Intensive Care, Accident and Emergency.

The Medical Committee should generally meet once a month at a set day of the month and time, with a fixed agenda.

The role and responsibilities of the Committee are:

- To promote the clinical interests of the hospital and ensure a high standard of care.
- To consider ways and means of effecting improvements so as to bring about higher degree of efficiency, effectiveness and economy in the running of the hospital, its departments and sections.
- To formulate plans for growth and development of the hospital, review proposals for upgrading its services, and establish priorities in the context of budgetary constraints.
- To recommend major changes in organizations structure and rules and regulations of the hospital in so far as they have a bearing on patient care services, teaching and clinical research.
- To approve inter-departmental operational policies relating to the admission and care of patients and utilization of facilities.
- To grant clinical privileges to individual doctors on the advice of the concerned head of department.
- To receive reports from various technical committees constituted in the hospital to oversee specific activities.
- To advise the Hospital Administration on important decisions concerning the hospital and welfare of patients, community and staff.

QUALITY COUNCIL/QUALITY ASSURANCE/MEDICAL AUDIT/ PEER REVIEW COMMITTEE

A central Quality Council or Quality Assurance Committee is advocated to coordinate, monitor and review the quality assurance activities in the hospital.

Membership of the committee includes:

Hospital Committees

- CEO / Hospital Director *(Chairman)*
- Quality Assurance Officer *(Secretary)*
- Principals of Medical and Nursing Colleges
- Hospital Administrator
- Medical Superintendent
- Nursing Superintendent
- Heads/Representatives of Divisions of Medicine, Surgery, Pediatrics, Obstetrics and Gynecology, Laboratory
- Heads/Representatives of Departments of Radiology, Anesthesia, A and E
- Chief Pharmacist
- Medical Records Officer.

The role of such a Quality Council is:
- To determine the objectives, set priorities and approve plans for quality assurance activities in the hospital.
- To receive periodical reports from the Quality Assurance Officer on activities carried out, risk management initiatives, mortality audits, infection control, length of stay, utilization review, patient satisfaction surveys, etc.
- To advise on policies and rules to effect improvements in quality of patient care and safety of staff.

A central Medical Audit/Peer Review Committee is a thing of the past and is currently not advocated. This is because the technicalities of care between one discipline and another are so diverse that it would be inappropriate for a clinician from one speciality to opine on the quality of care rendered by another unrelated speciality. (For example, it is difficult for an Urologist or Internist to speak on authority on the shortcomings associated with a neonatal death. Instead, it would be more appropriate that neonatal mortality statistics and detailed case-review be discussed at scheduled meetings involving Obstetricians, Neonatologists, Pediatric Surgeons and Nurses specialized in these areas.) For that reason, and because audits must be conducted in a scientific manner free from administrative action, it has become customary to assess quality of care (through mortality audits, maternal deaths, peer review, utilization review, medical records review, etc.) on a Divisional/Departmental basis. Rather than a central committee, the clinicians, nurses and diagnostic staff involved with the care of the concerned patient/s should meet on a periodical basis to review the adequacy and competence of care provided and to agree on measures to be taken to improve the same. The role of the Hospital Administration is not to actually perform the audits but, through the Quality Assurance Office, to ensure that such audits are carried out on a regular on-going basis.

MEDICAL RECORDS COMMITTEE

Membership of this committee includes:
- Medical Superintendent *(Chairman)*
- Medical Records Officer *(Secretary)*
- Quality Assurance Officer
- Nursing Superintendent or her representative
- Senior clinician representatives of the Divisions of
  — medicine
  — surgery
  — pediatrics
  — obstetrics and Gynecology
- Statistical / Health Information Officer.
  The Committee generally meets once in 2-3 months.
  The Committee's terms of reference are:
- To review medical records for timely completion, clinical pertinence and overall adequacy for patient care, education and research, administrative and legal purposes.
- To review medical records to ensure that they reflect the condition and progress of the patient, to justify the diagnosis, warrant the investigations, treatment and end results.
- To approve the format of the complete medical record, forms to be retained or discarded, and order of arrangement of forms in the patient's file.
- To approve the various forms for requisitions, reporting, record of clinical data, certificates, etc. and thereby promote standardization of form size, form contents and design, patient demographic data, appropriate color coding, and reduction in number and variety of forms.
- To determine the retention policy for the patient's file and various other records and registers.
- To advise the Medical Records Department on policies in relation to clinical requirements.
- To review plans and programmes of the Medical Records Department with regard to staff, space, facilities, and in-service training.

THEATER USERS' COMMITTEE

The members of the TUC include:
- Head, Division of Surgery / Chief Surgeon *(Chairman)*
- Operation Theater Manager / Nursing Officer *(Secretary)*
- Medical Superintendent
- Quality Assurance Officer
- 5-6 senior clinical representatives from the Departments of Cardio-thoracic Surgery, Dental Surgery, General Surgery, Genito-urinary Surgery, Obstetrics and Gynecology, Ophthalmology, Orthopedics, Otorhinolaryngology, Pediatric Surgery, Plastic Surgery, Neuro-Surgery
- 1-2 Anesthesiologists
- Nursing Officer, Surgical Wards
- CSSD Manager.

The Theater Users' Committee should generally meet once a month.

Its terms of reference include:
- To formulate policies for theater utilization by different departments, prepare a department-wise standing schedule/roster for use of theaters for elective surgeries, set guidelines for priority allotment of theater/s for emergencies, and ensure most effective use of facilities, staff and theater time.
- To advise on the general staffing pattern and training programs specific to theater staff.
- To advise on equipment and instrument requirements for common use in the theater.
- To rationalize the use of sutures, dressing materials, surgical devices, consumables and theater linen so as to achieve standardization and restrict the range of varieties and sizes used by the various clinical departments.
- To monitor critical incidents which occur in the theater and institute risk management measures to reduce their frequency, seriousness and risk.
- To take note of post-operative infection, unscheduled patient returns to the theater, cancelled surgeries, non-functioning equipment and other factors that inconvenience patient care.
- To monitor standards of theater practice as it applies to the health and safety of staff working within the theater environment.
- To ensure that records relating to theater utilization and materials used are properly maintained.

BLOOD UTILIZATION COMMITTEE

The membership of the Blood Utilization Committee includes:
- Head, Department of Haematology and Blood Transfusion *(Chairman)*
- Blood Bank Officer *(Secretary)*
- Medical Superintendent
- Nursing Superintendent
- Quality Assurance Officer
- One senior clinical representative from each of the Divisions of Medicine, Child Health, Surgery and Obstetrics and Gynecology
- Pediatric Oncologist and Haematologist
- Adult Oncologist and Haematologist
- Senior Technologist in Blood Bank.
  The Committee generally meets once every 3 months.
  The Committee's terms of reference are:
- To establish broad policies for blood transfusion therapy in the hospital and thereby promote the adequacy, safety and effective use of blood and blood products.
- To audit blood use, with particular attention to the relevance of blood requests, crossmatched/transfused ratio, blood wasted, statistics on transfusion reactions and other adverse events.
- To establish a maximum blood ordering schedule whereby blood availability is ensured for scheduled interventional procedures but is not specifically allocated.
- To provide clinician feedback to the Blood Bank and advise on improvements desired by clinical, nursing and other staff.

INFECTION CONTROL COMMITTEE

Membership of the Nosocomial Infection Control Committee includes:
- Head, Department of Clinical Microbiology *(Chairman)*
- Infection Control Doctor / Officer *(Secretary)*
- Infection Control Nursing Officer
- Medical Superintendent
- Nursing Superintendent
- Quality Assurance Officer
- A senior clinical representative from each of the Divisions of Medicine, Surgery, Pediatrics and Obstetrics and Gynecology
- Community Health Doctor.

The Infection Control Committee meets once a month though urgent meetings will be warranted at times of infection outbreaks in the hospital.
The terms of reference of the Committee are:
- To institute appropriate control measures to minimize nosocomial infection in the hospital.
- To supervise the functioning of the Infection Control Team and its activities and effectiveness.
- To write, review and update periodically various infection control policies including those related to surveillance of hospital related infection, disinfection and sterilization of hospital appliances and surgical devices, safety of staff, universal precautions, isolation of patients, inoculation injuries, management of wastes, laundry and linen.
- To review hospital infection related statistics prepared on a monthly basis and recommend specific actions to be taken by the infection control team, various departments and wards, and specific staff.
- To educate through lectures, symposia, workshops and seminars medical, nursing and ancillary staff, patients and their attendants regarding nosocomial infection, their prevention and control.
- To ensure that notifiable diseases are adequately reported and communicated to the appropriate authorities.
- To ensure regular supply of appropriate equipment, consumables and drugs required to effectively control nosocomial infections.
- To supervise staff health and recommend procedures for protection of staff against nosocomial infection, ensuring their vaccination, periodical check-ups and application of universal precautions.
- To ensure that the various hospital contractors (e.g.: cleaning, catering, pest control, laundry, etc.) abide by the terms of their contracts in aspects related to control of infections, use of detergents and disinfectants, and general hygiene of the hospital.

CARDIO-PULMONARY RESUSCITATION COMMITTEE

The CPR Committee consists of the following members:
- Head, Department of Anesthesia *(Chairman)*

- Nursing Officer, In-service Education *(Secretary)*
- Medical Superintendent
- Nursing Superintendent
- Quality Assurance Officer
- One senior clinician representative from each of the Divisions of Pediatrics, Medicine, Surgery and Obstetrics and Gynecology
- A senior clinician representative from Adult ICU, Pediatric ICU, Neonatal ICU, and Accident and Emergency department.

The Committee meets once every 2-3 months.

The role and responsibilities of the Committee are:

- To develop and regularly review policies and procedures for cardio-pulmonary resuscitation.
- To develop standards and indicators for monitoring effectiveness of CPR procedures at the hospital.
- To institute a system for recording and evaluating every resuscitation incident, prepare periodical reports on appropriateness, efficiency and outcome, and make necessary recommendations for improvement.
- To plan, coordinate and oversee Basic and Advanced Cardiac Life Support training courses, by certified trainers, for medical, nursing and paramedical staff.

TUMOR BOARD

Hospitals that provide treatment and long-term follow-up in Oncology need to have clear protocols for staging and management of patients with cancer. Nevertheless, such hospitals should also have a Tumor Board to discuss newly diagnosed cases that warrant multi-specialiaty advice in formulating a plan of therapy: surgical, chemotherapy and/or radiotherapy.

The core members of the Tumor Board include:
- Head, Department of Oncology *(Chairman)*
- Surgical Oncologist *(Secretary)*
- Adult and Pediatric Oncologists
- Radiologist
- Histopathologist
- Radiotherapist.

The above core members of the Board may deputize representatives from their respective departments to attend meetings convened in their absence.

Additionally, the Consultant in charge of the respective patient (Surgeon, Gynecologist, Pediatrician) should also be invited to the meeting to present the specific case.

The member-secretary is responsible for scheduling cases to be discussed and for recording decisions of the Board.

The Board generally meets once a week and additionally when necessary.

The terms of reference of the Tumor Board include:
- Setting up guidelines and protocols for management of routine Oncology cases.
- Advice to treating clinicians on treatment modalities applicable in nonroutine and multi-disciplinary cases, especially when multiple treatments are involved.
- Reviewing norms regarding staging and management.

PHARMACY AND THERAPEUTICS COMMITTEE

The role of the Pharmacy and Therapeutics Committee is to oversee the prescribing practices in the hospital and thereby ensure rational therapeutics.

The members include:
- Medical Superintendent *(Chairman)*
- Chief Pharmacist *(Secretary)*
- Nursing Superintendent
- Quality Assurance Officer
- One senior clinical representative from each of the Divisions of Medicine, Surgery, Pediatrics and Obstetrics and Gynecology
- Representative from Anesthesia / Critical care medicine
- Microbiologist
- Clinical Pharmacist / Drug Information Pharmacist
- Pharmacist in-charge of Medical Stores.

The Pharmacy and Therapeutics Committee generally meets once a month and additionally when necessary.

The Committee's terms of reference are:
- To serve in an evaluative, educational and advisory capacity to the medical staff, pharmacy and administration in all matters pertaining to the purchase, stocking, distribution, prescription and use of drugs.
- To develop the hospital formulary and recommend on a periodical basis drug formulations to be added/deleted on the basis of their relative therapeutic merits and safety.

- To ensure a proper system for prescribing and dispensing of narcotics and controlled drugs.
- To develop guidelines for the hospital antibiotics policy and review on a periodical basis the use and misuse of antibiotics.
- To establish programs and procedures to promote rational prescribing practices and cost effective drug therapy.
- To initiate and direct drug use evaluation programmes and studies, and review the results of such activities.
- To monitor and evaluate adverse drug reactions and make appropriate recommendations.
- To recommend policies and procedures for drug evaluation and clinical trials and consider requests for such drug trials on hospital patients.
- To plan suitable educational programmes for hospital professionals on matters related to drug use.

CONTINUING PROFESSIONAL EDUCATION COMMITTEE

In a teaching hospital medical and nursing staffs are invariably exposed to educational programmes and clinical research and thus have an opportunity to keep in touch with the changing trends in healthcare technology. In a nonteaching hospital, to avoid professional decay, there is need for a group of enlightened and interested individuals to provide such scientific stimulus. This is often formalized through a committee, which will not cater only to doctors (as in CME) but to all categories of hospital staff.

Membership of the Continuing Professional Education Committee could include the following:
- An eminent and up-to-date clinician *(Chairman)*
- In-service education Nursing Officer *(Secretary)*
- A representative from each of the Division of Medicine, Surgery, Pediatrics and Obstetrics and Gynecology
- Medical Superintendent
- Nursing Superintendent
- Quality Assurance Officer
- Personnel / Human Resources Manager.

The CPE Committee generally meets once a month. Its scope of activities include:
- To advise on, plan, coordinate, monitor and evaluate programs for continuing professional education of hospital staff of all categories.

- To review the implementation of in-service training programs, make necessary recommendations and monitor action taken.
- To establish and implement policies and procedures relating to research and publication activities in the hospital and related ethical issues.
- To establish and implement policies and procedures regarding academic leave.
- To ensure the availability and maintenance of teaching and conference facilities including audio-visual aids and lecture/seminar rooms.

PURCHASE COMMITTEE

In the matter of purchases, every care must be taken to safeguard the interests of the institution. No supplier or staff member should be allowed to profiteer at the expense of the hospital. Purchase decisions, especially those relating to major cash outflows, should therefore be decentralized. Beyond making buyer-vendor collusion more difficult, Purchase Committees also ensure that, wherever indicated, all concerned are consulted and the best choice is made.

There may be separate Purchase Committees in the hospital for drugs, for laboratory supplies, for medical equipment, for general supplies, for catering/housekeeping/laundry/maintenance contracts, etc. Depending on the purchase and inventory replenishment system adopted by the hospital, these Committees may meet relatively infrequently or at periodic (e.g.: bi-weekly or monthly) intervals.

Members of a Purchase Committee include:
- Hospital Administrator *(Chairman)*
- Head, Purchasing Section *(Secretary)*
- Medical Superintendent
- Concerned technical heads—Chief Pharmacist, Chief Laboratory Technologist, Clinician/s using the equipment, etc.
- Concerned engineer – Electrical engineer, Biomedical engineer, etc.

The responsibilities of the Purchase Committee include:
- To ensure that all transactions are above-board and in the interests of the hospital.
- To oversee the tender process including purchase specifications and opening of quotations.

- To review comparative statements of offers received, shortlist preferences and advise on negotiations.
- To maintain confidentiality.

APPOINTMENTS COMMITTEE

Selection and appointment of staff should be candid and merited. Appointments Committees ensure openness, absence of favouritism, involvement of the concerned superior/s, and review of the applicant from varied perspectives.

There will invariably be separate Appointments Committees in the hospital for recruitment of doctors, nurses, technicians, administrative and support staff.

Members of such Appointments Committees include:
- The CEO/Hospital Director (for senior staff)
- Hospital Administrator
- Medical Superintendent
- Nursing Superintendent
- Personnel Officer
- Concerned Head of Department
- Technical Expert/s where indicated.

Section 5: The Clinical Services

CHAPTER

16

The Medical Staff Organization

...*In December 1919, the American College of Surgeons (predecessor of the Joint Commission on Accreditation of Hospitals) adopted the following five criteria, which became known as the Minimum Standard:*
1. "That physicians and surgeons privileged to practice in a hospital be organized as a definite group of staff... inclusive of... the 'regular staff', the 'visiting staff', and the 'associate staff'.
2. That membership upon the staff be restricted to physicians and surgeons who are (a) full graduates of medicine in good standing and legally licensed..., (b) competent in their respective fields, and (c) worthy in character and in matters of professional ethics; that in this latter connection the practice of the division of fees, under any guise whatever, be prohibited.
3. That staff initiate and, with approval of the governing board of the hospital, adopt rules, regulations, and policies governing the professional work of the hospital; that these rules regulations, and policies specifically provide: (a) That staff meetings be held at least once each month...; (b) That staff review and analyze at regular intervals their clinical experience in the various departments of the hospital...; the clinical records of patients, free and pay, to be the basis for such review and analyzes.
4. That accurate and complete records be written for all patients and filed in an accessible manner in the hospital......

5. That diagnostic and therapeutic facilities under competent supervision be available for the study, diagnosis, and treatment of patients, these to include, at least (a) a clinical laboratory......; (b) an X-ray department......"

The above principles, proclaimed almost a century ago, form the basis even today for the Medical Staff Organization in hospitals all over the world.

MEDICAL STAFF: WHAT IS DIFFERENT OR UNIQUE?

- Doctors are the most **dominant decision-makers** in the hospital. It is they who decide whether patients are to be admitted or not, what investigations and treatment are to be carried out and when the patients are to be discharged. Their patient care related decisions have wide ranging implications on technology, manner of functioning of the hospital and costs. Their performance and idiosyncrasies can make or break the reputation of the hospital. Given the right climate—which is the fundamental role of management—doctors can perform medical marvels, relieve human suffering and take the hospital to new heights never dreamt before. In contrast, not handled well, doctors can be reduced to the position of mere employees concerned only with permanency, ego status and monetary compensation. Decisions taken by the hospital administration affect doctors' motivation and attitude to work, which in turn influence the quality of patient care. It is hence important to involve doctors in decision making wherever possible: planning of new facilities, change in rules and policies, acquisition of new equipment, introducing new management concepts, controlling usage of consumables and drugs, revenue generation and cost control.
- It must be remembered that Medicine is a science, best left to medical professionals. Nontechnical staff should, therefore not dabble in and influence the practice of medicine. In fact, one of the most important objectives of the medical staff organization is **self-governance**. It is the senior doctors who should be involved in setting up the code of practice, medically related policies and procedures, treatment protocols, etc. and it is they who should regulate its implementation. The role of hospital administration in so far as medical staff are concerned is a global one and not patient specific—to support the medical staff organization, to

provide the best environment especially with regard to ancillary and support services, to ensure smooth and efficient running of the hospital.
- Beyond the medical profession being another avenue to satisfy human needs, having chosen medicine as a career, doctors are aware of the **self-sacrifice** expected of them. Doctors know that theirs is not a 9 to 5 operation, that can be shut down on weekends or when they are on leave; they are aware that medical emergencies cannot be postponed to suit convenience, that emergency care must be provided irrespective of the patient's ability to pay. The hospital administration must in turn recognize that doctors' services cannot be abused just because of the avowed humanitarian approach. Even not-for-profit hospitals have an obligation to compensate doctors fairly, especially to attract and retain the best talent. There are moves to limit the number of working hours per week of junior doctors (who traditionally have been known to work on 36-hour continuous shifts when on duty) and to compensate doctors for overtime work as for other occupations.
- In hospital practice, a doctor does not function in isolation but as a team member. As different doctors have to manage the patient during the course of a hospitalization episode or over several outpatient encounters, **continuity of care** must be ensured through proper patient documentation in medical records, firm adherence to procedures and treatment protocols, and written instructions to be complied by other doctors, nurses, paramedical and support staff.
- Being exposed to a patient's innermost secrets, doctors have an important moral obligation to maintain **confidentiality**. This must be supported by all other staff of the hospital who come in contact with medical information.
- Doctors are bound by rules of conduct. The Medical Council of India published its **Code of Medical Ethics** which includes general principles/responsibilities, duties of physicians to their patients, duties of the physician to the profession at large, professional services of physicians to each other, duties of physician in consultation, duties of physician in cases of interference, duties of physician to the public, disciplinary action, list of offences. The UK General Medical Council, in its July 1998 document on Maintaining Good Medical Practice, has more

specifically spelt out the responsibilities of doctors as members of clinical teams in hospital practice.

Objectives of the Medical Staff Organization

- To ensure that all patients admitted to the hospital, treated in the OPD/A and E, or through community extension services receive the best possible care.
- To initiate, periodically review and implement rules and regulations for governance of medical staff.
- To provide means whereby medico-administrative issues are discussed with the Hospital Administration and Governing Board.
- To establish and maintain high professional and ethical standards by means of review, analysis and evaluation of quality of medical care being rendered.
- To provide opportunities for high standard of in-service education.
- To foster an atmosphere of study and clinical research subject to the hospital's philosophy, financial limits and professional capabilities of staff.
- To develop community health services supportive of total community development.

Nature of the Organization

The medical staff organization may be formal/tight or informal/loose depending on the nature of the hospital and the clinician-hospital relationship:

- A rigid, *formal* medical staff structure occurs in the case of large, specialist, well-reputed, teaching hospitals, having mostly full-time salaried clinicians, who are organized into departments and units.
- A relatively *informal* medical staff organization is associated with small, for-profit, nonteaching hospitals where senior clinicians are mainly part-time/visiting. In this latter scenario, Consultants may have their own arrangements with the hospital, and the medical staff organization is more like an association of doctors bound by a set code of conduct. However, even in such loose structures, there could be some elements of the more formal model.

The characteristics of a formal medical staff organization include:

Clinical Committees

The structure, function and relationship of Committees play an important role in the medical staff organization. The main body that governs the practice of medicine in the hospital is the Medical Committee. Reporting to it are various committees:
- To regulate and monitor the quality of care:
  — medical Bylaws Committee
  — quality Assurance Committee
  — infection Control Committee
  — pharmacy and Therapeutics Committee
  — utilization Review Committee
  — blood Utilization Committee
  — credentialing Committee
  — tissue Review Committee
- To liaise between various users of a service:
  — medical Records Committee
  — theatre Users' Committee
  — cardio Pulmonary Resuscitation Committee
  — tumor Board
  — intensive Care Committee
  — diagnostic Services Committee
- To undertake specific tasks:
  — continuing Medical Education Committee
  — disaster Management Committee
  — medical Planning Committee
  — ethics and Research Committee

The structure and functions of the more frequently constituted committees have been detailed in the chapter on "Hospital Committee" elsewhere in this book.

The Chief of Medical Staff

He may carry this title or the more popular designations of Medical Director or Medical Superintendent. He may be a full-time medical administrator or an administrator-cum-clinician. In the former case, he may be also the Chief Executive Officer of the hospital or he may be only in-charge of medical administration, reporting to the CEO. If he is part administrator part clinician, he takes on the role more of a well-respected clinician, heading the medical establishment perhaps for a fixed tenure, with less direct involvement in day-to-day administrative matters, which are relegated to a Hospital Administrator.

The job requirements and duties of the Medical Director/Superintendent have been detailed in the chapter on "The Hospital Administrator—Role and Responsibilities" elsewhere in this book. In summary, he:
— should have knowledge of administration, rules and regulations;
— should have high level of leadership capability;
— is overall responsible for efficient functioning of clinical and ancillary services, and quality of care;
— is administratively responsible for medical and paramedical staff;
— is responsible for all matters having medico-legal implications.

Clinical Directorates

Some large specialist hospitals tend to be organized on the basis of their major service lines for several reasons:
- In keeping with the concept of 'span of control', rather than the Medical Director having to directly deal with 15-20 clinical departments, more effective supervision is ensured if these services are grouped into 4-5 allied specialities;
- It is more economical to share resources (e.g.: resident doctors, nurses, medical secretaries, hospital beds, OPD facilities, equipment, surgical devices, etc.) for activities which are common to a group of allied specialities and sub/super-specialities;
- Particularly with respect to very small clinical departments, certain activities (e.g.: quality assurance, clinical meetings, training of junior doctors, conferences, etc.) are more effectively carried out with a larger group;
- By dividing the hospital into such revenue/cost centers, it is possible to formally involve doctors in management and make them financially accountable for their clinical decisions, control over usage of resources, revenue generation and cost control. Through clinical budgeting, it is possible to set up a financial system whereby each directorate earns revenue for the service it provides and pays other directorates or the hospital for the services it utilizes. Doctors thereby become cost conscious and take more rational decisions relating to patient care. Involvement

in decision making, and management of its own affairs, including clinical audits, are also more motivating for the doctor and is consistent with the currently recommended management technique of devolution of powers.

In NHS Trust Hospitals in the U.K. a clinical division/ directorate could include 5-8 allied clinical departments (e.g.: Division of Medicine comprises of Internal Medicine, Cardiology, Gastroenterology, Endocrinology, Nephrology, Neurology, and Respiratory Medicine). In the US a clinical department, analogous to a directorate, could entail several divisions or super/sub-specialities.

A clinical directorate is generally headed by a clinician, perhaps elected for a 3-year term. Assisted by a manager and a nurse administrator and supported by an office set up, such a Head/ Director/ Chief/Chairman would generally be responsible for:
- Management of all medical, nursing and paramedical staff of that directorate and including their recruitment, performance, discipline;
- The appropriate working of the concerned specialities and level of care provided by staff of the directorate, quality assurance, utilization review;
- Raising of revenue through provision and expansion of services, including marketing and contracting;
- Control of costs through economical use of resources;
- Decisions related to procurement of equipment, drugs, surgical devices and medical consumables.

Though clinical directorates operate with fair degree of independence, they should function within the framework of broad policies laid down by the Hospital Management. Otherwise a situation could arise with mini-hospitals within a hospital, and the CEO and Hospital Administration being unable to exercise control and coordination over the hospital as a whole.

Speciality and Sub-speciality Departments

Each major discipline/speciality (e.g.: Medicine, Surgery, Pediatrics, Obstetrics and Gynecology, Laboratory Medicine, Anesthesia and Intensive Care, etc.) is a distinct clinical entity and so functions as a separate department. Further, depending on the extent that super/sub-specialities are developed in that hospital, they may be organized into independent clinical departments or they may function within the umbrella of the related major speciality as 'areas of clinical interest'.

114 Hospital Administration

The number and size of clinical departments depend on:
- The hospital size/bed complement;
- The quantum of workload (average inpatient occupancy, outpatient visits, number of major and minor surgeries, working hours per week, frequency of duty rota, teaching and research commitments, etc.);
- The number of specialities and super/sub-specialities functioning independently in that hospital;
- The number of clinicians required in each speciality or super/sub-speciality proportionate to its quantum of workload;
- Statutory requirements or norms prescribed for teaching hospitals (e.g.: Medical Council of India, University);
- Management plans to develop and give importance to particular services.

Each clinical department is managed by a senior clinician of that speciality/super-speciality, who may be appointed for a fixed tenure or on a permanent basis. The job-description and responsibilities of a head of department are detailed in the chapter on "Hospital Organization—Structure and Function" elsewhere in this book.

Clinical Units

Considering the nature and quantum of workload, and for better team cohesiveness, a clinical department may be sub-divided into two or more units. The staffing complement of each clinical unit depends on:
- Number of its outpatient sessions per week, and number of outpatient visits per session;
- Its bed strength, bed occupancy, inpatient admissions, bed turnover interval;
- Type and number of diagnostic and therapeutic procedures;
- manpower required to run the on-call / duty rota which may be 1 in 3 days (or 1 in 4, 1 in 5);
- teaching and other commitments.

Ideally, to ensure optimum bed/doctor ratio and high staff productivity, a 'general intake' unit should be allotted about 30 beds and have a staffing complement of 1 Consultant, 1 Sr Registrar, 2 Registrars and 2 SHOs. The Consultant clinician heads the unit, reports to the department head and is responsible for the smooth and efficient functioning of the unit.

Medical Staff Hierarchy

For the effective functioning of the medical staff organization and execution of work procedures, the doctors in each department/unit are organized in the hierarchy of Consultant, Senior Registrar, Registrar, Senior House Officer (and Intern in a teaching hospital). Although the job description of these medical staff may vary slightly from hospital to hospital, and from speciality to speciality, in general their responsibilities are as below:

- Consultant (Clinician with 7-10 years postgraduate experience; also called Professor/Assoc Professor in teaching hospital):
  — he reports to the department head, routes official correspondence through him, and keeps him informed of relevant clinical and administrative matters;
  — he administers and manages staff of the unit, supervises their performance, ensures that they keep him informed of relevant issues, and delegates to them activities they are qualified and competent to do in accordance with their clinical privileges;
  — unless independent admission/treatment privileges are also granted to a subordinate doctor of the unit, it is the Consultant who bears final responsibility for the care extended to all patients treated by the unit whether as outpatients or inpatients;
  — the above ultimate clinical responsibility covers accuracy of diagnosis, interpretation of results, administration of drugs, prompt attention, need for and proper performance of all diagnostic and therapeutic procedures whether personally carried out by the Consultant or not;
  — beyond his presence at the hospital during its official working hours, he should be accessible at all times and respond promptly when summoned in emergencies, especially when he is on-call;
  — in consultation with the head of department, he ensures adequate consultant cover in his absence, including during off days, holidays and when he is on leave;
  — he provides outpatient consultation, attends to interdepartmental references, and examines inpatients as warranted;
  — he ensures that records of patients treated by his unit are legible, up-to-date and correctly reflect the patient's condition and response to treatment;

- he ensures that the patient is given a written report at the time of inpatient/outpatient discharge from the hospital or back-referral to the primary physician;
- he meets with the members of his team and other relevant staff to periodically audit the quality of care extended by the unit;
- he ensures that staff under his charge comply with service regulations, hospital policies and procedures, and treatment protocols;
- he imparts on-the-job training to his subordinates;
- he participates in clinical committees, education and research activities of the hospital and carries out other administrative responsibilities entrusted to him.

- Senior Registrar (Clinician with 5-7 years postgraduate experience; also called Junior Consultant, Reader or Assistant Professor):
  - he reports to his head of clinical unit and, through him, to the Head of the department;
  - he works under the supervision of the Consultant;
  - he supervises Registrars, Senior House Officers and Interns subordinate to him;
  - unless another Consultant has been nominated to provide cover, he heads the clinical unit in the absence of the Consultant;
  - he assists the Consultant head of unit in administering the unit, supervises the performance of subordinate staff, ensures that they keep him informed of relevant issues, and delegates to them activities they are qualified and competent to do in accordance with their clinical privileges;
  - he provides outpatient consultation, attends to interdepartmental references, and examines inpatients at least once a day (and more frequently when warranted);
  - he independently carries out diagnostic and therapeutic procedures in accordance with his approved clinical privileges;
  - he ensures that records of patients treated by his unit are legible, up-to-date and correctly reflect the patient's condition and response to treatment;
  - he prepares and verifies medical reports, death reports and medico-legal reports issued by the unit;

— when on-call, he is readily accessible to provide telephonic advice and be immediately summoned to the hospital when required;
— when on-call, he carries out evening rounds on all new admissions and critically ill patients;
— he coordinates the clinical audit, teaching and research activities of the department/unit;
— he carries out all other duties as may be assigned to him by the Consultant.

- Registrar (Clinician undergoing postgraduate training or with 1-3 years postgraduate experience; also called Specialist, Lecturer, Tutor, Senior Resident): The Registrar
  — reports to his head of clinical unit and, through him, to the head of the department;
  — works under the supervision of the Consultant and Senior Registrar;
  — supervises Senior House Officers and Interns subordinate to him;
  — is generally the senior most doctor on duty in the hospital after normal working hours, and so takes on-the-spot decisions on behalf of his unit, but he is expected to keep his superiors on-call informed, and immediately summon them when warranted;
  — examines all inpatients at least once a day and more often when clinically warranted (e.g.: after surgery, when patient critical, etc.)
  — admits patients from the outpatient and A and E departments in accordance with the protocols of the unit;
  — independently provides routine outpatient consultation and attends to routine interdepartmental references, but keeps his superiors informed of all cases that merit their attention;
  — initiates interdepartmental references in consultation with his superiors;
  — requests for investigations, follows up on results, prescribes medication, and assists his superiors at diagnostic and therapeutic procedures;
  — independently performs diagnostic and treatment procedures which he is authorized to do in accordance with his clinical privileges;
  — verifies and countersigns discharge certificates prepared by his juniors;

— prepares medical reports and certificates which require authentication by his superiors;
— participates in teaching and research activities of the unit.
- Senior House Officer (Clinician with basic medical degree; also called Resident Medical Officer): The Senior House Officer
  — reports to his head of clinical unit and, through him, to the head of the department;
  — works under the supervision of the Consultant, Senior Registrar and Registrar;
  — supervises Interns subordinate to him;
  — clerks patients and is responsible for initiating and updating the admission record, progress notes, operation notes, discharge summary, leave and death certificates;
  — follows up on results of investigations requested;
  — follows up on instructions of his seniors with regard to scheduling and preparing patients for diagnostic and therapeutic procedures;
  — assists his superior staff at diagnostic and therapeutic procedures;
  — prescribes medications to inpatients and outpatients in accordance with departmental protocols and instructions from his seniors;
  — participates in training and research activities of the unit.
- Medical Intern (Medical Student who has completed the final year examination and is undergoing the one year mandatory preceptorship):
  — he works for 2-3 months in various departments in accordance with his internship programme;
  — since he is under training, he is not authorized to practise independently;
  — he is not authorized to prescribe medications, issue medical certificates or certify deaths;
  — he examines and clerks inpatients and outpatients, writes admission, progress and procedure notes, discharge summaries;
  — he draws blood samples for investigation;
  — he follows up on results of investigations requested by the unit;
  — he assists his superiors at diagnostic and therapeutic procedures;

— he participates in training and research activities of the department.

Employment Categories of Medical Staff

Senior House Officers, Registrars and Senior Registrars generally are full-time salaried employees of the hospital. The employment relationship that Consultants have with the hospital may vary from hospital to hospital:

- Full-time, salaried, without private practice. This is common in teaching centres of excellence, some Government and mission hospitals and industrial hospitals. A nonpractising allowance is additionally offered. It is, however, difficult to police the implementation of this policy. Often clandestine practice exists when the salary is inadequate and management turns a blind eye.
- Full-time, salaried, with geographically limited private practice at the hospital (in the evening), home or clinics, outside the normal working hours of the hospital. This is common in Government and voluntary hospitals.
- Full-time, part-salaried, partly allowed a percentage cut from the amounts collected from patients in private wards. Sometimes there may be a restriction that the private patients of the Consultant should be admitted to that hospital only.
- Part-time, part-salaried, allowed unrestricted private practice. In addition to the nominal salary paid by the hospital, the Consultant may be given a percentage cut on consultations, daily visits and procedures carried out on private patients. Some hospitals even pay a commission on certain investigations requested by the respective Consultant or his clinical unit.
- Honoraries. This had been in vogue in some State Government hospitals but is being progressively discontinued. It also persists in some hospitals in the voluntary sector. Such Consultants have the same privileges as a salaried Consultant but do not receive a monthly remuneration. They may receive payment in proportion to the income generated by them for the hospital, but more often than that, they collect their fees from the patients referred from their private practice.
- Fee for service. The Consultant is only on the hospital panel to be called in whenever needed. This is seen in many for-profit

hospitals. The whole or portion of the amount collected from the patient towards consultation and procedures are passed on to the Consultant. In some cases, the Consultant may collect the fees directly from the patient.

These are but a few of the arrangements that exist for Consultants. The actual agreement, quantum and form of compensation packages are many—limited only by the imagination of the doctor, management and financial consultants.

BYLAWS, RULES, REGULATIONS APPLICABLE TO MEDICAL STAFF

One of the most important functions of the Medical Staff Organization is to develop and adopt bylaws, rules and regulations to establish a framework for self-governance of medical staff activities and their accountability to the management.

Major elements of these bylaws include:

Appointment of Clinical Staff

There must be a procedure to fix and annually review the medical staff positions. The manner of filling the positions should be specified: by internal promotion through proper channel, advertisement, review of applications on file, special invitation, visiting staff, locum staff. The appointment process should clarify the method of verifying qualifications and clinical competence, selection interview, role of the credentials committee, term of appointment, medical fitness. Reappointment should be contingent on past performance and hospital need.

Clinical Privileges

To guarantee a high level of care there must be a mechanism to ensure that each clinician will operate only within the limits of his competence as judged by his qualifications and training and as verified by his Consultant or Head of Department. Thus there must be a mechanism in the hospital to periodically examine the credentials of each member of staff—from the senior most to the junior most in each speciality—and grant, renew or revise clinical privileges for each doctor. These privileges lay down the limits or boundaries of practice and confirm what each doctor is authorized to do independently or under supervision. Clinical privileges cover: outpatient consultation, inter-departmental references, inpatient admission, list of common and higher level diagnostic and therapeutic procedures, list of surgeries and other invasive procedures, prescription of select antibiotics and controlled drugs, etc.

Performance Review

The hospital bylaws should specify the frequency and manner of appraising the performance of medical staff. Appraisal is generally done by the clinical head of unit and is subjected to review by the head of department. Such evaluation should detail the performance of the appraisee, behavior of the doctor, competence, etc. The Quality Assurance Department may additionally be able to draw up the performance profile of clinical heads of units: workload, utilization indicators, operative results, length of stay, risk management indicators, prescribing practices, revenue generation, etc.

Service Rules

The hospital will have its employee standing orders or service rules. These need to be reviewed and more specifically applied to medical staff. The rules should detail out the general conditions of employment, retirement age, working hours, holidays, arrangements for on-call, on site availability on duty days, prompt attendance for emergencies, code of behavior, general duties and responsibilities, acts considered as misconduct, disciplinary process, process of appeal, requirement to participate in departmental meetings and other official forums, leave entitlements and leave procedure, service benefits, nature of approval prior to undertaking external commitments, regulations prior to making statements on public media.

MEDICO-ADMINISTRATIVE POLICIES AND PROCEDURES

The Medical Committee and Hospital Administration should agree upon the medico-administrative policies and procedures that need to be complied with by the medical staff. Salient issues in this regard relate to:
- Outpatient system for booking, appointments, referral and back-referral, outpatient procedures

- Daycare Unit policies and procedures
- Inpatient admission policies and procedures
- Emergency treatment irrespective of patient's ability to pay
- Medico-legal formalities
- ICU and CCU admission and operational policies
- Policies for cardio-pulmonary resuscitation, labelling of patients not for resuscitation, certification of brain death, discontinuation of ventilatory support
- Policies relating to trauma resuscitation, multi-organ trauma
- Inter-department referrals for consultation or take over
- Patient billing policies
- Patient consent, Patient rights
- Medical records documentation, medical reports and discharge summaries, retention policy
- Reporting of critical incidents and risk management issues
- Use of single rooms free of charge for patient isolation and on other medical grounds
- Reporting of notifiable diseases
- Drug prescribing policies, adherence to drug formulary, use of controlled and narcotic drugs
- Equipment and drug trials conducted in the hospital
- Medico-ethical and bio-ethical principles governing clinical research, induced abortions, in vitro fertilization, sex determination, Organ transplants from live and cadaveric donors, etc.

CLINICAL PROTOCOLS:

As stated earlier, hospital care centres on team approach. Continuity of care must be assured irrespective of the physician who is currently managing the patient.

- In order to ensure such a unified approach to patient care management, each department should write up protocols for:
  — routine work-up of patients;
  — common diagnostic and operative procedures carried out;
  — management of ailments where treatment regimens are fairly standardized (e.g.: in asthma, tuberculosis, malaria and its complications, leprosy, HIV infection and AIDS, uncomplicated epilepsy, myocardial infarction, duodenal ulcer, snake bite, etc.).

Techniques in 'managed care' go a step forward. Through professional consensus the most clinically effective and cost efficient mode of management for common clinical conditions are agreed upon. Flow charts with specific milestones are then developed to ensure compliance, monitor progress and detect divergence. In this manner the treatment goals can be achieved without delaying the length of stay and increasing costs.

Section 6: The Nursing Services

CHAPTER
17

Nursing Service

*...Of all categories of hospital staff,
the best organized and
most compliant are invariably the nurses...*

Nursing care is extremely important for good patient outcome. More so in a hospital set up. While physicians plan the treatment and perform the diagnostic and treatment procedures, it is the nurses who spend more time caring for the patient and looking after all his needs throughout the hospital stay. The success of patient care and the reputation of the hospital depend to a large extent on the efficiency and the *tender loving care* extended by the nursing staff. Ensuring high level of nursing care is, therefore a big challenge for the Hospital Administrator.

Nurses constitute a large proportion of the total number employees in any hospital. Nursing is the single largest department of the hospital. Further, due to the close work relationship with ward support staff, generally the Nursing service also manages ward clerks, medical orderlies, porters, and sometimes, even cleaners and other housekeeping staff. The sheer magnitude of the Nursing department necessitates strict compliance with the conventional principles of organizational structure and function. Fortunately, this is not a problem in most hospitals.

OBJECTIVES OF THE NURSING SERVICE:

- To organize the nurses in a manner so as to render high quality of nursing care consistent with the philosophy and objectives of the hospital.
- To support and assist the physicians in medical care and carry out procedures prescribed by medical staff, as consistent with nurses' training and expertise.
- To establish and implement the philosophy, standards, policies, rules and procedures for the smooth and efficient functioning of the nursing service in the hospital.
- To delineate the responsibilities and duties of nursing officials and various categories of nursing personnel.
- To estimate the requirements for nursing personnel, advise on appointment of adequate and competent nurses, and establish policies and programmes for their orientation, placement, on-the-job training and supervision.
- To estimate the need for facilities, equipment and supplies and implement a system for evaluation and control within the administrative and financial framework of the hospital.
- To develop and maintain a system for recording patient care and administrative nursing data.
- To organize and oversee the functioning of wards and other specialized service areas (such as outpatient department, operation theatre, day-care unit, etc.) which are generally managed by nurses.
- To ensure healthy work environment, close collaboration and mutually supportive relationship between nursing and other departments and services in the hospital.
- To establish a good rapport between nurses and patients, patient attendants and visitors.
- To periodically appraise the performance of nurses and carry out regular nursing audits which are necessary to maintain and improve the standard of nursing care.
- To carry out in-service training and thereby augment and update knowledge and skills of nursing staff.
- To train student nurses and provide facilities for advanced training of nursing and other personnel.

THE NURSING ADMINISTRATION

The Nursing Office

Staffed by senior nursing officials and secretarial/clerical staff, the centralized Nursing Office is responsible for administration and coordination of the hospital nursing service. Beyond pursuing the general nursing service objectives cited above, the organizational and clerical activities of the Nursing Office include:
- Formulating rules and regulations applicable to nurses, including their working hours, code of conduct, discipline, reporting system, appraisal;
- Developing and periodically revising nursing policies and procedures related to patient care in general and nursing care in particular;
- Receiving periodical reports from the nursing units;
- Maintaining record of nursing service activities and compiling reports, plans and budgets as and when required;
- Selecting and assigning/reassigning nurses to various wards and specialized service areas depending on vacancies/need and abilities/interests of the staff concerned;
- Monitoring shift/duty rosters, attendance and leave of nursing staff;
- Maintaining personal records of nurses;
- Dealing with professional and personal problems of individual nurses and attending to their welfare;
- Investigating incidents, complaints, allegations of misconduct pertaining to nursing staff;
- Clearing departmental requisitions;
- Transmitting information and instructions, and liaison with other departments and with the hospital administration.

Nursing Superintendent

Also called the Director of Nursing, Principal Nursing Officer or Matron, the Nursing Superintendent generally reports to the Chief Executive Officer. Being the head of Nursing, she should:
- Be a well qualified nurse, preferably with a post-graduate qualification in Nursing Service Administration or one of the nursing specialities;
- Have 10-15 years previous experience in senior nursing positions in medium/large sized hospitals;

- Have an impressive personality and strong leadership qualities;
- Be able to communicate effectively;
- Have the drive to generate ideas and plans and follow them up to their full implementation;
- Work in full harmony with the Medical Superintendent, Principal of the Nursing College and other senior officials of the hospital.

Her role and responsibilities include:
- Organizing and administering the nursing service;
- Planning the delivery of nursing care in accordance with the philosophy of the hospital and the medical staff requirements, and implementing the approved plans;
- Developing and monitoring rules, policies and procedures relating to nursing services;
- Coordinating activities of various nursing units;
- Delegating to the Asst Nursing Superintendent and Nursing Officers specific tasks and responsibilities;
- Assisting in the selection of qualified, competent and appropriate nursing personnel;
- Staffing the services adequately and, depending on the workload, making periodical adjustments in staff deployment;
- Supervising nursing staff in general and senior nursing officials in particular;
- Continuously evaluating the efficacy of nursing care provided to patients;
- Ensuring high level of performance, discipline and work ethics by nursing staff;
- Approving shift/duty rosters and leave especially of senior nursing personnel;
- Establishing and maintaining harmonious and effective relationships with other departments in the hospital and with the College of Nursing;
- Monitoring upkeep of facilities and usage of supplies;
- Preparing reports, plans and budgets for the nursing service.

Deputy/Asst Nursing Superintendent

Functioning in staff position, a Deputy/Asst Principal Nursing Officer is usually delegated with responsibility for specific activities, under the overall charge of the Nursing Superintendent. In large hospitals, there may be two deputies, each responsible for a group of nursing units, in which case they function in line position. Additionally, each of them may be placed in charge of certain activities of the Nursing Office.

Duty Nursing Officers

Also called Night Supervisors, these senior nurse executives, by rotation, provide on-the-spot cover for the Nursing Superintendent and the Unit Nursing Officers outside normal working hours. A Duty Nursing Officer is responsible for the following:
- She works on 8-12 hour shift duty, on nights and on weekends;
- On starting her shift, she takes over from the Nursing Superintendent and from the Unit Nursing Officers any specific matters to be followed up on;
- She receives shift ending reports from each ward;
- She carries out rounds to supervise the functioning of all wards, with special emphasis on the care administered to critically ill patients and new admissions;
- She is kept informed of all critical incidents occurring in the hospital during her shift;
- On being intimated of any problem that nurses encounter with respect to the medical, ancillary and support services, she takes action to resolve the same;
- She informs the Nursing Superintendent, Medical Superintendent and/or Chief Executive Officer any major problem that warrants their immediate attention;
- She compiles a report of the shift and hands over to the next Duty Nursing Officer or Nursing Superintendent on completing her duty.

Unit Nursing Officers

The wards and specialized service areas of the hospital are grouped into nursing units for more effective supervision and management of day-to-day affairs. Depending on the major clinical specialities, there may be Unit Nursing Officers (also called Asst Nursing Superintendents, Departmental Sisters) for Medical, Surgical, Maternity, Pediatrics, Psychiatry, etc. Unit Nursing Officers are also appointed for specialized service areas like Operation Theatres, Critical Care, Accidents and Emergencies and Outpatients, Infection Control, In-service Education, etc. A Unit Nursing Officer should

have advanced training and post-graduate certification in the respective area. Her responsibilities include:
- Consistent with the hospital philosophy and the nursing objectives, and in consultation with the Nursing Superintendent, she plans the organization and delivery of nursing service for her respective wards / specialized services areas;
- She interacts with the concerned senior physicians to promote effective delivery of patient care services in the respective areas;
- She allocates and re-allocates nursing and support staff to the wards/services within the nursing unit, approves their monthly duty rota, annual leave roster, leave applications;
- She periodically appraises the performance of staff under her charge and recommends them for training, promotion, disciplinary action, etc.;
- She approves ward indents for patient appliances, nursing materials, surgical consumables, hospital linen, stationery;
- She ensures that her nursing and support staff comply with the nursing, clinical and administrative policies and procedures;
- She performs daily rounds to inspect the working of her unit, to supervise the staff, and to take note of or resolve day-to-day affairs;
- She is kept informed of all critical incidents occurring in the unit;
- She liaises with the Nursing Superintendent and with the Hospital Administration for the smooth and efficient running of her unit and she keeps them informed of relevant matters;
- She participates in administrative, teaching, research and quality assurance activities of the Nursing Department.

Nursing and Support Staff at the Ward Level

Ward Sister

An important link in the managerial chain, the Ward Sister (also called Head Nurse, Ward Nurse) is responsible for the effective functioning of the ward. She is generally a nursing graduate with 5-7 years experience as a staff nurse. Post-basic certificate in the related speciality and a course in Nursing Administration are added assets. Reporting to the Unit Nursing Officer, a Ward Sister's duties encompass:
- Ensuring compliance of administrative, nursing and medical policies and procedures relating to ward management

(e.g.: admission and discharge formalities, rules applicable to inpatients, regulating patient attendants and visitors, nursing protocols, infection control, isolation policy, verifying payment prior to patient discharge, linen and laundry policy, waste disposal, maintenance, etc.);
- Good patient relations and public relations;
- Safeguarding cleanliness of the ward;
- Proper upkeep of ward materials (infrastructure, furniture, fixtures, equipment, policy manuals, registers and files, notice boards);
- Indenting, custody, controlling use, maintaining records and periodical checking of inventory (equipment, narcotics and dangerous drugs, surgical consumables, linen, general supplies, patient records);
- Supervising the nursing care plan for inpatients;
- Accompanying senior doctors on ward rounds and following up on patient care instructions relating to nursing, ancillary and support services;
- Indenting patient diets;
- When indicated, performing activities as a staff nurse;
- Orienting new staff;
- Assigning staff nurses to inpatient groups/cubicles;
- Supervising staff nurses, ward clerks, medical orderlies and cleaners assigned to the ward;
- Preparing the monthly duty rota for ward staff, recommending leave requests, recording attendance, reporting absence from work;
- Coordinating and facilitating work of other staff (such as doctors, medical record staff, X-ray/lab technicians, dieticians, social workers, physiotherapists, etc.);
- Cooperating with nursing tutors in assigning activities to student nurses, arranging demonstration of procedures, supervising student and intern nurses;
- Reporting and investigating critical incidents and staff and patient complaints;
- Accompanying nursing and hospital executives in their ward visits;
- Participating in professional and hospital activities.

Staff Nurses and Midwives

In a hospital set up, Staff Nurses undertake varied functions:
- Bedside nursing care as per physician orders and nursing care plan;
- Communicating and interacting effectively with patients and their attendants, families and visitors to promote the patient's comfort and speedy recovery and to resolve any patient-hospital problems;
- Assisting doctors during patient examination, surgery, anesthesia, invasive procedures;
- Attending to ward routines—maintaining patient and ward records, stocking and replenishing drugs and other supplies, assisting at other ward management activities;
- Screening ambulatory patients—well baby clinics, immunization, monitoring growth charts, antenatal and postnatal clinics;
- Health promotion and disease prevention—health education, diabetic screening and education, follow up of patients with communicable diseases, monitoring staff health, nosocomial infection control;
- Performing procedures—first aid, wound dressing, suture removal, catheterization, phlebotomy, dialysis, normal vaginal delivery, cardio-pulmonary resuscitation, administering chemotherapy;
- In-service education—orienting new staff, assisting in training of student nurses;
- Community health.

Ward Clerk

At least on the routine day shift, it is extremely useful to have a trained medical records clerk at the ward level to relieve nurses from routine clerical and administrative tasks, such as:
- Attending phone calls, passing on messages;
- Updating bed occupancy, effecting admission-discharge-transfer transactions, updating patient data on the computer, following up on investigation results, retrieving computerized information;
- Pasting results in patient file, assembling forms within a patient record, deficiency check, coding, liaison with medical records department;

- Typing patient discharges;
- Upkeep of ward registers;
- Maintaining records relating to diet indents, general supplies, drugs, surgical consumables, ward equipment;
- Follow up of routine ward activities – contacting ancillary and support staff, repairs, supervising ward cleanliness, etc.

Aides/Orderlies

A competent medical orderly too can be of considerable assistance to nurses with respect to routine mundane tasks, such as:
- Cleaning and tidying patient beds, changing bed linen;
- Lifting, turning, transferring and portering patients;
- Bathing and shaving patients;
- Transporting laboratory specimens, collecting X-rays;
- Inter-department messenger work;
- Collecting ward supplies.

Non-nursing Duties

As mentioned earlier, nurses are highly compliant. And they do not complain too much. In fact, "for the patient's sake", they most willingly shoulder multifarious duties, including doubling up as physician's secretary, ward clerk, medical orderly, porter, billing clerk, cashier, caterer, medico-social worker, record keeper cum statistician, housekeeping or laundry supervisor, pharmacist, medical store purchase clerk, etc. Though nurses probably perform these tasks with great efficiency—thus inducing doctors and hospital administrators to reward their reliability with more such duties—it must not be forgotten that clerical and nontechnical functions detract nurses from their principal role, leaving very little time for nursing care. It is, therefore important that the Nursing Administration be vigilant and resist attempts to burden the nurses with nonnursing duties, with the ensuing risk of compromising patient care.

Determining the Nursing Complement in a Hospital

Justified or not, the most frequently cited reason for poor service in any area of work is "shortage of staff"! Considering the personalized nature of nursing care and its importance for patient recovery, it is all the more important not to give room for such an excuse. How many nurses, therefore, should a hospital employ?

There is no ready formula to determine the nursing complement relative to the hospital size. The number of nurses depends on several factors:
- Nature of the hospital;
- Patient case-mix, high/intermediate/low dependency patient profile, intensiveness of nursing required, number and complexity of clinical procedures;
- Patient turnover, ward occupancy, permanent and variable staffing;
- Hospital design and layout, visibility, number of single rooms;
- Automation in patient appliances;
- Availability of nursing support personnel;
- Personnel policies—working hours for nurses, leave days (public holidays, annual/maternity/casual/sick leave) permitted, absenteeism rate, compensatory off or overtime payment, provision for part-time help, time spent for staff development;
- Nursing assignment system – case method, functional nursing, team nursing, modular nursing, primary nursing;
- Nursing care hours per patient day, unproductive nursing hours;
- Staffing schedule - straight or split shifts, duration of shifts, block or cyclical scheduling, shift rotation cycle, maximum continuous days/nights on duty desired to avoid tiredness, rest days following night duty, etc.
- Staffing norms, such as for:
  — critical care (ICU, CCU, NICU, OT recovery) - 1 nurse per bed
  — high dependency - 1 nurse per 2 beds
  — low dependency - 1 nurse per 3-5 beds depending on acuity of care
  — operation theatre - 1 scrub nurse and 1 circulating nurse and 1 anesthetic nurse per table
  — delivery suite - 1 nurse per delivery room.

Objective review by the Nursing Administration of the above factors, comparison with other hospitals/wards of similar size and technology, and possibly time motion studies help in arriving at the *number of full time equivalent (FTE) staff nurses required per shift in each ward* or area of activity. Once this basic staffing pattern is agreed upon, it is possible to calculate the ward nursing complement allowing for night-offs, weekends, holidays, absenteeism, staff development, etc., and thereby arrive at the total nursing complement required for the whole hospital. One possible way, which has been found to work effectively, is illustrated below:

(Example, to estimate the nurses required for a 30-bed ward if it is desired that a nurse, working on a 6-week rotating schedule, does 6 days morning duty for 2 weeks, 6 days evening duty for 2 weeks, 7 continuous night duties, 7 continuous day/night sleeping offs and 4 weekend offs:

Total nursing working hours for the ward:
7 hours morning shift (7.30am - 2.30pm) x 6 day week x 5 FTE
+ 7 hours morning shift (7.30am - 2.30pm) x 1 day weekend x 3 FTE
+ 7 hours evening shift (2.00pm - 9.00pm) x 7 days x 3 FTE
+ 10 hours night shift (8.30pm - 8.00am less 1.5 hours rest) x 7 nights x 3 FTE
= 588 man-hours per week or 3528 hours per 6-week cycle, where each shift-block begins on a fixed day of the week, say Monday.

Working hours per nurse comparing to other office staff: 8 hours per day x 6 days per week x 6 weeks per cycle = 288 hours.

From the above, the number of nurses required to cover all shifts given the above FTE staffing pattern = 3528 divided by 288 = 13 nurses.

To this add allowances for holidays, sickness, leave replacement = 3. Hence, the nursing complement for the ward may be fixed at 16 staff nurses.)

Nursing Bylaws, Rules, Policies and Procedures

The nursing bylaws regulate the organization and self-governance of the nursing service within the larger framework of the hospital set-up. The bylaws spell out:
- Objectives of the nursing service in consonance with the hospital objectives;
- Nursing organizational chart, hierarchy and relationship between the various categories of nurses;
- Criteria for holding a nursing position in the hospital, full-time employment, part-time employment, visiting/ private nurse and the fundamental rules and obligations governing each category;
- Responsibilities and powers of key nursing executives;
- Various statutory committees and meetings held by the nursing establishment;
- Performance appraisal process;
- Quality assurance and nursing audit process.

Nursing Service

Rules and regulations that govern the Nursing Service include:
- Employee service rules related to working hours, holidays, leave regulations and procedures, code of conduct, disciplinary process;
- Duty schedule, shift pattern, reporting time for each shift, overtime, compensatory offs, overtime payment;
- General patient interactions—admission, discharge and transfer formalities, orientation of patients, handing/taking over patients, patient and public relations, dealing with patient attendants and visitors, isolation of patients, patient ethics, confidentiality, consent, witnessing wills, custody of patient valuables, reporting absconding cases;
- Nursing documentation—nursing care plan, nursing notes, medico-legal formalities;
- Reporting critical incidents, adverse reactions to drugs, infusion, transfusion;
- Medication—dispensing and documentation of inpatient medication, mixing medication from two vials, insulin administration, skin testing, rules relating to storage and administration of narcotics and controlled drugs, DDA cupboard, reporting incidents of breakage/loss/unused narcotics, medication errors;
- Indenting, stocking, usage, control of surgical consumables and general supplies;
- Accountability for equipment, inventory, appliances;
- Inter-relationships with other departments—doctors, laboratory, x-ray, CSSD, medical records, dietary, laundry, housekeeping, maintenance, security, cashier.

As nurses working in a hospital generally come from diverse backgrounds and schools of training, there is a special need to have a written manual documenting the method of performing common clinical nursing procedures. Salient policies and procedures in this regard relate to:
- Basic nursing—bed bath, mouth care, enema, tepid sponging, application of cold compress, prevention and care of pressure sores, steam inhalation, care of the unconscious patient, changing patient positions, patient movement, lifting and transfer of patients, preparation of body after death;
- General nursing procedures—wound care, suture removal, suction, oxygen therapy, urinary catheterization, bladder wash, gastric lavage, intravenous cannulation and therapy,

blood transfusion and dealing with reactions, intra-pleural drainage, tracheostomy care, nebulizer therapy, stoma care, bandaging, application of binders and splints, skin traction;
- Preparation of patients for surgical and other invasive procedures, skin preparation, post-operative care;
- Tests—urine collection, bedside investigations, glucometer readings, phlebotomy, collection and despatch of swabs and other laboratory specimens,
- Maintaining nursing records—monitoring vital signs, neurological observation, Glasgow coma scale, nursing notes, input output record, nursing care plan;
- Infection control—hand washing, nontouch dressing technique, disinfection and sterilization, universal precautions, innoculation injuries, wastes disposal, dealing with infectious wastes, laundry;
- Safety of patients, staff and visitors—electrical safety in the hospital, nosmoking especially in unsafe environment, disaster management, evacuation during a fire,
- Activating CPR, basic cardiac life support;
- Assisting at various procedures—bone marrow aspiration, lumbar puncture, pleural aspiration, abdominal paracentesis, liver biopsy, endoscopy, dialysis;
- Health education of patient and family.

Nursing Meetings

It is common for the Nursing Superintendent, Asst Nursing Superintendent, Duty Nursing Officer and Nursing Officers to meet briefly every morning for handover, review of the patient census, and communication of important/urgent matters to be followed up on.

The Nursing Administration, Principal of the Nursing College, Duty and Unit Nursing Officers, Clinical Instructors, and Ward in-charges should meet once every 2-3 months to:
- Review policies and procedures relating to safe and efficient nursing practice.
- Ensure uniformity in nursing and administrative practices across the hospital.
- Identify problems relating to ward management.
- Discuss frequently occurring incidents and problems relating to patients, staff, public.

- Obtain feedback on the inter-relationship of nursing with clinical, diagnostic, ancillary, and support services.
- Respond to clarifications from individual members.

The CEO, Medical Superintendent, Hospital Administrator, Medical Records Officer, Chief Pharmacist, Head of Stores, CSSD In-charge, Dietician, and Head of Housekeeping may be invited to participate in such meetings when deemed necessary.

Nursing Audit

Concepts and techniques of quality assurance are discussed in detail in a separate chapter in this book. Suffice it to note here that, striving for quality nursing care, through continuous and periodical audit activities, is an essential function of nursing management. It is, therefore, important for the Nursing Administration to:
- Set up clear standards for measuring and monitoring performance;
- Carry out concurrent audit to review input and process factors of nursing care;
- Perform retrospective review of patient care through chart audit that focuses on patient-care outcomes;
- Collaborate closely with the Quality Assurance Department in hospital-wide QA programmes aimed at monitoring and improving the overall quality of patient care.

Section 7: Specialized Service Areas

CHAPTER
18

Casualty Services

What is the area of service in the hospital, which is often neglected but requires considerable improvement? Undoubtedly, it is the casualty service. It is often no-man's land. Serious concern has been expressed regarding the inadequacy of casualty services, throughout the country, whether in the Government or voluntary sector. It is often part of the outpatient department. Yet, the requirements are different.

Casualty service brings about an interface between the hospital and the community, which is emotionally surcharged. The casualty department provides the first impression on the patient, relatives and friends who come along with the patient. The first impression must be a positive one. Quick and competent care can save lives and also reduce the severity and duration of illness. Yet, not enough attention is paid to this important area of service.

In most hospitals, the organization of the casualty leaves a lot to be desired. The accommodation is generally poor. There is not enough appreciation of sepsis and cross-infection. The experience of the professional staff (medical and nursing) is very limited. Often juniors are in charge. The supporting services are inadequate. The equipment available is often of poor quality. The relationship of the casualty with other departments and wards is not close enough.

DEFINITION

The casualty services provide immediate, emergency diagnostic and therapeutic care to patients with:

1. injuries by accidents, or
2. sudden attacks of illness or exacerbation of the disease
These patients require immediate attention and treatment. Emergency patients receive resuscitation and life-saving treatment. The treatment provided must be immediate and competent. If the condition is serious, it can make all the difference between life and death. A person with minor injury, if treated promptly and properly, will be put back to work quickly. If the treatment is delayed or is not competent, the person can be out of job for a long time. Prolonged and expensive rehabilitation may be necessary to put the person back on the job. Hence a casualty service must avoid delay in attending to the management.

OBJECTIVES AND SCOPE OF SERVICES

1. Provision of immediate relief to and management of patients arriving at the hospital with acute medical and surgical emergencies, e.g., acute myocardial infarction, shock, status asthmaticus, acute abdomen, snake bite, etc.
2. Managing accident victims, providing first-aid, treatment of minor injuries and referred to appropriate speciality or hospital, in case specialized care is necessary and cannot be provided in this hospital.
3. Attending to all medico-legal formalities, including documentation of clinical condition and other particulars and intimation to and liaison with police.
4. Attending to patients coming outside the routine outpatient working hours, and
   i. Screening them for admission,
   ii. Observing them for short period to determine whether they need admission, or
   iii. Providing outpatient care.

Region/area

The extent of provision of casualty services depends on the background of the region or area. The requirement of services will vary between urban and rural, between cities and villages, between industrialized and agricultural areas. In the cities and industrialized centres, accident cases will require maximum attention. In all other areas, diseases affecting cardiovascular, pulmonary, gastrointestinal and other system will require attention.

Characteristics of the Hospital

A good casualty service requires the backup of all other services. This is possible in a hospital with such well-developed services. In the smaller hospitals and other health care institutions, emergency services must be provided but these will be limited. The service will be more in the nature of first aid and, where required, referral to institutions with better facilities.

Concept

The provision of facilities would also depend on the hospital's perception of the function of the casualty department. Our concept needs a marked change. We must consider the casualty as one of the most important areas of care and accord priority.

Analysis of Patients

In order to organize a satisfactory casualty service, the patient load must be analyzed.

In Hospital M with an outpatient load of 2,21,833, there were 18,947 casualty attendance. This represents about 9 percent of all patients coming to the hospital.

It is necessary to analyze this load further. How many are patients with injuries from accidents? How many are fractures (skeletal injuries)? How many general surgical patients, like those with acute abdomen? How many general medical patients, with acute attacks of bronchial asthma, high fever due to various causes, gastroenteritis and the like? How many were in shock? How many with suspected coronary thrombosis? How many with problems of ear, nose and throat or eye, whether they may be due to diseases, injuries or foreign bodies? How many with poisoning? A deep analysis will help to organize better casualty care.

Relationships

No casualty department is an island to itself. It must have close relationships with all other departments and units in the hospital; often, this is not the case. The Casualty Department is looked upon as one of nuisance, disorganizing other work. By its very nature of urgency, all departments and units must help in the work of the casualty. The medical officers in the casualty are frequently junior persons. They also do not know adequately the various parts of the hospital or the staff working in the hospital.

The casualty services of the hospital must build up good relationships with other emergency services in the area. This is especially so with respect to specialized centers and hospitals for trauma, neurosurgery, burns, infectious diseases and the like. Rapport with them will make referrals easier.

Policy

The hospital must formulate its policy regarding the casualty. This policy must be made known to all the staff in the hospital. The policy can be reviewed periodically (say, once in 6 months) and, if changes are needed, modifications must be effected and made known to all users.

The hospital must consider the use of gown and mask by all attending on the patient.

Planning

Not enough attention is paid to the planning of the casualty department. This is obvious when we look at the existing hospitals. While elaborate care is given to inpatients and outpatients, the casualty services remain the Cinderella and is often forgotten. Some makeshift arrangements are then made. The hotch-potch arrangement causes inefficiency and dissatisfaction. It leads to unnecessary morbidity and mortality.

Location

The Casualty must be located in front, so that it is easily identified and approached by the patients and vehicles. Avoid cross traffic.

There is need for diagnostic and investigative services, like radiology, clinical laboratory and blood transfusion services. They must be situated close-by. Priority in the use of these facilities must be given to patients from casualty.

Accommodation

Have separate entrance for the casualty. It must be wide. This should not be used by anyone else except those attending the casualty. It would be good to have separate entrances for patients brought by ambulance and for others. Provide adequate space for the services. This would include:

Reception and waiting There is need for receiving patients who may come by ambulance, other vehicles or walking. There must be space for stretchers, trolleys and wheelchairs. It must be made possible to get these items as needed, easily without cross traffic. Unloading must be large and designed for easy maneuverability of stretchers and trolleys.

The waiting area must be large, cheerful and clear. There is need for toilet facilities. There will be a receptionist's desk in addition to seats for the patients and persons accompanying. It would be best to provide for registration of the patient at the casualty itself.

There must be cubicles for examination and treatment. These must ensure privacy. 'Clean' and 'dirty' cases must be separated. The cubicles must be large enough for easy movement. It would be ideal to have a separate room for isolation of patients.

The treatment rooms should provide for treatment of shock. The number of cubicles will depend on the number of users. A medium sized hospital should have 2-3 examination rooms and an equal number of treatment rooms. They must be provided with enough couches, tables and chairs for examination and treatment.

The examination and treatment rooms must have sinks, washhand basins, towels and bins (covered) for disposal of used materials.

There must be rooms for the Casualty Medical Officer and nursing station.

Operation theatres must be provided. Depending on the policy of the hospital, there can be a minor operation theater (minimum requirement). But, if the hospital policy is to deal with all emergencies needing the operation (outside the usual operating time in the regular operation theaters) in the casualty, a major operation theater must also be provided. The operation theaters must have ancillary rooms—an anteroom, changing room and scrub area.

There is need for observation beds. The number will depend on the type and number of patients needing observation. It would be a wise policy to restrict the period of stay in the observation ward for a maximum of 24 hours. The patient should be sent home or admitted to the regular wards within that period. Casualty observation ward should not be used as overflow ward, to accommodate excess patients.

Adequate toilet facilities must be available for the staff and patients. Washing place must be provided.

There is need for a store.

The concept of avoiding sepsis and cross-infection must be present always. There is always the possibility of spreading infection. All procedures must be carried out with the important requirement of preventing cross-infection. The rooms must be washed frequently. Sterile instruments, preferably supplied from the central sterile supply and clean/sterile linen must be used. Regular bacteriological monitoring must be carried out—environment, instruments and staff. Swabs must be taken regularly and action taken promptly as determined by the results of the bacteriological examination.

It would be preferable to have sliding doors, as much as possible. The doors must be wide, allowing free passage of trolleys.

A public telephone must be available nearby.

The entire environment should be airy and cheerful. Enough light and ventilation should be provided.

Emergency lights must be fixed in all important areas to offset power failures. It would be good to connect all the electrical installations to the standby generator.

Clean, aesthetic, sign boards must be kept in all areas, informing and directing the people.

All surfaces of the inside of the building should be washable. The flooring should be hard wearing like Kotah or Wadi stones. The walls should have washable tiles, preferably in light, pleasing shades, at least to a height of 5 feet above the floors.

Staffing

Adequate, qualified and experienced staff must be available. The number will depend on the case load. All the staff must be given training in handling casualty patients.

Medical

There should be 24 hour coverage by Casualty Medical Officers. They will be in the nature of general duty doctors with a minimum of one year's experience as senior house officer, preferably in the same hospital. The appointment may be for a period of 3 years in the first instance and continued, if services are satisfactory.

The Casualty Medical Officer must be under the guidance of a senior doctor, preferably the Resident Medical Officer, who will be on call at any time of day or night. The Senior Medical Officer is responsible for arranging for the duty roster, supervision of the work and conduct of the Casualty Medical Officer and for ensuring correct and complete documentation.

The services of specialists must be available as required. The hospital must have a policy whereby the specialists will give priority to calls from the casualty.

Nursing

The Casualty must be under the overall supervision of a Ward Sister, who is senior and experienced. She would see to the upkeep of the casualty, including availability of all equipment, instruments, linen, etc. All equipment must be maintained in good working condition. It should be the duty of the Ward Sister to ensure proper working condition.

The ward sister will ensure that standard procedures are followed by all.

Cleanliness will be ensured. Asepsis will be insisted on. Steps will be taken to make sure that cross infection is avoided.

It will be the duty of the ward sister to see that all emergency medicines are available all the time.

There will be staff nurse and, where there is a school of nursing, nursing students. A well-maintained casualty is one of the best places for training. The student can acquire a high order of knowledge, skills and attitude.

Helpers

There is need for persons to transport patients, help in the upkeep of the place and maintaining cleanliness.

Equipment

All necessary equipment for the management of all emergencies must be available without delay. *Time is of essence*. There must be equipment for resuscitation and treatment of shock. Items like blood pressure recording apparatus, suction, transfusion stand, etc., are standard items. Ambu bags, laryngoscopes and similar items should be checked for proper working. There should be X-ray viewing boxes or lobbies in the casualty medical officer's room. Instruments (adequate in numbers and type) must be available. They are preferably supplied sterile from the Central Sterile Supply. Sterilising in the casualty may be necessary but is only second best.

Furniture

The furniture must be adequate but the space should not be cluttered. Space must be available for free movement of the patients and staff.

Stainless steel dressing stools, dressing trolleys, chairs for dressing and similar furniture will help in maintenance of cleanliness.

Medicines

All emergency and life-saving medicines must be available. They should be on a carefully designed emergency trolley.

There must be either piped in oxygen supply or sufficient number of oxygen cylinders (small size) on trolleys.

The operation theatre should have all necessary equipment, instruments and medicines for the administration of anesthesia, operation procedures and postoperative care.

Records

Proper recording is essential in all cases. This is necessary when questions are raised regarding management of the patient and for follow-up. Where treatment has been given free, it must be recorded so. This will be useful, especially when returns regarding free treatment provided are asked for by Government. The records will also help in quality control.

The records include:
1. Patients' register
2. Patient's case record
3. Medico-legal register
4. Police intimation book
5. Wound certificate register
6. Brought-in-dead register
7. Notifiable diseases register
8. Patient valuables book

9. Doctors' call duty register
10. Casualty incident report book
11. Other common registers for indents, etc.

Medico-legal

A proportion of the patients, especially with bodily injury due to accidents, will be medico-legal. When in doubt, it is best to treat as medico-legal. All records must be complete and kept in safe custody. Entries must be made in the appropriate registers and police informed. Do not delay in commencing treatment, just because the police has not arrived.

One vexing problem is that of giving evidence in court in medico-legal cases. If a designated person, like the Resident Medical Officer, is assigned this duty, it will be easier. He or she will develop sufficient expertise over a period of time to deal with the situation.

Health Education

The casualty provides a golden opportunity for providing health education. Often there is waiting time and time available with the doctor and nurse.

There must be signs declaring 'no-smoking'. There can be many charts for health and patient education.

When patients with injury due to drunkenness by himself or the driver of the vehicle are brought, there is an opportunity, to demonstrate effectively to those who brought him, the ill effects of drinking.

If patients with gastroenteritis are brought, health education on the need for proper drinking water and sanitation can be given.

The opportunities are many and they must be used effectively.

Common Management Problems

1. Poor quality service:
   - Incompetent doctors and / or nurses
   - Staff not trained to handle emergencies
   - No written policies and guidelines.
2. Prolonged waiting time:
   - Staff unable to cope with multiple emergencies, presenting simultaneously.
   - Communication delay when other doctors are summoned.

3. Poor public image:
   - Lack of courtesy
   - Inadequate amenities.
4. Improper documentation, esp. in medicolegal cases.

Evaluation

Periodic evaluation of the effectiveness of the service must be made. This can be done by review by the staff and also by getting the opinion of the public. Surveys can be made with properly designed questionnaires and also by looking into complaints. Once evaluated, corrective action should be taken promptly to the extent possible. Weaknesses in providing quality, quick care must be avoided and strengths built upon further.

Instructions to Casualty Medical Officers

1. The Casualty Department functions throughout day and night on all days including Sundays and general holidays.
2. The Casualty Medical Officers will work under the general supervision of the Resident Medical Officer or other Senior Medical Officer assigned this responsibility. Hours of work will be so regulated that there is complete coverage. No casualty medical officer on duty will leave his or her post until relieved by incoming casualty medical officer, nor be away from casualty, without having made specific arrangements to be contacted on the ward visited. The post should be covered by another medical officer during his or her unavoidable absence. He or she should, when leaving, also inform the staff nurse on duty.
3. In case the casualty medical officer cannot come on duty due to illness or accident, he or she should (as early as possible) contact the Resident or Senior Medical Officer by telephone.
4. All patients coming to casualty will be examined. Those requiring emergency treatment will be given prompt attention and admission, if necessary. Other patients will be prescribed medicines and advised to come to outpatient clinics on the following day. All examinations and treatment will be entered in appropriate card, while an entry should also be made in casualty register in the handwriting of Casualty Medical

Officer. Entries should be legible and carefully recorded as these documents are referred to in medico-legal cases.
5. Serious emergencies will be treated without delay and out of turn; the services of other senior house officers may be called for attending to emergencies and resuscitation of collapsed patients. All other patients should be treated in order of arrival. An explanation should be given to other patients who may be affected by the change in order of examination.
6. All accidents (road or industrial), suspected cases of assault and injury and poisoning cases should have their details recorded in accident register and be duly signed. Name and address of person bringing in the patient together with the registration number of the vehicle involved, if any, should be carefully noted. Particular care should be taken to note such names, addresses and registration number of vehicles in case of persons who claim that they were passers-by and have brought the patient. Patients should be warned against giving money or valuables to such persons. The Resident or Senior Medical Officer will be notified in all cases of serious accidents particularly in (a) medicolegal (b) multiple fractures, and (c) poisoning cases. Unless the injury is minor, all medico-legal cases should be admitted, particularly head injury and poisoning cases.
7. The following types of cases will be offered first aid or emergency treatment and ordinarily directed to other hospitals: (a) assault cases, (b) major burn cases (c) cases of dog bite requiring anti-rabic treatment (d) infectious cases (e) severe head injuries (f) cases of spinal fracture with neurological deficit, if adequate facilities are not available in the hospital. In serious cases of assault or injury, treatment will not be delayed or refused. The services of the surgical department will be called for urgently. No case will, however, be moved in case of head injuries, if there is any likelihood that patient will die on the way. In case of stab wounds and other serious injuries where it is felt that proper care may not be available elsewhere, the cases will be admitted and Resident or Senior Medical Officer informed.
7a. The police should be contacted on the phone in case where a dying declaration may have to be taken.
Do not wait for the police, to start treatment.

7b. Casualty Medical Officers will inform the Resident or Senior Medical Officer concerning accident cases treated in casualty and not admitted or refusing admission. This also applies to cases transferred to other institutions.
7c. All poison cases are admitted, no matter how trivial they may appear to be.
8. No patient should be kept unduly long in the Casualty.
9. All cash and valuables found on unconscious patients will be collected immediately, in the presence of attendants or persons bringing the patient. Then they will be handed over to patient's relatives and receipt taken or alternatively kept by nurse and the same noted in a book.
10. Where children are brought in as result of an accident, treatment will be started and an attempt made to contact their parents. The aid of the police may also be utilized for this purpose.
11. Members of Police department who come to enquire about accident patients should be treated with courtesy. The Casualty Medical officer will grant permission for the police to take a statement from the victims of accident if they are satisfied that the injured are in a fit state to make them. All enquiries by accredited members of the Press will be referred to Resident/Senior Medical Officer.
12. The clothes of assault cases who are admitted as inpatients will be handed over to staff nurses to be kept carefully.
13. The stomach-wash in case of poison cases will be retained in a labelled bottle for a period of two months.
14. The Casualty Medical Officer will satisfy himself that there are adequate medicines in the casualty for emergencies and bring any deficiency to the attention of Sister-in-charge, Casualty Department.
15. Drugs prescribed for all patients will ordinarily be for 1-2 days as treatment can be reviewed in the outpatient department clinics.
16. In case of disasters such as large fires or accidents, the number of patients admitted will be adjusted against vacant beds and surplus directed elsewhere. The Casualty Officer will inform the Resident Medical Officer and call upon all the senior house officers and other doctors available to assist in casualty.

CHAPTER
19

Disaster: Be Prepared

Disasters, large and small, are fairly common. Our attention has been drawn to the calamity which befell the nation at Latur and Osmanabad districts in Marathwada region of Maharashtra. An estimated 12,000 died in the earthquake. Many more were injured, physically and mentally.

DISASTERS

A disaster is a sudden, great misfortune. It is the situation arising from the event where disruption of great magnitude occurs in:
- Life (human, animal and plant); and
- Life supporting systems (water, air, food).

Disasters have been classified as 'natural' and 'man-made'. There is a complex relationship between them.

Natural Disasters

Earthquakes, floods, cyclones, landslides, droughts, etc.

Man-made Disasters

Riots and violence, terrorism, accidents (chemical, nuclear, transport), dam collapse, building collapse, food poisoning, fires, etc.

Man-made disasters are caused by human failures or accidents or violence. Sometimes, a clear distinction between man-made and natural disasters may be difficult.

In an earthquake, the poor construction of buildings can contribute significantly to loss of life and damages. The failure of authorities to warn people adequately and of people to respond promptly can contribute to the increased loss of life and damages. Fires may or may not be started by people. Every health care institution must be prepared and ready to tackle the crisis situation developing as a result of the disaster in its area. The Hospital Administrator must anticipate the crisis. It can save death and misery. The sudden increase in demand on the services of the health care facility must be met.

PLAN OF ACTION

A plan of action to effectively manage any crisis should be worked out in anticipation. Absence of a plan will add to the chaos and confusion which will come on whenever large numbers of people are affected. That will paralyze the services to be provided by the institution. What would have been possible ordinarily would become almost impossible. All the concerned people, the hospital administrator, medical, nursing and other personnel, the victims, the relatives and the public become frustrated. Lives may be lost unnecessarily because of lack of preparedness.

A hospital administrator must be ready, to the extent possible within the resources available, to manage the crisis as and when it occurs. The hospital administrator should always be in control of the situation, foreseeing what could happen and be prepared to meet the situation.

Different Types of Crisis

Certain areas are more prone to certain types of disasters, for example, cyclones, earthquakes, fires, etc. East coast of India is prone to cyclone, the Himalayan ranges to earthquakes. The needs to be met would also depend on the size of the city, town or village and the population and presence of other health care institutions in the area. The past experience will help. Specific action plans can then be drawn up apart from general preparedness.

Steps to be Taken

The action plan should give the various steps in handling crisis. This would give the personnel and the activities, in the proper sequence. As the health care institution tackles problems, the experience will help in reviewing the plan to make it more effective and efficient.

Crisis Team

The Hospital Administrator must develop a crisis team. The members of the team, consisting of doctors, nurses, paramedicals and supportive staff and others should be carefully selected and trained. Each one must be aware of his/her responsibilities, what to do and whom to contact, should they need assistance.

This crisis team should be capable of being assembled quickly, at any time of day or night. Hence, in the selection of people, priority should be given to those who are available easily and live close by in the campus, in the neighbourhood, having telephone connections and own transport.

The crisis team should be able to secure the help of others in the area. This would include practitioners and other volunteers, skilled and semi-skilled. A donor list of people willing to donate blood at short notice should be ready, with their correct addresses and telephone numbers.

Linkages

Crisis management in disasters might involve large numbers and specialist requirement beyond what is available in the particular institution. Hence, linkages must be formed and be in place for proper referral system.

Training and Reinforcement

The crisis team needs training and retraining. Some members of the team may leave and new persons will have to be inducted. They will have to be trained and assigned responsibilities. As they have to work with the team, they will have to be trained with the team.

Rehearsals are necessary periodically to ensure that the plan will work smoothly, should disaster strike. The members of the team should always be in peak condition.

Leadership

There is need for a unified authority. One leader should be identified, who will issue instructions. Those instructions must be followed; otherwise, there will be confusion and conflict.

It is also necessary to decide beforehand, who will be the leader, in the absence or inability to function of the designated leader.

The leaders should be available at the control station always. The leader should not run around. His or her duty is to coordinate and supervise the activities, ensuring that the plan is being carried out efficiently. He/she should be available to give advice and instructions. The leader motivates and encourages the crisis team to give their best.

The leader should ensure that there is proper communication:
  i. Between the members of the team,
 ii. With the anxious relatives and friends of the victims,
iii. With the public,
 iv. With the authorities, and
  v. With the media.

Usual Sequence

1. Information received at the health care institution.
2. The team leader and members of the team are informed.
3. The team gets ready and is in position with all the necessary facilities.
4. Victims are received.
5. Preliminary examination and sorting (triage).
6. Brief documentation.
7. First aid is given to all, attending to those seriously injured first. Observation—investigations—diagnosis—treatment.
8. Referral, where necessary.

Hospital Administrator should always be at hand, even if he/she is not the leader of crisis team. The Administrator's presence lends support to the team. And he/she is ready to ensure that the entire hospital and its resources are at the service of the afflicted.

Psychosocial Consequences

Our focus is always on the physical aspects of disasters: the loss of life, physical injuries and damages to property. It is seldom on the psychosocial effects.

The emotional reactions may be:
  i. Immediate, during the disaster; and
 ii. Occurring after the event (soon after or later).

Immediate Reactions are to

  i. Physical injury,
 ii. Exposure to extreme danger,
iii. Witnessing death of close ones,
 iv. Traumatic experiences of helplessness and hopelessness,
  v. Separation from near ones, and
 vi. Need to choose between helping others and fighting for own survival

The adaptation reaction may not function properly:
- Paralyzing anxiety;
- Uncontrolled flight behavior; or
- Group panic.

The immediate post-disaster reaction or "disaster syndrome" may be present in 25-75 percent of the victims, during the first hours or days following the event.

Reactions After "the Event"

1. People feel numb or relieved, often with strong positive feelings about having survived; later stress effects may show.
2. Intense feeling of anxiety (frightening memories of the experience).
3. Nightmares.
4. Post-traumatic stress disorder.

Occasionally, the symptoms may not appear for several months. Spontaneous recovery occurs in the majority of the cases. All these reactions may cause perceptions of being physically ill and may need health care: physical and psychological. Facilities must always be available in the right place. Certain equipment and materials should be earmarked for dealing with disasters. They must be checked periodically. It must be ensured that they can be used without any delay.

Oxygen cylinders, full with pressure gauge, flow meters and tubing for connections, spanner for opening. Stretchers, wheelchairs, trollies, splints. Medicines (verified for date of expiry); IV fluids, with giving sets; blood collection and giving sets. Dressing and sutures materials, gauze (sterile). Instruments (sterile). Ambulances and other transport.

CHAPTER 20

Outpatient Services

The outpatient services provide the main linkage of the hospital with the community. The outpatient department interacts with the neighborhood. Efficient outpatients produce a favourable public image.

The outpatients are becoming more and more important. Ambulatory care reduces dislocation of work, is cheaper and at the same time gives access to the various investigative and diagnostic facilities of the hospital.

OBJECTIVE AND SCOPE OF SERVICES

1. Provision of general medical services to outpatients on scheduled/unscheduled basis:
   - Preventive and promotive services (immunization, screening, antenatal clinics, well-baby clinics)
   - Curative (consultation, investigations, therapeutic procedures, speciality services)
   - Follow-up of discharged patients, chronic illnesses, post-natal clinics, and
   - Rehabilitative (physiotherapy, occupational therapy; prosthetics and orthotics).
2. Family Welfare Service; counselling.
3. Health education.
4. Medical, nursing and paramedical education.

Location

1. Near the main roads and close to main hospital entrance, but with sufficient space to provide for parking, etc., and to prevent noise and dust pollution.
2. Separate from inpatient wards and other departments, but connected with them

- Can function more efficiently in terms of scheduling and communications,
- Easier for patients to find their way around,
- Less patient and attendant traffic through central hospital,
- Kept closed when not in use, and
- Easier to expand, should a need arise.
3. Disadvantage of physically separate outpatient and inpatient departments:
    - Certain specialized diagnostic facilities may be available only in the inpatient section of the respective speciality thus inconveniencing patients,
    - Some outpatient facilities are required for use also by inpatients,
    - A separate facility may require duplication of certain services that could otherwise be shared, esp, satellite laboratories, and
    - Distance between inpatient and outpatient facilities may cause inconvenience to doctors who have responsibilities in both areas.
4. OPD should be close to:
    - Medical Records
    - Laboratory
    - Radiology
    - Pharmacy

    It should be adjacent to Casualty.
5. Preferable to have OPD of all specialities in same building to facilitate cross-references between various specialities.

Physical Infrastructure and Facilities

The number of patients availing of facilities in the OPD varies with the situation, e.g., distance from the centre of the town, other nearby health care facilities and the services provided. Generally, we should provide for every bed, 2-3 outpatients and for every outpatient, 2-3 attendants; thus 4-6 persons visiting OPD per bed. Recommended size of OPD: 2-3 sq ft per OPD attendance. The Bureau of Indian Standards, while laying down norms for a 30 bed hospital, has suggested that out of the total hospital area of 60 sq metres per bed, the entrance zone should be 2 sq. metres per bed, the ambulatory zone 10 sq metres per bed and diagnostic zone 6 sq.metres per bed.

Outpatient Services

Public Areas/Facilities

a. Entrance
   - Easily accessible
   - Ramp and steps
   - Wide door
b. Foyer
   - Reception, enquiry
   - Sign boards, layout plan
   - Bay for trolleys, wheelchairs
   - Public telephone
   - Toilets
c. Registration
   - Counters for centralized registration of fresh and repeat visits
   - Control desk for sub-registration at respective service area
   - Retrieval of lost cards
   - Cash counters.
d. Facilities for health education
   - Posters
   - Pamphlets
   - Audiovisuals
e. Waiting area with seating accommodation
   - At foyer
   - At each bank or tier of consultation/treatment rooms.
f. Corridors, at least 7 ft wide.

Clinically Related Facilities

a. Layout of consultation cubicles:
   - Double-loaded single corridor with rooms on each side of the corridor
   - Double corridor for accessibility from opposite sides of the room for patients and doctors respectively
   - Triple corridor with two rows of examination-treatment rooms on each side of a staff corridor.
b. Configuration of consultation and examining room:
   - One consultation room (office) and two examining cubicles per doctor
   - Combined consultation/examination room with a curtained cubicle for patient to undress.
c. Rooms for specialized examination:
   - Refraction
   - Audiometry

158 Hospital Administration

- Electrocardiography
- Dental chair and equipment

d. Treatment rooms:
   - Injections
   - Dressings
   - Minor procedures—incision and drainage, suturing, suture removal, wound debridement
   - Plaster room

e. Recovery room:
   - At least 2 beds required if patient collapses during a procedure
   - Resuscitation facilities.

f. Clean and dirty utility rooms.

Ancillary Facilities

Many of them depend on the type and size of the hospital.

General		
a. Medical records	Centralized	Combined Op and IP record
		Separate OP record
	Decentralized	For each discipline
b. Clinical Laboratory	Single centralized sample collection area, attached bleeding facility and toilets	
c. X-ray and ultrasound		
d. Pharmacy		
e. Physiotherapy and Occupational Therapy	- gymnasium - heat therapy - hydrotherapy	

Specialized	
f. Gastrointestinal endoscopy laboratory	- sigmoidoscopy - gastrofiberscopy - colonofiberscopy
g. Pulmonary function laboratory	- spirometry - bronchoscopy
h. Neurological laboratory	- electroencephalography - electroneuromyography
i. Cardiac laboratory	- echocardiography - computerized stress test treadmill

Administrative and Supporting Facilities

a. Office of
   i. OPD in-charge—Asst Nursing Superintendent
   ii. Public relation officer/Enquiry officer

Outpatient Services 159

    iii. Security officer
    iv. Medico-social workers
 b. Cash counters
 c. Store room
 d. Toilets

Problems in Functioning of OPD

Patient Complaints

a. Prolonged waiting time
   - Too many patients in relation to doctors
   - Doctors busy elsewhere in the hospital at the time of OPD
   - Doctors come late, or absent from OPD for prolonged durations
   - Delays for registration, collection of laboratory specimens, payment, because
     — procedure not streamlined for efficiency
     — lack of sufficient helpers especially during peak hours
     — bottlenecks because of nonavailability of consultant, laboratory results delayed/misplaced
     — patient referred by registration staff to wrong consultant
     — critical equipment shortage, out-of-door X-ray, ECG, etc.
b. Dissatisfaction with quality of service:
   - Doctors do not spend sufficient time with patient, possibly due to heavy workload
   - Lack of undivided and uninterrupted consultation, especially by senior doctors
   - No privacy, especially in the larger hospitals
   - Advice given by doctors not clear
   - Consultation only by junior inexperienced doctor
   - Too many investigations ordered, resulting in unnecessary repeat visits
   - Unfamiliarity with procedures to be followed to avail service, especially to carry out laboratory/X-ray investigations after consultation
   - Improper guidance of procedures to be followed, location of departments
   - Multiple service points (instead of a single-window concept) often located distantly from each other
   - Certain specialities may not function on same day, necessitating a revisit of cross-reference advised

c. Dissatisfaction with amenities:
   - Insufficient/unclean toilets
   - Lack of seating accommodation
   - Poor transport facilities to hospital
   - Poor security, theft
   - Erratic power supply and absence of electric generator connections to departments like ophthalmology, dental surgery, ENT which need electricity for routine work
   - Absence of female attendant when lady is being examined by male doctor.

Doctors' Complaints

a. Heavy workload, each doctor in a large general hospital having to see about 50 patients per morning
b. Since time of commencement of OP coincides with time doctors report for duty, there is not enough time to finish inpatient rounds (particularly of post-operative patients) prior to attending OPD
c. Excess clerical work—OP records, filling of multiple requisition slips, replying to reference letters, absence of secretarial help
d. Nonavailability of patient's records or results of investigations advised at previous visit. Doctor required to liaise with MRD, laboratory and radiology departments for duplicate reports, clarifications, etc.

Medical Records

a. Misplacement of records:
   - Not returned by consultant
   - Wrongly filed
   - Reports not available
   - Taken by patient
b. Records not properly filled up
   - Lack of continuity in care by multiple providers, with possible effect on quality of recording
   - No standardized record format and disagreement as to content, qualitatively and quantitatively.

Solutions for Effective Functioning

1. *Reduce overcrowding and minimize patient waiting time.*
   a. Screening and disposal of minor illness patients by general duty doctors, thus reducing load on specialist clinics

b. Appointments system to spread out the reporting time of patients: either 'individual' or 'block' appointments. The block appointment system calls for a certain number of patients to be present at a given time so as to provide a sufficient pool of patients; thus the physician will at no time find himself idle and it limits the pool to the capacity of the waiting room.
   c. Application of queuing theory modules of operations research whereby the waiting time can be estimated by noting the patient arrival rate per hour, service rate per hour and number of servers. By effecting changes in these parameters and in the queue system it is possible to substantially reduce patient waiting time to acceptable levels.
   d. Special clinics at different timings, especially during afternoon hours—e.g., well-baby clinic, diabetes clinic, leprosy/T.B. follow-up, super-specialist clinics etc.
   e. Increasing the hours of OPD services, evening OPD services.
   f. Synchronize functioning of ancillary facilities with OPD workload such that the laboratory, radiology and pharmacy are open and adequately staffed during peak hours when patients referred from the OPD arrive for these services. Also these departments to remain open for a longer duration as compared to OPD.
   g. In built organizational arrangement to deploy doctors and other staff from less busy areas to the OPD and ancillary service departments if and when queue exceeds certain limits.
2. Improve guidance of patients and facilitate easy understanding of hospital procedures and routines:
   a. Information graphics and signage system; name boards, pictorial representation of services provided, direction signs, color coding of different service areas.
   b. Effective enquiry and reception services
   c. Hospital volunteers, guides.
   d. Procedural instructions to be printed on reverse of investigation requisition slips.

Data Required for Planning, Monitoring and Control

Volume

   i. Clinic/departmentwise statistics of new and repeat visits on monthly and yearly basis.

ii. Percent changes in new and repeat visits over years in relation to availability of doctors, registration staff. In case of part-time consultants, determine full-time equivalency with number of individuals represented in parenthesis.
iii. Fluctuation in visits by days of the week (or month)—average, high, low.
iv. Determine adequacy and utilization of clinics from clinic schedules of preceding year to determine the number of hours the clinic was in session, estimate number of rooms used per clinic session, multiply number of session hours by number of rooms to arrive at number of scheduled hours, and divide this by number of patients seen or average service time to evaluate adequacy of rooms. Further, by estimating actual room hours scheduled and dividing by potential room hours, it is possible to determine the percentage of clinic efficiency rate.

Utilization and Vital Statistics

The number of people who account for total annual visit volume determines utilization (average number of visits per person per year). This figure should be broken down by vital statistics of the population (age and sex) and by service. Such information helps in deciding staffing, program planning, etc.

Visit Levels

Several types of levels of visits depending on specialty:
- New appointments—walk-in, scheduled
- Short follow-ups
- Annual physicals, well-child checkup, immunization
- Complex treatments.

Although visit volume may remain stable, utilization, staffing, distribution and amount of revenues may change significantly.

Cost and Revenues

- Direct patient care costs—salaries, cost of supplies consumed
- Indirect patient care costs—utilities, free-care.

Those costs should be broken down by service and matched with revenues of respective services. As far as possible, each service should be self-supporting; else cross-subsidy system to be developed.

CHAPTER 21

Day Care

...Day surgery is now considered the best option for fifty per cent of all patients undergoing elective surgical procedures though the proportion will vary between specialities... The Royal College of Surgeons of England, March 1992.

WHAT IS DAY CARE?

Day care is a concept in healthcare delivery by which a patient is admitted to a hospital for a few hours for a prescheduled surgery or for an invasive or high-risk diagnostic/treatment procedure. The admission is on the premise that the patient requires post-procedure observation or nursing care during the recovery period. Such a patient is not considered an inpatient and is not counted in the inpatient census since:
— the length of hospitalization is less than one day—in fact the patient generally reports in the morning and goes home latest by the evening, there being no overnight stay;
— although the patient is admitted and records are maintained, the rules and procedures normally applicable to inpatients do not apply to such cases.

Day care, however, excludes minor procedures carried out in the Outpatient Department or Casualty/Emergency Department.

Benefits of Day Care

Day care has several advantages for the patient, in that it:
— minimizes disruption to the normal lives of patients and their families;
— avoids the distress associated with hospitalization, especially in children;
— decreases the procedure waiting period particularly if the delay is linked to long waiting lists consequent to bed shortage;

— lowers the risk of nosocomial infection;
— reduces the overall hospital bill.
— day care results in more effective utilization of hospital resources since: the scarce hospital beds can be better utilized for patients who will significantly benefit from hospitalization instead of blocking such beds with patients who merely require post-procedure observation and nursing care;
— there is a higher operative throughput as prescheduled surgeries need not be cancelled due to beds booked for such elective cases being occupied by acute/emergency admissions;
— there is better organization of work as separate manpower and operative resources can be earmarked for day surgery and for acute inpatient work;
— it reduces hospital expenditure (related to beds, ward nursing personnel, night stay, diet, etc.); in government hospitals, such savings can be re-deployed for improving facilities and for increasing the number of patients treated;
— for-profit hospitals stand to gain from day care since higher patient revenue is generated through procedures rather than by prolonging the length of hospital stay.

What Does Day Care Planning Set out to Achieve

- It ensures that patients for day care are adequately screened and cleared in advance, thus avoiding unnecessary cancellation of operation lists and scheduled procedures.
- It strives to develop protocols to ensure that patients are scheduled for procedures after being properly prepared, are assured adequate post-procedure care and follow-up, are confirmed to be fully fit prior to discharge, and are given clear written instructions to adhere to thereafter.
- It streamlines administrative procedures relating to bed booking, admission, retrieval and dispatch of medical records, movement of the patient, payment and discharge.

Organization for Day Care

There are three possible models:

Day Care Unit

This is the ideal situation where the hospital has a purpose-built self-contained unit with its own reception, observation beds, theater/s, recovery area and administrative facilities. A roster by which specified days/sessions are allotted to various clinical teams enables clinicians to schedule their day care patients and utilize the facility efficiently without compromising on their inpatient and outpatient commitments.

Day Care Beds

Another option is to earmark a part or full ward exclusively for day care admissions and to utilize the operation theaters and other facilities common to the hospital. This has the advantage that the respective theaters are more geared to cope with procedures specific to their specialities and surgeons can schedule their day cases as part of their normal surgical lists. The arrangement works efficiently so long as there is under-utilization of beds and operative time. It must, however, be acknowledged that surgeons will always give more importance to acute/emergency/major surgery than to relatively minor and intermediate type of procedures that are undertaken as day care surgery. Hence, as inpatient resource utilization increases, day care patients will encounter delays, postponements, cancellations and less clinical commitment.

Mixing Day Care Patient with Inpatients

This system involves utilizing inpatient beds in wards of various specialities for day care patients admitted to the respective specialities. Beyond the advantages associated with the aforesaid system, there is an additional advantage that the ward and nursing staff of each speciality are more competent to handle patients with procedures specific to that speciality. However, the drawbacks associated with the former system become more obvious, and with time, this method proves unsatisfactory, as it is impossible to reserve beds for relatively less important day care patients when there is need to accommodate emergency admissions and more serious elective cases. Thus day care pre-planned admissions or surgeries will often have to be cancelled resulting in patient dissatisfaction, wastage of scheduled theater time, and last minute disruptive postponements that may never materialize.

Facilities of a Day Care Unit

In March 1992, the Royal College of Surgeons of England, through its Commission on the Provision of Surgical Services spelt out clear guidelines for day care surgery. This report also details the facilities desirable in a model day care unit:

Easy access to the exterior, adjacent car park, ground floor, distinct from the inpatient, emergency and outpatient areas, lockable when not in use at nights and on weekends. If an integrated unit is not possible, the day care ward should be located close to the operation theater designated for day care surgery.

Optimum efficiency is achieved with 2 dedicated operating theaters and a workload of 12 cases per theater day supported by a 20-bed ward.

The anesthetic room, operation theatres and recovery areas are as for any other operative set up. Additionally, the theater should be suitable for performing common operations in various surgical disciplines. It must hence have facilities such as blackout (for ENT and Ophthalmology), compressed air, image intensifier and plaster room (for Orthopedics), control of ambient temperature (for Pediatric Surgery), laser, laparoscopic and cystoscopic equipment (for General Surgery, Urology and Gynecology), etc. The theatre should also be equipped in case the minor surgery unexpectedly develops into a major one necessitating resuscitation, monitoring and ventilatory support.

The day care ward should have facilities, equipment, staff and protocols to cope with post-surgical care and complications (even resuscitation) related to various operations performed. Additionally, it should also be equipped and staffed to perform various medical procedures and provide post-procedure care in super-specialist interventional procedures. The ward facilities should include male, female and pediatric cubicles with changing room, lockers for patient clothes and valuables, toilets, etc.

Ancillary and support facilities include: patient reception and admission office, cashier, day unit office, staff changing and rest room, nurses' station, doctor's room, pantry, equipment store, clean and dirty utility, etc.

Scope of Work

Although a speciality-wise list of day care surgeries is included in the Royal College of Surgeons guidelines, it is up to the individual clinicians and hospitals to formulate their own list keeping in mind the local situation, capabilities and patient characteristics. The type of day care procedures include:

- Invasive diagnostic/treatment procedures in Internal Medicine, Pediatrics, Cardiology, Oncology and Radiology (e.g.: blood transfusion, bone marrow aspiration/biopsy, chemotherapy, pleural biopsy, pleural/peritoneal tap, venesection for cor pulmonale, liver biopsy, angiography, angioplasty, colonoscopic polypectomy, bronchoscopic biopsy, radiology, nerve blocks for pain relief, etc.) performed on ambulatory patients, which would otherwise necessitate hospitalization.
- Minor and intermediate surgical procedures in ENT, Dental Surgery, General Surgery, Gynecology, Ophthalmology, Orthopedics, Pediatric Surgery, Plastic Surgery, Urology, which are not associated with significant post-operative complications and which do not require post-procedure observation for more than a few hours.

Operations unsuitable for day surgery are those that are associated with significant incidence of postoperative complications, involve major blood loss, or often cause post operative pain requiring prolonged intravenous analgesia. Further, operations for day surgery should not exceed 1 hour in adults and 30-40 minutes in children.

Patient Selection

The following criteria may be used as guidelines in selecting an outpatient for day care surgery:

Physical Status

Except for the condition for which the procedure is indicated, the patient should otherwise be 'fit and well'. Suitable day care patients are those in classes 1 (normal healthy patient) and 2 (minor systemic disease not interfering with normal activities) of the American Society of Anesthesiologists ASA classification. Patients who have imperfectly controlled diabetes, chronic respiratory or cardiovascular disease should be excluded.

Obesity

Patients who are too obese, with body mass index (BMI = Kg weight/ m^2 height) more than 34 should be excluded from day surgery. Patients for laparoscopy should have a BMI < 30.

Age

Children less than 6 months of age and elderly patients more than 65-70 years should not be booked for day care surgery.

Social Circumstances

Patients for day surgery should have a relative or friend to drive them home and look after them for 24-48 hours. The patient should stay within one hour's drive of the hospital, and should also have access at home to a telephone, indoor toilet and bathroom.

Pre-Anesthetic Clearance

All day care patients who will require general anesthesia should be cleared in advance either by the Pre-anesthetic Clinic at the hospital or by a senior Anesthetist of the referring hospital as per the protocol laid down.

Pre-procedure Advice to Patients

Prior to being scheduled, the patient or guardian should receive explanation about the surgery/procedure and his/her informed consent should be obtained in the prescribed form and included in the respective medical record. The patient should also be advised about the need for an attendant, and driving and activity restrictions during the post-operative period.

The clinician who schedules the procedure should provide the patient with a memo documenting the booking particulars—patient name, name of procedure, date of procedure, clinician who will perform the procedure, reporting time. The patient will be advised that the booking stands cancelled if he does not report in time. The booking should also specify if any specific matters need to be attended to by the day care nursing staff when the patient reports (e.g. lab/X-ray tests, specific preparation of operation site, etc.).

Patients should also be advised that if, for any reason, they wish to postpone or cancel the surgery/procedure, the Day Care Unit office should be notified at least 48 hours in advance. This office will then liaise with the concerned Clinical Unit and inform the patient of the revised appointment date.

The payment formalities (financial estimate, payment of advance, final settlement procedures) should be made known to the patient so that there is no delay or inconvenience on the day of the procedure.

It is sometimes advisable that patients make a prior visit to the Day Care Unit to familiarize themselves on where to report and any other requirements/formalities to be complied with.

Patients for day surgery who will be administered general anesthesia should be given clear written instructions that they must not eat solid food for 5 hours before surgery. They may drink clear fluids upto 2-3 hours preoperatively.

Responsibilities of the Day Care Staff

Based on the bookings effected, the Medical Records Department retrieves the patient's file, updates the investigation reports and sends the same to the Day Care Unit on the day prior to the scheduled procedure.

Once the patient is admitted, it is the responsibility of the Day Care staff to verify the patient's understanding of the procedure, consent, presence of an attendant, arrangement made to take the patient home, and post-procedure requirements. The patient and procedure site are then prepared, special instructions complied with, clinician notified, pre-medication given if prescribed, and patient sent to the operation theatre or facility where the procedure is to be performed.

All clinical and nursing notes for the patient will be documented in the concerned medical record.

Following the procedure, the Day Care staff are responsible for observation, providing nursing care and complying with post-procedure instructions of the Clinician.

Discharge and Post-procedure Advice

The general discharge criteria include the following:
— stable vital signs
— alert, orientated
— comfortable, pain-free
— able to get up, walk and dress without assistance
— able to tolerate oral fluids, minimal nausea/vomiting
— accompanied by responsible adult.

Prior to discharge, the clinician responsible for the procedure should have satisfied himself that the patient is fit for discharge, and should take into consideration any post-surgical complications that could arise such as haemorrhage, residual effects of local anesthesia, urinary retention, etc. Patients who develop complications or are not fit for discharge should be admitted, though the incidence of such cases should normally not exceed 2-3 percent of patients.

At the time of discharge, patients should be provided discharge medication and a written discharge summary documenting the procedure carried out and instructions to be adhered to by the patient. These include: pain control medication, other medication, restriction in activities, phone number to contact and where to report in case emergency review required (for bleeding, persistent pain, nausea or vomiting, or any other complication), arrangements for dressing or suture removal if required, follow-up appointment.

As following any surgery, bed rest and light diet promote recovery and wound healing. Till they have fully recovered from the effects of anesthesia (at least 48 hours) and pain medication, patients should be advised not drive, operate heavy machinery, consume alcohol and nonprescribed drugs, or sign legal documents.

Management Issues

The Day Care Unit is generally headed by a senior clinician, though the day-to-day administration is delegated to a Ward Nurse. The nurse staffing requirements for the operation theater and recovery area are as for any other operation theater set up. The number of nurses for the day care ward depends on the turnover and complexity of cases undertaken. Beyond nurses, the Day Care Unit requires medical orderlies, medical record clerk for admissions and secretarial staff for the day care office.

It is the responsibility of the Unit and the Hospital Administration to periodically monitor day care productivity and quality of work in terms of the following indicators:

— average number of patients treated per day;
— average number of surgeries performed per theatre session;
— proportion of day care surgery to total surgery speciality-wise;
— percentage of day care patients who cannot be discharged but require admission;
— percentage of patients who report at the emergency department with complications, and percentage of such patients who require admission;
— nonattendance rates;
— patient feedback and patient satisfaction surveys.

CHAPTER 22

The Operating Department

...Because of the high investment in infrastructure, equipment and personnel, perhaps the most important yet most difficult aspect about managing an Operation Theater relates to maximising utilization of available theater time...

WHAT IS THE OPERATING DEPARTMENT?

An operating **department** is a unit consisting of one or more operating suites together with ancillary infrastructure for the common use of these suites, such as changing rooms, reception, recovery area, circulating space, etc. An operating suite is a self-contained unit inclusive of the operating theater and its own ancillary areas, namely anesthetic induction room, preparation room, scrub-up and exit area. An operating theater is the room or twin-theater in which the actual surgical procedure is carried out. However, the operating department is often loosely referred to as the operation theater or OT.

OBJECTIVES OF THE OPERATING DEPARTMENT:

- Provision of an ideal environment for conducting surgery:
  — promoting a high standard of asepsis,
  — ensuring proper care and comfort of patients,
  — providing optimum conditions of work for staff.
- Establishment of rules, procedures, work-flow and protocols for the smooth and efficient functioning of the department and performance of operative procedures:
  — defining operative sessions and allocating theater time to various surgical teams/consultants based on need,

— fostering a high degree of work discipline,
— streamlining general routines to be adhered to,
— ensuring care and availability of equipment and facilities,
— promoting optimum utilization of theater and staff time.
- Prevention of iatrogenic complications:
  — ensuring a high standard of safety and safeguarding patients and staff from environmental, operative, anesthetic, radiological and other hazards,
  — caring of patients in the immediate post-operative recovery period.

Issues in Theater Design

Centralisation

Gone are the days when it was thought advisable to build speciality operation theater/s within the confines of specific clinical departments (like an A and E OT, Gyne OT next to the Delivery Suite, Cardiothoracic theater in the Cardiothoracic block, etc.). With centralisation of all theaters into a single Operating Department it is possible to ensure:
— flexibility in allocation of theater time to various specialities depending on actual need;
— nonduplication and greater economy in use of common facilities (patient reception, change rooms, stores, recovery area, etc.), personnel (anesthetists, scrub and recovery nurses, theater technicians, etc.) and materials (especially standby equipment and surgical consumables);
— better supervision of procedures related to sterility, theater discipline, efficiency of work flow;
— availability of a theater for immediate use in dire emergencies related to any speciality.

Location

In the past, the Operating Department was often located in the top floor of the hospital so to separate it from the general hospital traffic and air movement. Further, this made ventilation easier as air-conditioning plants were invariably sited on the roof. However, with better hospital design and building technology, these constraints have been overcome. More important now is the need to locate the OT in close proximity to the post-surgical ICU, surgical wards, CSSD and cardiac interventional laboratory.

Zoning

The Operating Department is segregated into four distinct zones so as to ensure a high work discipline, promote asepsis and thereby minimize nosocomial infection.

— the outermost *protective zone* is the entrance area for patients, staff and supplies where normal hospital standards of cleanliness apply and where normal everyday clothes can be worn. This zone is maintained at a small positive air-pressure relative to the general hospital corridor and includes the waiting room for patients' relatives, OT reception and control room, staff change rooms and toilets, trolley bay and patient transfer area, storerooms, and sometimes a mini-cafeteria.

— inner to this is the *clean zone* where all patients, staff and supplies must have undergone a cleaning/changing routine to enter. The clean area serves to isolate the operating rooms from the protective zone and to allow changed staff to move from one sterile part of the Operating Department to another without re-entering the protective zone or passing through any non-clean area. The clean zone is maintained at a positive air pressure slightly higher than the protective zone. It includes the preoperative patient waiting area, recovery room, plaster room, blood storage and frozen section lab, mobile X-ray unit and dark room, staff lounges, offices for anesthetists and OT sister, anesthesia store, work room for unsterile theater instruments.

— the innermost area is *aseptic* or *sterile zone* where conditions are as near sterile as possible. This zone is maintained at the highest air-pressure so as exclude entry of air from the other zones. All staff who might handle exposed instruments in this zone must be scrubbed and gowned. The aseptic zone includes the operating room, scrub room, anesthesia induction room and theater supply room for sterilized instruments. If there are twin theaters, the two operating rooms should be effectively isolated from each other. The sterile zone communicates with the dirty corridor or disposal area through an inter-lock hatch system.

— the *disposal zone* has an air pressure less than the sterile zone. It includes room/s where used instruments, suction bottles, waste materials and soiled linen are temporarily stored before being collected for disposal or for cleaning and sterilization. The disposal zone may also include the dirty wash up room, disposal corridor and janitor's closet.

Number of Operating Rooms

This is dependent on several factors:
— surgical bed complement (The formula by HMC Macaulay and RC Davies in 1966 in Hospital Planning and Administration, WHO, Geneva, is possibly the best guideline: The number of operations per day can be estimated by dividing the number of surgical beds by the average length of stay of surgical patients. One can then determine the number of operating rooms required. For example, if there are 150 surgical beds and the average length of stay for surgical patients is 5 days, it can be expected that there will be about 30 operations per day. Considering that an average of 6 operations can be performed per day in one theater, about 5 theaters will be required. Adding 1 theater to be always reserved for emergencies, approximately 6 theaters will be required for 150 beds, i.e., a rough norm of 1 OT for 25 surgical beds);
— expected number of surgeries per day (on an average, 2-3 major and 3 minor operations may be performed per day per theater); approximate duration of surgical procedures performed, as dependent on the type of speciality and number of major surgeries;
— range of surgical specialities, especially those which require a dedicated OT (e.g.: cardiac, neurosurgery);
— whether day surgery is integrated into the main OT or not; emergency surgery workload;
— normal working hours for the theater, whether there is a routine second shift, number of operating days per week;
— theater efficiency and minimization of downtime between surgeries.

Operation Theater Size, Features and Facilities:

— the optimum size is 18 x 18 feet, though cardiac and neuro theaters may require operating rooms of 500-600 sq. feet to accommodate a large surgical team and special equipment.
— the floor to ceiling height is generally 10-11.5 feet. The walls should ideally have a finish of laminated plastic, vinyl sheet or epoxy resin type of paint. Tiles are not recommended due to the

crevices in between. The walls should be impervious to moisture, be washable and be able to withstand repeated application of detergents and disinfectants in general use. OT walls are generally of smooth matt finish, pale color, joint-less and the paint should not allow build-up of static electrical charge.

— the floor should be easily washable, nonstaining, impervious and moderately electro-conductive to minimize danger of explosion due to static spark.

— OT doors should be wide enough to allow frequent movement of patients, equipment, staff, and materials. It is important that doors to an OT be kept closed so as to maintain the positive-pressure difference between the sterile and clean zones.

— lighting is of three types: The general lighting is by fluorescent tubes, recessed in the ceiling, which provide even illumination without glare. For illumination of the operating area, a ceiling suspended shadow-less light is required with an intensity of 1000 lumen per square foot on the working plane and 300 lumens per square foot at the bottom of a narrow deep cavity. A satellite light for additional lighting or for a simultaneous second surgery is often provided. OT lights should be adjustable in any position in relation to the operating area. Filters are incorporated for color correction and for heat absorption. Certain lights have provision for battery back up in the event of power failure or malfunction of the main lamps. The third type of lighting is the headlamp used by surgeons for specific lighting of deep cavities.

— an efficient ventilation system should ensure supply of cool/heated (65-75^{0}F or 18-21^{0}C) humidified (50-60%), fresh, passed through HEPA (high efficiency particulate air) filter which are 99.8 percent efficient at the 0.5-1.0 micron level, and delivered in a vertically downward flow. The pressure grading should be highest in the sterile zone, gradually diminishing towards the clean, protective and disposal zones. There should be no movement of air from one OT to another.

— the general facilities of an operation theater/room include: pendant with outlets for piped gases, suction, compressed air, electricity; clock for lapsed time; operation table; diathermy machine; anesthetic machine, ventilator, monitoring equipment, defibrillator; instrument trolleys. Individual specialities have further specific requirements: blackout for ENT, ophthalmology and arthoscopy; compressed air lines, image intensifier

and plaster room for orthopedics; high ambient temperature for neonatal and pediatric surgery; laproscopic and minimally invasive surgical equipment for general surgery, cardiothoracic surgery, gynecology; laser equipment, operating microscope, etc. for ophthalmology, vascular surgery, general surgery, neurosurgery. Other general theater equipment include a high speed sterilizer, fire fighting equipment, patient transfer trolleys, etc.
— communication: for ease of communicating instructions and messengering, each operation theater/room should be connected to the control room through hotline or stentophone. The control room should also be given intercom over-ride facility for immediate access to the ICU, blood bank, radiology, histopathology and surgical wards. A closed-circuit television system with bi-directional speech facility enables recording and live display of surgical procedures at a remote loation (e.g., auditorium or classroom) elsewhere in the hospital. This helps in restricting the number of medical students and others entering the OT.

Theater Materials

Linen: Linen used in operating theaters should be of a strong close-weave material having a pore size of about 10 microns which prevents skin particles from escaping. Though green is most often used, white, blue or grey materials are also preferred, as they are restful to the eyes. The requirements of linen vary from hospital to hospital depending on the number of operations per day, type of surgeries, number of OT personnel, use of disposable surgical gowns, etc. Swabs used in the theater should contain radio-opaque markers.

Instruments

Surgical appliances and instruments depend on the various specialities. There are general packs for common surgeries and specific packs for specialized procedures. It is the responsibility of the concerned surgeon to set out the standard list of instruments generally required, and to specify in advance if any particular instrument is additionally required for a specific surgery. The theater nurse responsible for the specific theater/speciality should thereafter arrange for the indenting, stocking, use, care, condemnation and replenishment of instruments.

Surgical Consumables and Drugs

So as to avoid duplication and date-expiry, surgeons and theater nurses should take particular care to standardize surgical consumables that are common across specialities. This especially applies to suture materials, staples, gauze, dressings, catheters, endotracheal tubes, drains, syringes. Individual surgeon preferences and pressure from suppliers can result in too much of a variety than is surgically justified, to the detriment of the hospital and the costs of patient care. The Anesthetist is generally responsible for administration of drugs in the OT and so will specify what is to be indented and stocked.

Theater Records

The most important record to be maintained is the central OT register. This computerized or manual register generally documents the operation serial number, patient's name, hospital number, age, sex, admitting ward, pre-operative diagnosis, type of anesthesia, surgical procedure performed, major/intermediate/minor type of procedure, tissues removed, date and time of starting and finishing surgery, name of surgeons and anesthetist, scrub nurse. Additionally, each theater may maintain a register documenting further details of the surgery performed, consumables used, anesthetic particulars, swab count, etc.

Theater Staffing

The OT Manager

The Operating Department Manager is usually the OT Nursing Officer. At times, for reasons of cadre seniority, leadership and enforcement of discipline, the Chief Surgeon or Chief Anesthetist may be designated as overall in-charge of the OT. Even so, it is the OT manager who sees to the day-to-day running of the theaters and who should ensure:

— efficient management of the control room and theaters;
— availability of facilities, equipment, instruments and nursing staff for scheduled surgeries and emergencies;
— proper care and maintenance of equipment;
— theater cleanliness and sterility;

— adherence to work discipline (changing, timeliness of clinical and other staff, theater 'ritual', universal precautions);
— replenishment of consumables;
— maintenance of operation theater records;
— reporting of iatrogenic complications;
— liaison with other departments and with the administration.

Staff

It pays to designate a senior nurse, of the cader of Ward Sister, to be responsible for the smooth and efficient functioning of each operating theater/room. This Nurse, who should only rarely double up as a scrub nurse, is responsible for management of the theater including care of facilities, equipment and instruments, replenishment of consumables and drugs, deployment of staff, maximising utilization of theater time and minimizing downtime between surgeries. Besides her, 3 nurses are generally required per theater - a Scrub Nurse, Circulating Nurse, and an Anesthetic Nurse. A Theater Assistant or Nursing Aide may be additionally provided for every two theaters to assist in patient transfer, patient positioning, messengering. For the recovery area, it is necessary to have a nurse-patient ratio of 1:1 and so the nursing complement will depend on the throughput and time patients remain in the immediate post-anesthetic recovery unit.

The Theater Users' Committee

The OT Committee can play a major role in streamlining the running of the OT and liaison between various specialities. The membership of this Committee and its terms of reference are detailed under "Hospital Committees" elsewhere in this book.

Management Problems Specific to the OT

Poor Utilization of Theater Time

This is perhaps the most important and perennial problem that vexes Hospital Administrators and Clinicians. The reasons for poor time keeping are many:
— failure to schedule elective surgeries in a proper manner;
— late arrival of patients because of absence of patient consent, inadequate pre-operative preparation, pending laboratory or

X-ray investigations, lack of blood, nonavailability of porters to transport the patient;
— late arrival of surgeons because of their commitments at other hospitals, ward/outpatient work, emergencies involving other patients, general unpunctuality;
— staffing difficulties like shortage of doctors/nurses, inadequate domestic staff to clean the operating room between surgeries;
— last minute cancellations which prevent re-scheduling of other patients;
— critical equipment out of order, non-availability of an essential consumable;
— poor coordination with other departments, especially frozen section and mobile X-ray.

Organizational Problems

— The large number of staff from various departments entering the OT daily makes it more difficult to enforce theater discipline and compliance with theater routines. For example, it does become embarrassing for the OT manager to pull up senior surgeons (for improper changing or hand-washing, non-punctuality, nonadherence to universal or safety precautions), but such situations are not infrequent and result in major work conflicts.
— the stressful nature of OT work precludes a serene work atmosphere. Tense situations therefore lead at times to unreasonable behavior on the part of doctors, nurses and others.
— nurses are made answerable for the inefficiencies of others— delays in repair of equipment, consumable stock-outs, improper patient preparation, patient delays, etc.

Economy

The Operating Department is a place of high capital investment and high recurring expenditure. Hence every attempt must be made to increase throughput and control use of consumables. It is also important to account for all consumables and drugs used for each patient so as to recover the costs – a difficult and laborious task for OT staff who have other priorities, but a crucial factor in ensuring economy.

CHAPTER

23

Diagnostic Services

Scientific health care management requires the help of many diagnostic investigations. The Hospital Administrator will find requests for many new tests and procedures. These require more and more equipment and trained and skilled personnel. The Administrator will have to take decisions regarding these newer tests and equipments. The departments providing diagnostic services can be *centers of high income and expenditure.*

The Diagnostic Service Departments include the professional and technological departments, which assist in the diagnosis and proper management of the patient or health problem. They include:
1. Clinical laboratory, with its subdivisions of clinical pathology, clinical chemistry, microbiology, histopathology and blood bank.
2. Radiology, with its subdivisions of radiodiagnosis and, where available, ultrasound, computerized tomography and nuclear medicine.
3. Specialized laboratories for investigations like electrocardiography and, where available, electroencephalography, electromyography, endoscopy and respiratory functions.
4. Laboratories for testing speech and hearing.

Unique Features

Organization

The size and scope of service depend on:
- i. size of the hospital,
- ii. its geographic situation,
- iii. characteristics of the care provided by the hospital, and
- iv. association with other medical centres.

Staff

The staffing pattern generally:

i. The chief of the service is usually a medically qualified person with postgraduate qualifications in the appropriate subject like Pathology/Clinical Pathology. He/she functions as administrative chief of the department and as a specialist concerned with the quality of the services provided.
ii. Medical and nonmedical technologists responsible for supervision and coordination of work, providing technical assistance, quality control and record keeping.
iii. Technicians whose duties involve preparation of the patient, drawing the sample, performing the analysis, carrying out the procedures and reporting the result.

The departmental set-up may be centralized or decentralized with separate sections. Hospitals may establish laboratories in several areas for common OPD requests (blood counts, urine examination, chest X-rays, etc.). Even with a centralized set-up, for work outside the routine working hours, it is usual to provide for emergency set-up so that the entire department does not have to function.

Centralization

Advantages

1. Nonduplication of equipment and facilities.
2. Routine tests can be done faster and more economically, by 'batching'.
3. Larger volumes make automation feasible.

Disadvantages

1. Delays (transportation of patient/sample).
2. Large volumes of work may lead to compromise in quality.

Decentralization

Advantages

1. Rapid availability of results.
2. Specialized procedures in certain areas, e.g., for neonates.
3. Less inconvenience to patients.
4. Essential for critically ill patients.

Disadvantages

1. Lack of adequate supervision and control.
2. Wastage of consumables.

Physical Facilities

Location

Diagnostic service departments should have easy accessibility to outpatients and inpatients, close to lifts and staircases and should be compact. There must be easy access to wheelchairs and stretchers.

Areas of Activity

These will include administrative area (space for chief of service, secretary, clerks, conference), work area (rooms grouped by functions, modular design, movable partitions and standardized benches), service area (washing, sterilization, media preparation, storage), and patient area (reception, waiting, toilets, sample collection, recovery).

One important aspect, within the department of Radiology, is the flow of traffic. The primary planning is based on patient traffic (accessibility, promptness of attention, comfort, convenience, privacy, proper examination, easy exit). Secondary planning relates to work flow (progressive movement to facilitate completion, reporting, despatch, filing). Technician traffic must be minimized (minimum of personnel, maximum efficiency, minimal fatigue). Supervision by technologist or specialist must be planned (interviewing and examining patient, supervision of work by the staff, reporting).

Space

The space requirements vary with the size and type of hospital and the services rendered. It is good to remember that the number of procedures increases with time, even when the patient load is stationary. It is necessary to provide for expansion.

Equipment

There is high level investment, with the tendency towards more and more automation. This ensures speed, accuracy, less use of consumables and less manpower. It is essential to avoid duplication and redundancy. The equipment must always be maintained well. There is need to enter into service contracts and preventive maintenance. Adequate stock of consumables must be maintained. There must be service and trouble shooting manuals.

Resuscitation

The patient may collapse during investigative procedures. It is, therefore, necessary to have emergency drugs (preferably on a trolley), and resuscitation equipment. These must be checked for satisfactory performance, date of expiry, etc., at weekly intervals.

Occupational Hazards

Care should be taken to protect all personnel from radiation (lead impregnated wall/glass, lead aprons, personnel monitors, safe handling provisions) in the case of Radiology and from infections (hepatitis B) in clinical laboratory.

Nature of work (peculiar to diagnostic service departments)
1. Majority of work is undertaken during routine working hours. But emergency services are required beyond them. Scheduling is possible as the volume of work is mostly predictable, esp., the specialized procedures. Workload correlated well with inpatients admissions and number of outpatients visits.
2. Productivity can be standardized.
3. Generally, a few tests account for the greater part of the workload (e.g., haemoglobin, total and differential count and erythrocyte sedimentation rate in haematology and glucose, blood urea nitrogen, sodium and potassium in clinical chemistry). These require priority in automation.

Inter-relationships with Other Departments

It is necessary to maintain cordial relationships with other departments, who are the users. There should be good rapport between the clinicians and the staff of the service departments. Conflicts might arise because of nonadherence to policies and procedures (on either side), abuse of 'emergency', patient not prepared properly, delay in reporting and lack of reliability of results.

Management Problems

The most important problem is lack of trained manpower, especially the chief of service. Among others are allocation of work and resources, setting objectives (range of tests, reporting time), quality control, budgetary control, ordering of supplies, wastage and breakage.

The hospital administrator should ensure that all necessary resources are available to ensure smooth running of the service departments. Malfunctioning of these departments affects not only them but also every area of patient care.

CHAPTER 24

Medical Records

..."*Clear, concise, accurate history of the patient's life and illness, written from the medical point of view... and in its true form is a complete compilation of scientific data derived from many sources, coordinated into an orderly document by the Medical Records Department and finally filed away for various uses, personal and impersonal...*"

Dr. Malcolm T. MacEachern,
former Director of Hospital Activities of
the American College of Surgeons

OBJECTIVES OF MEDICAL RECORDS

Patient Care Management

- A patient's record chronologically documents the patient's condition, course of illness, investigations performed, treatment administered, clinical progress and significant patient-provider interactions during each episode of care.
- The file can be used to objectively review and monitor the patient's response to treatment so that appropriate additional or corrective measures can be taken.
- The instructions documented in a patient's file serve as a means of communication between the physicians and other health professionals caring for the patient. This is essential for continuity of care.
- Perusal of a medical record enables health professionals involved in subsequent care in gaining insight into the patient's previous condition/s and response to treatment. Complete record of previous hospitalization and investigations avoids repetition of examinations, patient discomfort and expenses.

Quality Review

- The patient's record serves as a basis for evaluating the adequacy and appropriateness of care.

- It enables the institution to evaluate the performance and competency of its health professionals, as also in medical audit, negligence related enquiries and risk management.
- Patient records are used in surveys by licensing and accrediting agencies in evaluating care and in determining compliance with standards of the respective agency.

Legal Affairs

- The patient's or guardian's consent for surgery and for various high risk/invasive diagnostic and treatment procedures are filed in the patient's file and safeguards healthcare providers against libel and unauthorized transgression.
- The patient's record substantiates medico-legal issues pertaining to patient injury, accident, assault, criminal cases, insurance, workmen's compensation, wills, deficient mental state, confinement to hospital, etc.
- A patient's file provides data to protect the legal interests of the physician and the health care facility from negligence and malpractice claims.

Education and Research

- Medical records assist health professionals and students in clinical discussions, review of care, case studies, teaching, etc.
- They are indispensable as a database for medical research.

Public Health

- Medical data form the basis for reporting vital events (births and deaths), infectious and communicable diseases, and compilation of health related statistics.
- They help to identify disease incidence so that epidemiological plans can be formulated to improve the overall health of the nation.

Financial Reimbursement

A patient's file authenticates payment claims of the health facility, which is needed for processing payment claims from third party payers.

NATURE AND CONTENTS OF MEDICAL RECORDS

The Unit Record

There are two basic types of records consonant with the registration system adopted. In the unit record system, each patient has one file only, identified through a unique hospital number. All the data pertaining to that patient, recorded over repeated ambulatory, inpatient and emergency care episodes, are recorded in that single file. The antithesis to this is the serial record, where a separate file, under a different registration number, is maintained for each episode of inpatient care. A unit record contains the complete picture of the patient's medical history and therapy and obviates the need to separately call for records pertaining to earlier treatments. Though this is the best system and is advocated for most specialist hospitals, it must be acknowledged that combined/unit records can get too bulky, necessitating multiple volumes. Hence, in predominantly general practice ambulatory set-ups, the hospital may opt for separate outpatient and inpatient records. The patient's outpatient record, then serves as the unit record, and there will be a separate record for each hospitalization episode. The outpatient record will contain references of various admissions and copies of the related discharge summaries. If further details are required at the outpatient level, the relevant inpatient file can be requisitioned.

Format Types

Medical record format refers to the methodology adopted for recording patient data and the organization of the forms within the medical record. There are essentially three formats in use:

Source-oriented Medical Record

This is the traditional format, where the patient's record is organized in sections according to the categories of providers who record the data. Within each section the forms are arranged chronologically. The major advantage of this system is that, since notes and reports relating to each source are written and filed contiguously, it is easy for professionals belonging to the respective discipline to access the particular document, review progress and up-date information. The disadvantage is that it does not help in quick identification of all of the patient's problems when differently noted by the various healthcare providers. Nor is it possible, at a glance, to determine all the care (e.g.: medical, surgical, nursing, physiotherapy, etc.) being administered at a given time, since these are recorded in the respective provider-sections and not according to the problems of the patient.

Problem-oriented Medical Record

POMR, introduced by Lawrence L. Weed and Harold D. Cross in 1969, provides a systematic method of documentation to reflect logical thinking on the part of the treating physician who is expected to define and follow up each clinical problem separately. POMR contains four basic components: the data base, the complete problem list, initial plans, and progress notes. Elements of the database include the chief complaint, present illness/es, patient habits and social data, past history, physical examinations and base-line laboratory data. The problem list (titled, numbered and placed in front of the chart as a table of contents) summarises symptoms, abnormal findings and specific diagnoses that require management or diagnostic work-up. This list is constantly updated. Fresh additions can be listed, while changes are marked as "dropped" or "resolved" along with date of recording. The initial plans, numbered correspondingly to the problems addressed, delineate what is to be done. These fall into three categories: more information for diagnosis and management, therapy, and patient education. Progress notes, also preceded by the number and title of the appropriate problem, consist of one or more of the following elements given the acronym of SOAP: subjective symptoms, objective examination, assessment of current condition, and plan statements. POMR helps to: consider all the patient's problems in the total context; indicate clearly the goals and methods of treatment; facilitate medical education by documenting logical thought processes of the physician; and quality assurance, since data are organized and measurable. The major disadvantage is that POMR is quite complex and so requires substantial training of medical and professional staff.

Integrated Medical Records

Patient data, from all sources and all professionals, are listed in strict chronological order. Thus history and physical examination may be followed by a progress note, a nurses' note, a x-ray report, a physiotherapist's or dietician's note, a consultation, etc. The advantage of this system is that all information on a particular episode of care is recorded sequentially, thus providing a clear picture of the patient's illness and response to treatment. The disadvantage is that it is difficult to compare similar information (e.g.: serial blood pressure measurements and medication to control hypertension) as data are scattered over the record. At times only progress notes are integrated. This format has the following merits: quick assessment of the patient's progress is possible because current notes of all disciplines are together; the number of specialized forms is reduced leading to a less bulky record; the team concept of health care is encouraged.

Characteristics of a Good Medical Record

A properly written medical record is associated with good patient care while a poor medical record invariably indicates poor care. Characteristics considered essential to a good medical record include:

Appropriate Documentation

A medical record must contain sufficient and factual data, written in sequence of events, to clearly identify the patient, justify the admission and continued hospitalization, support the diagnosis, and warrant the treatment and end results. It should be detailed, complete and up-to-date to enable various attending physicians to determine the patient's condition at any given time, review response to past treatment procedures, and provide effective continuing care. Hospital and medical staff bylaws should explicitly state physician and nurse responsibilities in recording accurate and complete clinical information.

Signatures

Every entry must be authenticated with the name, in block letters, of the healthcare provider. Better still, there should be the signature and rubber stamp of name, designation and department of the professional recording the observation. All entries should also contain the date (and time, if relevant).

Abbreviations

Only authorized abbreviations and symbols are to be used.

Timeliness

It is imperative that entries be made as close as possible to the time of occurrence of the event being documented. Admission notes are to be completed within 24 hrs of admission, while records of discharged patients are to be completed within two days.

Legibility

The usefulness of the record depends on the legibility of entries. The following reports should be preferably typed: specialized investigation and treatment procedures, radiology, pathology, surgery, discharge summary and medical reports.

Correction of Errors or Omissions

Errors should not be erased or covered with correction fluid. Mistakes or wrong entries should be scored with a single line and should bear the individual's signature and date. Omissions should be rectified by entries after the last entry on that day, with an explanation for it being out of sequence.

Medical Record Forms with Final Order of Arrangement

The order of arrangement of case sheets is different at the ward level when the patient is under treatment and different after discharge. For this reason, some hospitals prefer to have a temporary folder to hold case sheets pertaining to the current inpatient episode, and on discharge of the patient, these forms are re-assembled and included into the patient's permanent unit record. The final order of arrangement in a unit record is generally as follows: patient identification sheet, summary of diagnosis sheet, followed by four sections with dividers for out-patient treatments, correspondence and medical reports, investigation reports on mount sheets, and inpatient notes filed episode-wise. An alternate practical method to filing forms in the unit record is to file all outpatient and inpatient doctor related case sheets in a chronological manner, while nursing and other forms can be filed in inpatient episode-wise.

Forms Design and Control

Well designed forms are easier to complete, ensure that all pertinent information is captured without default, reduce writing time, avoid duplication of information and ensure that the patient's record does not unnecessarily become bulky and unreadable. In order to achieve these objectives, the following principles should be adhered to:

Centralization

Individual physicians and departments should not be permitted to introduce forms without the approval of the Medical Records Committee or Forms Committee. This limits the introduction of multiple forms of a similar nature and at the same time ensures that other requirements of the hospital are met.

Standardization

Medical record forms should invariably be of the specified size to enable proper filing. Case sheets are of A4 size (210 mm x 297 mm), while investigation request/report forms are of B6 size (175 mm x 125 mm).

Design Principles

It is desirable that every form has a title, form number, page number if multiple pages involved, name and logo of institution, and patient identification data (name, hospital number, age, sex, ward) or place of inserting the patient's ID label. Forms should also contain instructions for users if not implicit, departments to be forwarded to if multiple copies involved, sufficient space to record all relevant data to be captured, space for approving signatures. While designing forms it is generally advisable to avoid heavy ruled lines, narrow margins, crowded entries, lack of symmetry, unconventional type styles or fonts, and too large or too small types. Attractive features include: frequent use of hairline rules, adequate margin space, neat arrangement of boxes, occasional use of shading, restrained use of colour. Line and vertical spacing should be appropriate for filling by hand or by typewriter/computer. Particulars to be filled in by different persons should be grouped together, related items should be sequenced, data on the form should be arranged to facilitate flow of writing, and vertical alignment should facilitate minimum tabular and marginal stops when typing.

Forms Appraisal

Periodical appraisal of forms should be carried out to review usefulness of each item of data to be recorded and duplication of same clinical data in multiple forms. This helps in combining certain forms, elimination of some data items or forms, and inclusion of omitted data.

INDEXES AND REGISTERS

Master Patient Index

This index lists all patients treated at the hospital on outpatient and inpatient basis. The index contents include: full name, address, sex, birth date, unit/hospital number, open outpatient episodes, particulars of each inpatient episode including dates of admission and discharge, result, name of consultant and serial number of inpatient registration. In case a patient loses his or her hospital number, computerized phonetic (soundex) query of master patient index helps to track down patients with similar sounding but differently spelt names, and thus avoids opening duplicate files for the same patient.

Disease and Operation Indexes

Disease index, maintained separately for each group of codes, generally lists the patient's hospital number, age and sex of patient, date of admission and/or discharge, end result of hospitalization, disease code, decimal digit expansion, operation code and name/number of physician, service/department. Operation index includes the diagnosis code, surgeon code, name and code of procedure/s, hospital days, post-operative days, discharge status, patient's hospital number, patient's age and sex. The nomenclature and classification system most frequently used is the WHO International Classification of Diseases 10th revision or ICD 9-CM for diseases, and ICD 9 or 9-CM for operative procedures. In some countries (e.g.: U.S.A., Australia, Nordic countries, U.K.), the above data are also compiled as Diagnosis Related Group (DRG) or Health Resource Group (HRG) codes for easier comparison of length of stay and for financial reimbursement.

Physician Index

This is a summary of activities specific to individual physicians. Maintained in a confidential manner through use of physician codes, this index provides data on trends in volume, activity profiles, mortality and morbidity statistics, complication rates, etc. to distinguish active from inactive members, and for quality assurance purposes.

Registers

Important registers which ought to be maintained on the computer include:
- Central patient admission and discharge register
- Ward admission and discharge register
- Operating room register
- Delivery suite register
- Births and Deaths register
- Emergency service / Casualty register
- Medico-legal cases register
- Wound certificate register
- Cancer registry: has 4 basic components: master index file, accession register, case files, follow-up file.

FILING METHODS, STORAGE AND RETENTION

Numbering and Filing Systems

Unit numbering is preferred over serial numbering particularly when the system of combined/unit records is used. Unit numbering entails assigning each patient a unique number at the time of the first visit to the hospital and using this number for all subsequent treatments. This unit number is used for all transactions even though each episode of outpatient treatment (one or several visits relating to that ailment) or inpatient hospitalization is given a different episode number. Each patient thus has a single file irrespective of the number of admissions and outpatient visits, and this record is filed according to the unit number. If the hospital opts for separate outpatient and inpatient records, the serial-unit adaptation is used. Here, outpatient records are filed as per the unit number while inpatient records are filed according to serial number. If the patient is readmitted, his record of the previous admission is brought forward and filed with the record of the recent admission, with a cross-reference in the folder of the earlier record indicating the file transfer. The patient's outpatient folder and master patient index list the serial episode numbers allotted for each admission.

Method of Filing

Any of the following three systems can be used depending on the expertise and resources available:

Straight Numeric Filing

It refers to filing of records in exact chronological order according to unit/serial number. It is easy to train clerks to file records in this manner and, since earlier numbers relate to older records, purging of inactive records is easier. The system, however, has the following disadvantages: Because all digits of the record number must be considered simultaneously, misfiling is high. It is then difficult to trace records wrongly filed. Secondly, the heaviest filing activity is concentrated in the area housing recent records, making it difficult for several clerks to file at the same time without getting in each other's way. Thirdly, it is not possible to divide the work equally and hold filing clerks responsible for specific sections, thus making it difficult to monitor the quality of filing.

Terminal Digit Filing

It is simple, accurate and increases the productivity of file clerks. The six digits of the unit number are broken up into the last two (primary) digits which are considered first. Records sorted out in this manner are taken to the respective primary section and segregated according to the middle two (secondary) digits, following which the record is filed as per the numerical order of the initial two (tertiary) digits. Although it is more difficult to train clerks to file in this manner, the advantages are many. Since only two digits are considered at a time, misfiling is substantially reduced. Secondly, the use of colour-keyed folders further reduces the scope for misfiling. Thirdly, since there are 100 primary sections, and new numbers are evenly distributed, the congestion that results when several clerks file active records in the same area is eliminated. Fourthly, clerks can be made responsible for a group of sections, thus distributing the work evenly and making it easier to monitor quality.

Middle Digit Filing

It maintains the numeric order of records while at the same time incorporates the advantages of terminal digit filing. Here the primary digits are the middle two, the digits on the left are the secondary digits, and the last two digits on the right are the tertiary digits. It is, however, more difficult to train clerks to file in this manner.

Medical Record Retention Policy

Lack of storage space is a perennial problem. It is hence necessary to have a firm policy for transfer of inactive records and further destruction after the period beyond which they will not be required. The point at which records should be shifted to inactive storage depends on the space available for active records, the yearly expansion rate of current files and the frequency with which old records are required. Destruction of records depends on the intensity of research, patient readmission rate, statutes of limitation and costs of microfilming or inactive storage. However, since records not in active use for more than 10 years are generally not required for clinical, scientific, legal or audit purposes, it has become customary to destroy such records provided the following conditions (stipulated by the American Medical Record Association in 1974) are complied with:
- The following basic information should be preserved while destroying records: dates of admission and discharge, record of diagnoses and operations, operative and pathology reports, discharge summary, birth and death certificates.
- Complete medical records should be retained of minors for the period of minority plus the applicable statute of limitations as applicable in that state.

- Complete medical records should be retained of patients with mental disability in a similar manner as for minors.
- Complete medical records should be preserved indefinitely when requested in writing by the patient, his physicians or legal counsel for an interested party.

Miscellaneous Records Retention

These again depend on their possible future use and the statute of limitations:

Nurses' Bedside Records

These have generally served their purpose after discharge of the patient. However, it must be noted that because nurses' notes are so well written up, they are the documents most relied upon during negligence-related enquiries. Nevertheless, since they contribute to the bulk of the inpatient folder, if storage space is a major limiting factor, after 2 years (depending on the statute of limitations) they may be removed from the patient's record and discarded.

Registers of Admission/Discharge, Birth/Delivery Room, Death, Medico-legal cases

These should be preserved permanently and possibly microfilmed.

Other Registers

They are of Operation, Admission/Discharge, Narcotics administration, Infection, X-ray, Daily census, Daily statistics, Monthly report: may be destroyed after 1-2 years of completion.

Disease and Operation Index

Though most hospitals can destroy these after 10 years, medical college hospitals may preserve these for 25 years.

Physician Index

Five years from the time of the clinician leaving the hospital generally suffices.

X-rays

Five years from period of inactive use.
With the progress of computerization in hospitals, tendency to store much of the above data live on the computer, moves towards paperless records, and the possibility to scan relevant case sheets of inactive records for on-line computer storage and retrieval, controversies surrounding the retention policy assume less importance.

HEALTH CARE STATISTICS

Daily Analysis

- Daily census of admissions, births, transfers in, transfers out and deaths compiled by ward and by speciality.
- Daily discharge analysis.

Monthly Reports

- Summary of outpatient visits (first and repeat).
- Summary of inpatient activity speciality-wise: number of admissions, discharges, deaths, hospital days, mean length of stay, bed turnover ratio, occupancy rate, mortality rate, operations, infections, specialized procedures.

Census

- Inpatient bed occupancy ratio:

$$\frac{\text{Total inpatient service days for a period} \times 100}{\text{Total inpatient bed count} \times \text{no. of days in the period}}$$

- Average daily newborn inpatient census:

$$\frac{\text{Total newborn inpatient service days for a period}}{\text{Total number of days in the period}}$$

Death Rates

- Hospital Death Rate (Gross Death Rate):

$$\frac{\text{No. of inpatient deaths in a period} \times 100}{\text{No. of discharges (including deaths) in the same period}}$$

- Net Death Rate (Institutional Death Rate):
$$\frac{\text{Deaths (incl. newborn) less those under 48 hrs for a period} \times 100}{\text{Total number of discharges (including deaths and newborn) less deaths under 48 hrs for the period}}$$
- Postoperative Death Rate:
$$\frac{\text{Total no. of deaths within 10 days postoperative for a period} \times 100}{\text{Total no. of patients operated upon for the period}}$$
- Anaesthesia Death Rate:
$$\frac{\text{Total number of deaths due to anaesthetic agents for a period} \times 100}{\text{Total no. of patients administered anaesthesia for the period}}$$
- Maternal Death Rate (Maternal Mortality Rate):
$$\frac{\text{Total no. of direct maternal deaths for a period} \times 100}{\text{No. of obstetric discharges (incl. deaths) for the period}}$$
- Neonatal Death Rate
$$\frac{\text{Total number of newborn deaths for a period} \times 100}{\text{No of newborn infant discharges (incl. deaths) for the period}}$$
- Perinatal Mortality Rate:
Intermediate (20-28 wks gestation or 500-1000gms weight) and late foetal (after 28 wks) deaths, plus neonatal deaths (less than 28 days), divided by births and foetal deaths for the period, multiplied by 100.

Caesarian Section Rate

$$\frac{\text{Total no. of caesarian sections in a period} \times 100}{\text{No. of deliveries (incl. caesarian sections) in the period}}$$

Infection Rates

- Hospital Infection Rate:
$$\frac{\text{Total no. of nosocomial infections in the hospital (or specific clinical unit) for a period} \times 100}{\text{Total no. of discharges (incl. deaths) in the hospital (or specific clinical unit) for the period}}$$
- Postoperative Infection Rate:
$$\frac{\text{No. of infections in clean surgical cases for a period} \times 100}{\text{Number of clean surgical operations for the period}}$$

RELEVANT MEDICAL RECORD TECHNOLOGIES

Computerization

The degree of computerization varies from hospital to hospital depending on the resources available and computer culture prevalent. Starting from the basic R-ADT (Registration - Admission Discharge Transfer) module, computerization has been progressively applied to various registers and indexes (particularly the patient master index, coding of diseases, operation and delivery register), compilation of statistics, chart location and tracking system, generation of laboratory and other reports, word processor applications for discharge summaries and medical reports, scanning of inactive records, risk management, etc. However, because of the innumerable variables involved in documenting history and clinical findings, the memory disc space involved especially for storage of ECG, x-rays and other graphics, legal issues relating to a computer printout versus a written and signed original document, the feasibility of paperless medical records is still something for the future.

Microfilming

Storage of medical records on microfilm achieves almost 98 percent saving in filing space and filing equipment, reduces paper handling, and protects records against loss, theft and manipulation. However, the costs associated with photographing, storing, reading and printing micro-records are high. Microfilming is therefore cost-effective only if the records are relatively inactive and if they are to be maintained for over 15 years. Although in U.S. courts microfilms may be admitted as primary evidence, this has not become universally applicable. Besides, most medical practitioners still prefer medical records in the original form.

LEGAL ASPECTS OF MEDICAL RECORDS

The exact applicability of laws relating to medical records differs from country to country depending on legislation, Government regulations and judicial pronouncements. However, the following principles are more or less universally applicable:
- The Governing Board, the Hospital Administration and the Medical Records Department are held responsible for the maintenance, safe custody and proper use of a patient's medical record.

- Patients, guardians and legal heirs have a right to change patient registration particulars (e.g.: name, parent's name, birth date, age, address) provided the request is made in writing and sufficient proof is advanced in this regard.
- The medical record is the physical property of the Hospital. However, this does not prevent the patient from submitting legitimate claims to see and copy the information therein. In fact, the U.K. Patient's Charter specifically grants patients the right to a copy of their hospital record. A similar claim has been upheld by the Mumbai High Court.
- The medical record, when applied as a personal document, is a **confidential** document. The hospital and the physician are generally prevented from releasing such privileged information without the written authorization of the patient. In the case of minors or the mentally incompetent, the legal guardian, and after a patient's death, the legal heirs can give authorization for release of information from the patient's file.
- Calling a physician as a witness for a patient in a trial, or when the patient brings legal action against his physician, relinquishes the right of the patient to confidentiality of medical information during court proceedings.
- The information contained in a medical record may be made available to another health facility if the same is necessary for the continuing care of the patient. However, if the patient's new physician (other than the physician who attended on him in the hospital) requests for an abstract, it is not to be given unless there is a signed authorization from the patient.
- Governmental agencies have no automatic right to a patient's record unless this right is exercised through Court.
- A patient may authorise disclosure by indicating in writing the name of individual or institution that may be given the information, purpose of information, and extent or nature of information to be released.
- Just because a third party (insurance firm, employer, etc.) is meeting the expenses of hospitalization, it does not have the right to the medical record or discharge summary unless the patient has authorized release of such information.
- Courts have the right to subpoena a patient's record. Such a record, when produced, can be admitted as primary evidence in legal proceedings.

- Quasi-judicial bodies such as Medical Councils have the right to summon for a patient's record when enquiring into professional misconduct or negligence.
- When releasing the original record as above, the Medical Records Department should safeguard against future tampering of data. The case sheets should be numbered, documented on the folder, a photocopy preserved in safe custody and acknowledgement secured while handing over the original.
- Accreditation bodies have the right to summon and review medical records as impersonal documents.

THE MEDICAL RECORDS DEPARTMENT

Organization

The Medical Records Department is considered as an ancillary service department. It is generally organized into 4 sections:
- Registration, Admissions and Appointments
- Medical Records Archive
- Inpatient Records Processing, and
- Release of Information and Statistics.

Staffing

The MRD is headed by a Medical Records Administrator/Officer/Librarian who has undergone formal training in medical records technology. The department head reports to the Medical Superintendent with respect to clinically related matters and to the Hospital Administrator with regard to administrative and legal issues. The department is additionally staffed by officers/librarians, statistician, technicians and clerks formally trained in medical records as also with clerks, registration assistants, secretaries and messengers who attend to routine administrative tasks.

Functions

The major responsibilities of the department include:
- Patient registration, booking of appointments, and initiation of medical record documents for outpatients, inpatients, emergency and day care patients.
- Filing, custody, storage, prompt retrieval, file track in/out, issue and transport of patient files to clinics and wards, collection of the file promptly after patient disposal;

- Authorized release of patient files for patient care, education research, administrative and legal purposes;
- Assembling and record deficiency check, discharge analysis, coding of diseases and operations;
- Maintenance of indexes and registers, cancer registry;
- Ensuring confidentiality of patient data;
- Implementation of the medical records retention policy;
- Reporting births and deaths, and notifiable diseases to state health authorities;
- Issue of birth/death notification certificates, medical reports, co-ordination and release of sickness and medico-legal certificates;
- Storage of medico-legal data and evidence, liaison with police;
- Monitoring bed occupancy, inpatient census, hospital service analysis, compilation of hospital statistics;
- Providing data for infection control, risk management, medical audit, quality assurance, utilization review.

COMMON PROBLEMS ASSOCIATED WITH MEDICAL RECORDS

Physician Related

- Entries in record are perfunctory, inadequate and do not reflect patient's condition and treatment given.
- Entries illegible, not traceable to respective doctor, not signed, not dated, use of inappropriate abbreviations.
- Iatrogenic complications not factually documented, nosocomial infections not reported.
- Timing/date of discharge differ from nurses' notes.
- Admission-discharge summary sheet incomplete and hence record cannot be indexed and filed.
- Non-return of records taken for research or case presentation.

Nurse Related

- Pages in record lack patient identification data.
- Wrong hospital numbers entered manually.
- Charts held up in wards, not returned following discharge.
- Census incorrect, especially transfers.
- Investigation reports not correctly filed, especially for patients transferred to other wards.

MRD Related

- Records misplaced, wrongly filed, unavailable when required.
- Patient files can get too bulky, covers are invariably tattered.
- Investigation reports not filed.
- Delay in coding and indexing.
- No follow-up on non-returned records.

THE MEDICAL RECORDS COMMITTEE

The objectives, composition and terms of reference of the Medical Records Committee are detailed under the chapter "Hospital Committees" elsewhere in this book.

THE HOSPITAL ADMINISTRATION VIS-À-VIS THE MRD

The Hospital Administration is responsible for:
- Ensuring implementation of decisions of the Governing Board relating to records to be maintained and any specific directions regarding how these records should be processed and stored.
- Ensuring implementation of decisions by the Medical Staff Committee and Medical Records Committee on matters pertaining to medical records.
- Compliance by the Medical Records Department of laws, regulations and standards laid down by state health authorities, courts, accrediting bodies.
- Safeguarding patient records against loss, defacement, tampering, unauthorized use, fire and water damage.
- Organising and ensuring the smooth and efficient functioning of the Medical Records Department by:
  1. Appointment of a qualified and competent department head
  2. Providing sufficient staff
  3. Delegating duties, delineating and clarifying accountability of subordinates
  4. Implementation of personnel policies, disciplinary action
  5. Harmonious working of the department with other departments of the hospital
  6. Providing equipment, space, facilities
  7. Financial management, availability of sufficient budget.

CHAPTER 25

Pharmacy

OBJECTIVES OF A HOSPITAL PHARMACY

The Objectives of a hospital pharmacy are to:
1. Make available all the drugs and pharmaceuticals needed for patient care (inpatient and outpatient), according to the hospital formulary: the right drug (effective, safe, with good benefit/risk ratio) in the right formulation and dosage. An efficient department should determine in advance and stock adequate quantities of drugs, at the same time avoiding idle inventory.
2. Disseminate information regarding drugs among the users, functioning as a Drug Information Centre.
3. Prepare certain medicines (usually intravenous fluids, mixtures and ointments) depending on the policy of the hospital.
4. Observe high standards of professional skill in dispensing medicines according to the prescriptions.

The Pharmacy Department needs special attention because:
1. It is an area of high investment, being usually next only to salaries and wages.
   In hospital M (1993-94), with a total expenditure of rupees two crores and twenty three lakhs, the salaries and wages were rupees eighty nine lakhs and the cost of medicines came to rupees forty five lakhs (20% of total expenditure).

The Pharmacy should be under good financial control.
2. The availability of the right drug in the right formulation at the time it is needed, is important for proper therapy and satisfaction of the users.
3. Leading causes of discomfort, disability and death are often preventable or treatable with drugs.
4. Mistakes can be disastrous, both in terms of morbidity and mortality.
5. There are many rules and regulations which must be complied with.

Functions of the Pharmacy

1. Purchase, storing, distribution and dispensing of quality drugs at reasonable cost to outpatients and inpatients.
2. Inspection of all pharmaceuticals in all the hospital services, for quality, availability, proper storage, date of expiry, etc.
3. Developing and maintaining information regarding all drugs, chemicals and biologicals (including quality, cost and sources of supplies) and making the information available to the medical and other staff of the hospital.
4. Ensuring that the pharmacy and the hospital conform to the relevant Acts, Rules and Regulations, (and esp., the Drugs and Cosmetics Act) maintaining all necessary registers and records.
5. Establishing and maintaining adequate accounting procedures for (i) pharmacy charges (ii) supplies (iii) concessions and free services.
6. Observing all the relevant rules and procedures for materials management as are applicable to drugs and other supplies in the pharmacy.
7. Furnishing reports of the activities, periodically and a comprehensive report annually.
8. Where the hospital policy is to have preparation of medications, undertake such preparation, with *adequate quality control*.
9. Carry out all such responsibilities with due consideration for ethics and human values.

PROBLEMS IN DRUG SUPPLY AND POTENTIAL FOR IMPROVEMENT

Among the problems are the purchase of irrational drugs, misuse of drugs, improper storage, expiration of dates, theft and high prices. Improvement can be effected by proper selection of drugs and the rational use, improved purchasing, effective dispensing practices, careful inventory control, better storage and improved security.

Drugs and Therapeutics Committee

For the efficient functioning of the pharmacy, it is necessary to bring together the *users of the service* (the medical and nursing staff), the providers of the professional service (the pharmacists)and the *administrators*. This is achieved by the Drugs and Therapeutics Committee.

Functions

1. Preparation of the hospital formulary (selection of drugs and their formulations) and periodical updating. Generic names should be used to the extent possible, at the same time ensuring quality.
2. Selection of manufacturers and suppliers.
3. Framing of the policy of the pharmacy and making known the policy to all users.
4. Development of pharmacy services (i) outpatient (ii) inpatient
5. Budget consideration
6. Periodical review of the functioning and management of the pharmacy.
7. Developing of drug information system.
8. Monitoring of adverse reactions.

What is the Optimum Composition of the Committee?

The composition and size of the committee would depend on the type and size of the hospital. The committee should be representative of all groups and yet be not too large to avoid difficulties in meeting frequently. For a medium-sized, general hospital, the following composition is suggested:
1. Medical Superintendent (Chairperson)
2. Administrator
3. (4) and (5) specialists in different disciplines.
6. Nursing Superintendent
7. Chief Pharmacist (Secretary)

How often to meet?

The committee should initially meet as often as needed to prepare the formulary.

The Drugs and Therapeutics Committee of hospital M had 28 sittings over a period of one year before the formulary was finalized.

Once the formulary has been completed, the committee may meet once in two months or so. It is better to meet at fixed times, on fixed days, say, the second Tuesdays of alternative months at

2.00p.m. This will help the members avoid conflict with other engagements. Also other users will know when the committee meets to review the formulary and consider new proposals.

Formulary

Care must be exercized in the preparation of the formulary. It should ensure *the Rational Use of Drugs*. The drugs and their formulations should be selected on the basis of (i) effectiveness in the given conditions, (ii) good benefit-risk ratio and (iii) cost-effectiveness.

There are about 60,000 drug formulations in the country with over 8,000 manufacturers, large and small, producing and marketing them. Many of these drugs are hazardous or useless. It is necessary to weed these out.

The Drugs and Therapeutics Committee may adopt different methods for preparing the formulary:
1. Review the existing list of drugs in the hospital, and after discussion on each, eliminate the useless, harmful and unnecessarily costly drugs; include those which are useful, beneficial and cost-effective.
2. Choose *de novo* the appropriate drug for each indication.
3. Use the WHO list of essential drugs and modify it as warranted. According to WHO only about 250 drugs are required. The Health Committee had recommended about half the number.
4. Use other hospital formularies and adapt them to fit into the requirements of the hospital (British National Formulary and other formularies such as those of St. Martha's Hospital, Bangalore and CMC Hospital, Vellore).

It is important to include all emergency medicines and antidotes against poisons, including snake-bites and overdoses of drugs.

Once the formulary has been completed and accepted, copies must be made available to all users. Only drugs included in the formulary should be stocked in the pharmacy. There must be mechanisms for periodically updating the formulary, with additions and deletions in the light of newer knowledge or requirements.

The formulary should give the indications, contraindications, side and adverse effects, special precautions to be taken, the usual dose and duration of treatment, and the cost. It would be better if the cost for the full (average) course is also given.

Style

The style of the formulary should be simple. The details given and the style of language used will depend on the type of the hospital pharmacy for which the formulary is meant. In all cases, simplicity and direct information and instruction are to be followed.

Size

The size of the formulary should be suitable for the health care services to be provided. In all cases, it should be pocket-sized; the formulary is more likely to be used and more frequently by the prescriber, if it can be carried easily.

Additions and Deletions

Any of the prescribers in the hospital must be able to request for changes (additions or deletions) in the formulary. This must be done in writing to the secretary of the Drugs and Therapeutics Committee giving the reasons; more efficacious; less side-effects; less costly, shortens the period of treatment/hospitalization; etc. If the Committee considers that this request is in the best interests of the hospital patients, the change will be effected. If more information is required, the same will be collected from suitable sources. The person requesting for the change may be invited to the particular meeting of the Committee to explain in greater detail.

All additions and deletions must be given in writing to all the holders of the formulary.

Revisions

The frequency of revision will depend on the circumstances. It is advisable to revise the formulary once in two years.

Purchase

Once the decision is taken as to the drugs to be stocked in the pharmacy, action has to be taken to get them. All the rules of materials management should be followed. These would include
- Levels at which stocks are to be maintained,
- ABC analysis –fast moving, moderately fast moving and slow moving,

Pharmacy   209

- Reorder levels,
- Lead or lag time, and
- Advantages of bulk order or bulk purchase.

Hospitals get special rates and advantage should be taken by purchasing from the manufacturers, distributors or stockists. The pharmacy should not accept the questionable practices of gifts for the purchase of a certain quantity of a particular brand.

Never go in for 'gifts'

Purchase should be made from reliable sources. Quality must be ensured. It is necessary to have a selection of suppliers.

One way of reducing cost is by group purchasing.

Another way would be by inviting competitive quotations, especially for the major items (costwise).

Orders

Except in an emergency, orders should be in writing. Write the order in a printed, duplicate order book. The order should clearly indicate the terms under which the supplies are to be made, including cost, period of supply, quantity and full specifications. Send top copy to the company; retain duplicate copy in the book in the pharmacy. In case of urgency, telephonic orders may be placed and confirmed in writing immediately thereafter.

Special orders will have to be placed for dangerous drugs. Excise rules will have to be followed in the case of spirit: getting a licence, transport pass, register of receipts and utilization of stock, opening of new stock only in the presence of the Excise Inspector and sending of returns of stock. Special measures have to be adopted for dangerous drugs and narcotic drugs, such as pethidine and morphine.

Goods Received Note and other stores records will be as for any stores, giving full details. Damages, if any, should be brought to the notice of the carriers and suppliers immediately.

One important requirement is to note the date of expiry Ensure that there is sufficient time for the drug to be used completely before the expiry date. Usually the suppliers take back the item, if they are returned reasonably before the date of expiry.

Use bin-cards Include details of the transactions (receipt, issue) – cost and tax, expiry date, unit price, re-order level, economic order quantity, and other relevant information.

Issues from stores are always to the dispensing part of the pharmacy. There must be written *indent* and signed issue and receipt.

Control of store Only designated persons should be allowed to enter the store.

Indents will be given by the user departments/wards in writing, preferably in duplicate, with full signature.

Gifts of medicines from abroad: A few organizations abroad give gifts of medicines free under various schemes. These are controlled under the Indo-German, Indo-US and the Indo-UK agreements. Hospitals can receive such consignments of medicines if they are registered under the terms of the concerned Agreement. The supplies may be made direct to the hospital or through organizations in the country. These medicines are free of customs duty. They have to be dispensed completely free to the patients without any discrimination based on religion, community, etc. No charges can be made to cover cost of transport, dispensing and other overheads.

These medicines received as gifts will be subject to the same stock control measures as those purchased. In addition, they require satisfactory proof of free distribution to the patients.

Avoid these gifts if possible. They can lead to problems like date of expiry over, difficulty in deciphering (different language) and keeping of records. The medicines supplied are often not the medicines we require.

Storage

The storage conditions must satisfy the requirements of the drugs maintaining their potency. This includes temperature (some drugs and biologicals require storage under proper refrigeration) and clean dry conditions (high humidity can be detrimental). It is necessary to have rotation of stock, so that the oldest material is used at the earliest. The principle is *first-in, first-out*.

An important requirement is to have a dated drugs register, especially with drugs having expiry dates. Examine the register at least once a month. Those likely to go out of date must be used or returned to the supplier. Out of date items should not be in the pharmacy.

Nagpur Times, 21 July 1988 Dr. Kolhe found that there were injections in the hospital like Stemetil, Batch No.206 which had its expiry date in August 1987.

In the larger hospitals, the bulk storage may be in one place, with the required quantities being moved periodically to the dispensing area.

Pilferage

One of the problems is pilferage. This occurs in many pharmacies. All action should be taken to prevent it, which can be on a large measure or on a small scale.

Free Press Journal, Bombay, 20 September 1988 Large-scale pilferage of essential drugs from the hospital's store is responsible for the continuing drug shortage at the Diwalibai Mohanlal Mehta Municipal Hospital, Bombay.

The plan of the pharmacy and its location should be such that pilferage and access by unauthorized persons is reduced.

Distribution

The drugs must be made available in the required dosages to the users (inpatients and outpatients). The dispensing to outpatients is simple, though different hospitals have slightly different systems. Every prescription must be checked for the correctness of the dosages and strengths (depending on the age and other conditions), the signature of the doctor and other criteria. It is ideal to have every prescription to be dispensed and checked by another pharmacist before the drug leaves the dispensary. The dispensing should be done with proper container, labelling and instructions.

As regards the stocks to be supplied to the wards, the procedures vary based on the policy, which must be worked out between the pharmacist and the nurses in charge of the wards. Whatever be the procedure adopted, there is need for a list of medicines and the stock level must be maintained in the ward.

The pharmacist must visit ward regularly to make sure that:

i. the socks are stored properly and in adequate quantity, and
ii. there is no excess.

It is necessary to have proper entries in registers and returns for controlled drugs like narcotics.

Preparations

Many pharmacies prepare mixtures, ointments, antiseptic solutions and lotions and intravenous fluids. In all of them, it is necessary to follow good manufacturing practice. There are many rules and regulations to be complied with. Quality raw materials must be used. There is need for cleanliness and dust-free atmosphere. Personal hygiene and clean overalls are important. The containers must be airtight and sealed to exclude moisture and dust. Where special ampules and other containers are required, they must be provided. There is need for correct labelling, giving full details legibly. The finished product must be appraised, particularly with regards to clarity, uniformity of colour, particles, sediments, etc.

Quality

The quality of the medicines purchased, stored and supplied must be good. There are very many spurious and substandard drugs in the market. They should be avoided.

The quality of the medicines depends on the raw ingredients and good manufacturing practices. Changes can occur between manufacture and consumption. They may be changes in colour, consistency and chemical identity.

Quality assurance must satisfy:

1. *Identity*: The correct ingredients must be present
2. *Potency*: The ingredients must be present in the correct quantities.
3. *Purity*: Drugs should not contain harmful ingredients or contaminants.
4. *Uniformity*: There must be uniform distribution of the ingredients.
5. *Bio-availability*: The rate and extent of absorption into the blood stream must give the intended effect.

Points to be kept in mind regarding drug quality:
   1. Loss of potency: Poor bio-availability; expiration date; improper storage.

2. Toxic degradation eg., tetracyclines.
3. Contamination.

How can we assess quality? Procedures to assess quality
1. Good manufacturing practices report
2. Inspection of factory
3. Laboratory analysis (routine)
4. *Testing by exception* done when there is a complaint.

Staff

Staffing depends on the services provided by the pharmacy. Allow only qualified pharmacists to dispense. The number will depend on the number of prescriptions and the type of medications to be prepared and/or dispensed, as also the number of hours the pharmacy is open. Usually, apart from the chief pharmacist, there will be one pharmacist for 50-100 beds. In addition, there is need for administrative staff.

Drug Information Center

The hospital pharmacy has the responsibility of collecting and supplying correct information regarding drugs available in the market to the users in the hospital. Many of the formulations available in the country contain banned drugs, hazardous drugs, irrational drugs or their combinations. Individual prescribers will not be in a position to be in the know of these facts; they are often fed with incomplete information by those interested in pushing their products.

There is need for a good, systematic library, with standard text books, journals, charts and other literature. Literature (scientific) from different sources must be collected, analyzed and kept. Retrieval of data is very important; classification and filing should be done properly.

The information on any drug should give its nature, indications, contraindications, side-effects, special precautions, formulation and dosage, duration of treatment and other particulars, in addition to its pharmacology, pharmacokinetics and bio-availability by different routes of administration. Information regarding incompatibility, drug interactions, advisability of administration in pregnancy, childhood and old age, and in renal, hepatic and other diseases must be available. Certain drugs crystallize and precipitate out when given with large volume parenterals. The centre must also have information on the comparative price of similar products. Books and journals on legislation and regulation of drugs should be available.

If the pharmacy is situated in a city or large town, a network can be formed so that comprehensive, combined information will be available. Smaller pharmacies can establish linkage with larger ones.

Monitoring of Adverse Reactions

Any adverse reaction to the administration of any drug (particularly parenterals) should be reported immediately to the pharmacy. The pharmacy should take appropriate decisions immediately. It maybe good to have a small (3 member) committee, who will report to the Medical Superintendent / Administrator.

It may be necessary to suspend the issue of the particular drug and report the matter to the supplier, manufacturer and drugs controller. The batch number and other details must be noted carefully. If formulations of the same batch are still available in the wards, withdraw them until cleared.

Prescriptions

The pharmacist should exercise professional skill and utmost care in dispensing medicines. It is necessary to ensure that the correct drug in the correct dose and formulation is dispensed. There are many drugs with closely similar names but entirely different action. Instructions for use, such as "before food" or "after food" must be given. When a particular brand (the ultimate aim will be to use only generic names) is prescribed and is not available and an equivalent one included in the formulary is available, it should be possible for the pharmacist to substitute it, preferably after informing the treating doctor personally or over the phone.

The pharmacist should inform the patient (particularly the ambulant patient) of the possible side-effects and adverse reactions. The pharmacist should also look for possible interactions, when more than one drug is prescribed. It is also good to consider particular situations, such as pregnancy, old age, young children, etc., when drugs likely to have adverse effects are present in the prescription.

The pharmacist will follow the hospital policies on drugs in general and dealing with prescriptions in particular.

PHYSICAL FACILITIES

Site

The pharmacy serves both inpatients and outpatients. The pharmacy is the last place usually visited by the outpatients; hence it must be located close to the exit (avoid cross-circulation). It is better to locate it near the regular traffic (if multistoreyed hospital, near the available staircase). This will ensure:
1 Easy access to the staff (and relatives of patients) from the wards,
2. Access to suppliers (from outside the hospital) to the store
3. Better security, reducing possibility of thieves breaking open and taking away costly or, even worse, narcotic drugs. The walls must be thick and strong, making it virtually impossible to break them down.

If the pharmacy engages in the preparation of sterile fluids, the area must be located in a dust-free area.

Size

The size depends on a variety of factors:
1. *Location of the hospital* In a city or large town, there will be many Chemists and Druggists stores. If the policy of the hospital allows it, they can supply medicines and other materials direct to the patient. In a small place, the patient will be more dependent on the hospital pharmacy.
   The location will also influence the quantum of stock. In a large town/city, supplies can be got at short notice. This reduces the size of the inventory.
2. *Type of the hospital* An acute care general hospital with a number of specialities will require large number and quantity of items, with greater turnover. A hospital catering for one particular type of patients (tuberculosis, leprosy, eye diseases, etc.) will have medicines necessary for their treatment (and emergencies); the number of items in the inventory will be less.
3. *Rational use of Drugs* Hospitals which stick to the rational use of drugs will have a smaller inventory, as the number of formulations will be much less; unwanted drugs will not be stocked.

Space

For a medium-sized hospital, there should be:
1. Three dispensing counters and one cash counter (separate)
2. Two store rooms, including standard and refrigerated stores,
3. Administrative offices with record keeping, filing, bin cards, registers etc.
4. Rooms for compounding and production, if undertaken,
5. Small library, and
6. Enough circulation space.

Equipment

1. Refrigerators, for storing vaccines, sera and other substances requiring refrigeration. The refrigeration must have recording thermometers, so that we are sure of the temperature inside.
2. Shelves (preferably with variable heights)
3. Filing cabinets, kardex etc.
4. Equipment for preparations of fluids, mixtures, ointments, etc., if such preparations are undertaken
5. Other equipment, and
6. Furniture.

For Intravenous Fluid Preparation

1. Storage for unused and returned bottles or bags to be filled,
2. Washing area, with bottle washing and other facilities,
3. Autoclaving area with sufficient machinery, power and other ancillaries,
4. Distilling area (for glass-distilled, pyrogen free water) with distilling plants of adequate capacity,
5. Filing and capping area, with appropriate machinery,
6. Inspection and quality control area and tables, with light etc.
7. Stores for storing (i) raw materials (ii) finished products, before despatch to the pharmacy, and
8. Room for pharmacist, records etc

In addition, there must be facilities for testing for chemicals, reactions, pyrogens and microbiology.

The area for preparation must be clean and dust free, preferably air-conditioned, with filtered air and laminar flow.

If ampule filling is to be done, facilities for the same must be available.

If ointments and mixtures are prepared, space and materials must be provided near the dispensing area. It is not desirable to prepare these lasting for a long time.

Q System In the larger hospitals, small barriers should be placed opposite the counters to facilitate the "Q" system.

Telephone A telephone connecting all patient areas and administration with facilities to dial outside the hospital is necessary. The telephone should be kept in the administration area and not near the dispensing counters.

Arrangement of shelves The drugs must be arranged systematically along the shelves, so as to make it easy for the pharmacists to identify them, take them and replace, as needed. Walking within the pharmacy should be reduced to the minimum. The commonly used drugs must be easily accessible and preferably pre-packed in the usually prescribed numbers.

24-hour service The hospital must decide on the policy regarding the hours the pharmacy is open. It maybe better to have the pharmacy kept open during the first two shifts or one shift with staggered times, with the largest number of pharmacists being available between 9.00A.M. and 3.00 P.M. There can be a night pharmacy (stocked with emergency drugs and small quantities of other commonly required drugs) close to, but separate from the main pharmacy.

Charges for Medicines and Accessories

It is necessary to fix reasonable charges for medicines and other supplies, dispensed from the pharmacy. There should be no loss; the cost and overheads must be covered. At the same time, the cost to patient should not be higher than the retail price charged in the market and no undue profit should be taken. The charges fixed should take into consideration certain concessions given by the supplier, e.g., supply of 10 additional (free)bottles of IV Fluid on purchase of 100 numbers. Many formulae can be evolved.

Accounts Keeping

Accounting procedures must be good. This applies to various facets:

Purchase Care has to be exercised in getting full benefits. Hospitals often get medicines at much lower rates. It is necessary to determine the purchase price, which should include all aspects such as sales tax, discount, additional numbers of bottles, etc., being given.

Costing It is essential to determine the amount at which the hospital will be making the drug available to the patients.

Calculating the Rate for Supply to Patients

Medicines Consider
Price, including tax
Overheads and handling charges (say + 25%)
Extra quantities given, if any (-)

If the total is equal to or less than the Maximum Retail Price (MRP) plus tax, the price is fixed at the total arrived at; if it is higher, the price will be fixed at MRP plus tax.

After calculating the rates, separate lists are prepared for:
1. Tablets and capsules,
2. Injections,
3. Syrups and drops
4. Ointments, and
5. Others

In alphabetical order, with dates, leaving sufficient columns for changes at later dates, following the principles of First in—First out.

Accessories

1. Generally include cost price plus a certain percentage for overheads (not to exceed MRP +tax), and
2. In the case of materials like gauze, etc., include cost plus adhoc amount.

Medicines Prepared in The Pharmacy

For medicines prepared in the pharmacy (e.g., mixture, ointments, IV fluids), the cost is calculated by including
- Ingredients cost,
- Cost of containers, labels, etc.,
- Electricity and water,

- Depreciation on equipment and building,
- Salaries and overheads, and
- Cost of testing and quality control.

To the above is added a suitable margin to cover skills involved and unforeseen incidents, such as spoiling, breakages, etc.

Payment

As far as possible, patients maybe asked to pay for the medicines at the time of dispensing.
1. It ensures a smooth cash flow.
2. Patients are generally more ready to pay in small amounts rather than a big bill at the time of discharge.

It is advisable not to put the words "Medicines once sold will not be taken back" or to display such a board in front of the pharmacy as what the pharmacy does is to dispense medicines and not to sell them. This may, however, lead to requests for refunds for unused medicines.

LEGAL IMPLICATIONS

There are many legislations and regulations concerning the pharmacy. It is necessary that the pharmacy follows all the rules and regulations.

Licence

In Karnataka, the Drugs Controller insists that the hospital must take a licence to prepare intravenous fluids and other medications. The Controller considers the preparation of these substances as 'Manufacture for Sale' and insists that the law for 'manufacture for sale' be complied with. A licence is required for the pharmacy.

Sales Tax

One vexing point of contention is Sales Tax. The commercial Tax authorities treat the pharmacy as dealer and demand payment as sales tax and turn over tax. The hospital cannot be considered as a dealer as it performs only a service in supplying the required medicines to the patients in the hospital on the prescription of the hospital doctor. This is similar to the dispensing by a private practitioner, which is exempt from tax.

Insurance

Have all the stocks in the pharmacy covered by insurance against theft, fire, etc. The premium involved is not large but all records must be complete and up-to-date. It is also good to have the persons (at least the person dealing with cash) working in the pharmacy covered by fidelity insurance.

Reports

Periodical reports must be made available to the hospital administration as determined by each hospital. Statutory reports must go to the Government.

The annual report must be made available to the administration. This would give an overview of the functioning of the pharmacy and the financial status. This should have taken into consideration the stock position as at the end of the year, so that the opening and closing balances can be struck.

Health Education

The pharmacy and pharmacists can be of great help in the matter of patient education and health education and, therefore, in helping people to attain and maintain health.

Section 8: Human Resources

CHAPTER

26

Personnel

INTRODUCTION

As an Administrator, you have to deal with people in your hospital. They have to carry out their functions for the achievement of the objectives. Managing people is your most important task. Motivate them. They represent the greatest asset of your hospital. Do we manage our human resources the way we should? Mismanagement of human resources contributes a great deal to the disintegration of the functioning of the hospital.

It is essential to:

1. Recruit employees, who are suitable, qualified and have the requisite skills, attitude and experience for the job and to fulfil the objectives of the hospital,
2. Retain such employees, ensuring that each employee is provided with a satisfactory work environment and favourable service conditions and gets job satisfaction,
3. Maintain good interpersonal and employer-employee relations, and
4. Ensure that the employees are aware of, subscribe to and follow the objectives of the hospital, dealing with patients with competence and compassion and believing in the dignity of the person under their care.

As an administrator (whether there is a personnel department or not), your effectiveness and success depends on how well you understand the people with you and their needs. As the lower levels of need (basic needs such as food and housing) are satisfied, they become less and less effective as motivators. The higher levels of needs (respect by others and self-status and self-actualization) become important. The Administrator must be able to understand the unfulfilled needs of the employees. The financial incentives have been the traditional motivators but non-financial motivators are required to meet the higher needs.

In the earlier days, workers demanded mainly wage increases, better working conditions, reduced working hours, rest periods and more holidays. These continue to be the most dominant demands even now, but to them are added many other demands such as fair and impartial selection, rational performance appraisal, objectives to be spelt out, proper job descriptions to be given, keeping pace with technological progress (sometimes opposing their introduction if they consider them as a threat to their continuation and promotion) and high performance from management.

Recruitment

We have to match the man and the job. Whether it is a new post (a new job) or a vacancy to be filled, we must review the job and its requirement. Search the need of the hospital. If it is to fill the vacancy, we must ask ourselves why the previous incumbent left. There can be a variety of reasons. Finding out the reason can help in a better choice. Often, enough thought is not given to the recruitment of personnel. More thought is given in the purchase of machinery and equipment. We devote a lot of time in the selection of a monitor—defibrillator costing, say Rs. 40,000/- and with a useful life span of 5 years. We do not devote even half the time in the selection of a Physician (salary, say, Rs. 50,000/- per annum) who is expected to be with us for the next 10-15 years or more. Getting a wrong person can be a colossal waste and detrimental to the realization of the objectives.

Selection

Selection of the right person is one of the most important activities on which depends the future of the hospital. Our task is to search and find the right person.

Selection may be made by promotion (wherever possible, higher level jobs should be given to current hospital employees; a promotion is to be considered in the same manner as new employment), or by advertisement or other methods, (such as invitation of a person whose name has been suggested by knowledgeable person). The advertisement must give factual information. In such cases, give details in an information sheet to be attached to the application form. People would like to know about your hospital. This will help people with similar objectives to apply and stop others from applying. Mismatches will be reduced. The information sheet would give the salary and other benefits, if any, and also describe the job. It must indicate what we expect and what the candidate can expect.

Interview

Selection is carried out usually after an interview. From the applications received, a short list is prepared. In some cases written and practical tests are given (these are ideal in the case of technicians, radiographers, stenographers and others where the number of applicants is sizeable and skills are important). Other methods of assessment like group discussions can be held.

The interview must be utilized more to bring out the potential. The application form would have given most of the information regarding what the candidate has done. Clarifications can be obtained during the interview. But maximum use must be made to bring out the ability of the candidate to perform the job well.

It is important to provide the proper environment for the interview. It must be friendly. The interview must be such as to have the candidate in a relaxed mood, to bring out the strengths and potential. The seating must be comfortable.

The number of interviewers must not be too many. If there is a large number, it overawes the candidate. Try to restrict the number to three or four. If there are more, perhaps it may be better to split the committee, with each group probing into specific, predetermined areas.

Hold the interview at the appointed time. It is not correct to make the candidates wait for an unreasonably long time. If there are many candidates, it may be good to give different timings. It is also necessary to give sufficient time for each candidate. Do not hurry through. If you have done your homework of shortlisting, every candidate deserves to be given sufficiently long time. How much is sufficient? It depends on the job.

Introduce the members of the board to the candidate. This would help the candidate to answer pointedly to the person who puts the question—to the professional expert in a professional manner and to the social scientist in the way relevant. Avoid disturbances, as far as possible, during the interview. Instruct the Secretary not to put through telephone calls, unless they are emergent and cannot wait.

Appointment

If the candidate is selected, an appointment letter, setting forth full details of appointment, job descriptions, salary, and other conditions like employees' service rules must be given. All appointments must be preceded by a medical examination and the person should be found fit for the job. Handicapped persons may be eminently suitable for certain kinds of work. Appointments should be on probation so that performance can be evaluated. The period of probation is usually one year. If there are quarterly evaluation reports, a fair and just assessment can be made.

Furnishing Bio-data

Every employee should furnish at the time of joining, in writing his/her correct bio-data; subsequent changes, if any, must be intimated and included promptly. The Personnel Department must verify them with the certificates in original.

An important entry will be the record of age. The best proof of age is the entry in the School leaving certificate. Other certificate may be accepted at the discretion of the management and an entry made at the earliest possible.

Subbamma, an aide in M Hospital, had not furnished her age at the time of employment. In the provident fund application, her age was shown as 40 years. At the end of 20 years of service, the hospital terminated her services, the age of superannuation being 60 years. She produced an affidavit stating that her present age is only 53 years. A dispute arose between the employee and the hospital.

Every employee should be issued an identity card, which must be produced on demand.

Confidential Record

A confidential file showing all relevant data, including performance evaluation is kept on all personnel. The performance evaluation reports are very important. The evaluation must be done carefully by the supervisors. Appointments to higher responsibilities, continuation, punishments, termination, etc., should be done considering the periodical appraisal.

Training

Once recruitment of appropriate person has been made, it is necessary to nurture him/her. He/she must be kept up-to-date with proper training. Such training programs may be of different kinds for different categories of personnel and conducted under different auspices. But it is necessary that the employee continues to update knowledge, skills and attitudes.

Take Care of Your People

The hospital must care for its employees as people, respecting their dignity. The attitude towards the employees will determine ultimate success. The response of every hospital employee should be:
 "The higher-ups here do not just view us as a means to an end, only paying attention to us when there is a job to be done. We are made to feel important—not just for what we are and the jobs we do, but also for who we are".

Employees' Problems

The employees will have problems. There must be a machinery for resolving employee's grievances, quickly and with fairness. There are various ways in which this can be achieved (grievance resolving committees with participation by representatives of management and employees; arbitration boards). It is a good idea to establish a direct line between the Administrator and the employee who has a grievance and seeks help. Do not interfere directly but ensure that the grievance is handled properly and necessary action taken without undue delay. If the grievance is not resolved at the departmental level, then there should be procedures for appeals to higher levels of administration. It is always better, for both parties —employee and management, to have the grievance resolved at the hospital, rather than have recourse to the labour department or court under the Industrial Disputes Act. Procedures there drag on with both parties being made to spend a lot of time with arguments and counter arguments. In the meantime, the relationships sour and suffer. Remember that you have to work together after the proceedings in the labour court. It is better to have an amicable settlement, if necessary through arbitration through an impartial person, acceptable to all.

In tackling a grievance, there is need for judgement, tact, patience, listening skills and control of emotions. Obtain the facts and take an impartial position. Most of the grievances will be solved.

Grievances can be of different types. If an employee feels injustice has been done to him or her, the employee feels aggrieved. Or it could be for monetary considerations. A person working as a helper observes that another person working in a similar capacity with similar qualification and experience is being paid Rs. 50/- more per month. The helper is aggrieved. Employees often see rewards (and salary) in a relative, rather than an absolute fashion. Often, it is not how much one gets but how much one is receiving compared to other people.

It could be that the persons are not in the same hospital but in two different institutions in the same town doing similar work. One is paid more than the other. What can happen? There is dissatisfaction and demand to be paid equally.

If a state of equity exists, the individual is usually comfortable with the situation.

Most often grievances arise from:
1. Misunderstanding,
2. Misinterpretation,
3. Discrimination, or
4. Violation of agreement.

Keep an open door policy. It should not be existent only in name but in actual practice as well. The employee with a grievance must feel free to come and discuss it without fear of repercussions.

Encourage group discussions. Let the staff come out with what they really think and feel. They should not feel inhibited.

Problem People

Every hospital has problem people. So you will have your share of problem people. They do not perform their job satisfactorily and hinder the objectives of the hospital.

Problem people may be (i) uncooperative (ii) poor in work performance, or (iii) those who break the rules and regulations or code of conduct very seriously and habitually.

Recognize such people and deal with them effectively. Dealing with problem people is not a simple affair. Try to understand why they behave in the manner they do.

Selvan is a laboratory technician. Even though he was not fully qualified, the administration promoted him to the senior post, because he was proficient in his work. Very soon thereafter, he began absenting himself often without leave and without informing, dislocating the work. He was rude to the co-workers and to the Chief of the Department. Warnings, censures, fines and loss of pay had no effect. The new Administrator was constantly asked by the Chief of the Department to dismiss the erring employee. The Administrator probed into the matter. The technician was skilful and competent in his work; when he was present he was productive and quality of work was good. It was found that the employee had become an alcoholic. Counselling and treatment were given. The employee became regular and behaved well.

Do not assign employees permanently to the problem category. Most often you can win them over. But a time may come when serious action has to be taken and the employee's services terminated. Such situations must be rare. When they do crop up, be firm.

Hospital K had a rule prohibiting private practice of any kind by its doctors. One Surgeon D broke the rule frequently by going to Nursing homes and operating there. The Administrator counselled him and then warned him. These had no effect. Disciplinary proceedings were taken and the doctor was discharged from service.

There are many factors which can affect the performance of employees and make them problem people. If the Administrator can identify these factors, it may be possible to resolve them and make the people co-operative and productive.

Knowledge and Skill

In order to perform well, it is necessary to be knowledgeable of the work expected of the employee. He must have also the skills to carry out the work efficiently. We may add that he must have also proper attitude. Only if he has the knowledge, skills and attitude appropriate to his work, will he be able to discharge his duties well.

Family

Many employees bring their family problems to work. It is difficult to disassociate the home and workplace. The adverse emotions affect the work. Enough attention will not be paid to work on hand; their interactions with fellow employees, superiors and subordinates are vitiated by their own worries and problems. The presence of a child with serious disabilities and handicaps can affect work, sometimes adversely and sometimes in a beneficial way. In the hospital situation, some of them exhibit much greater compassion, identifying themselves with the patients and their relations. Others resent and react in the opposite way.

Support from superiors

Superiors may not understand the needs of the employee. Support is not given but there is only fault finding. Sometimes incapable supervisors place the blame on the subordinates, who respond unfavourably and over a period of time, the subordinates become problem persons. Employee effectiveness is lost because there is no proper guidance or planning or organization. The employee becomes a victim of the situation.

Staff nurse Mary was posted to work in the children's ward. She loved children and liked the work but was being constantly found fault with by the Ward Sister. The performance appraisal was poor. After a few months, Mary began losing interest in her work. She was reprimanded and there was a recommendation to discharge her from service. At the meeting of the administrative committee, it was suggested that the Nursing Superintendent may transfer her to the Intensive Care Unit and try her for some more time. Mary did an excellent job under the new Ward Sister who was capable and kind. When the Ward Sister went away, Mary was promoted to that position.

Adaptability

Some employees cannot cope up with the changes in function. When new automatic equipment is introduced in the clinical laboratory, the existing staff may not adapt themselves to the new equipment. They can become problem people.

Sangeeta was a capable senior technician. The hospital bought an automatic chemistry analyzer. She did not want to be trained on the new machine, as she had difficulty in comprehending principles (though the actual working of the equipment was simple). She became moody and irritable. The situation became intolerable and she left the hospital.

Social values

Most of the work in patient care require a well developed sense of compassion. This is especially so in the hospitals in the voluntary, non-profit sector. People who tend to be aggressive by nature may find conflicts in the situation. Good performance may be affected, not because of lack of ability or interest but because of conflict of values.

Emotional make-up of the person can also affect the work, if it is not in harmony with the demands of the situation.

Health

Employees must be healthy—physically and mentally. Chronic illness will tell upon the performance. In course of time, they may become problem people.

Girija, a 44 year old supervisory nurse, had been a model nurse previously. But later, her work became poor. She was grumbling and quarrelling with the staff nurses and other employees. She was feeling tired and fatigued all the time. A medical check-up revealed that she had developed diabetes mellitus and hypertension. She improved remarkably in her performance with the institution of proper therapy and the problem disappeared.

Workplace

Some people are highly sensitive to the environment and climate. They can become poor performers, simply because their situation is not favourable.

Das was an upper division clerk in the District Health Office in Mangalore. He got a transfer (at his request for the education of his son) to a hospital in Bangalore. He was good in his work to begin with but gradually his performance became unsatisfactory. Other employees thought that he had used undue influence to get the transfer. They were hostile. He did not want to go to the hospital. Absenteeism increased. A friend advised him to consult a psychologist. With counselling, Das adjusted himself to the new environment and the problem became less.

Poor facilities for work and other substandard aspects of the environment can affect performance and turn an otherwise good worker into a problem person.

When dealing with problem people,
1. Control your emotions. Though not easy under many situations, it can be cultivated. Good behaviour begets good behaviour. Remember all can improve. Give opportunities to change for the better. Be genuine in what you say. Do not pretend to be too nice or too considerate.
2. Give importance to the individual's feelings. Understand his/her emotional needs.
3. Learn the other side of the story. Very often, there are many sides to the story. Try to understand the whole story.
4. Apply rules uniformly and consistently. They should not be arbitrary and discriminatory. They must be applied uniformly throughout the hospital.

Late coming was condoned in some departments but strict action was taken in other departments. The employees who were subjected to strict discipline felt that injustice was done to them, even though action taken was according to the rules.

Retraining

Why should we Retrain Personnel?

1. Personnel may be considered for higher and better positions. These require greater skills, knowledge, and competence to cope with the requirements of the higher positions.
2. The knowledge, skills and attitudes of personnel tend to decline with flux of time.
3. Personnel have to be retrained when they are shifted from one job to another.
4. Newer technology is coming up all the time. Persons who were trained on older technologies, find it difficult to cope up with the newer, more sophisticated ones, unless they are trained again on the newer technology.

It is important that the objectives of the retraining are made clear to the trainee. What is he/she expected to accomplish? The objective must be within the ability of the trainee. Feedback must be given at appropriate intervals. The objective must be challenging. Set a standard. The trainee can measure his performance against the standard.

Factors Affecting Retraining

Many factors affect retraining. Among them are:
1. Age: the younger person accepts change more easily.
2. Maturity: It does not refer to age but to his/her:
   - Capacity to set high but attainable learning goals;
   - Willingness and ability to take responsibility for learning; and
   - Previous educational levels and experiences.

The mature trainee will respond better to a more participative challenging and collaborative relationship.

Progress

Learning new skills may not make uniform, steady progress. Some make rapid progress followed by relatively minor improvements. This is the "learning plateau". Not much obvious progress is made during this phase. Learning plateau might discourage both trainees and trainers. If it is understood that this is a fairly normal experience, the participants will not be discouraged. Reassurance is necessary. Appropriate action should then be taken to ensure further progress.

Some Hints

   i. Make retraining situations as similar as possible to the work situation in terms of physical or psychological conditions.
  ii. Give trainees plenty of opportunities for practice and rehearsal of new skills.
 iii. Expose the trainees to a variety of situations where they can tackle the problems.
  iv. Ensure that the trainees become aware of the features of the work conditions.
   v. Show the value of the retraining to the work situation.

All retraining programs should follow the motto of "learning by doing" and "learning while doing".

Personnel Officer / Manager

All medium-sized and larger hospitals should have a qualified and experienced Personnel officer/Manager to co-ordinate the needs and interests of the hospital with those of the employees to provide efficient and economical health care service.

Responsibilities

1. Plans a comprehensive personnel program, within the overall personnel policy of the hospital and administers it, after approval by the Administrator.
2. Advises the administration on personnel problems.
3. Proposes changes in personnel policies, as necessary.
4. Develops procedures for recruitment of new employees and helps in their recruitment.
5. Interprets the philosophy, policies and rules and regulations of the hospital to the employees (especially the newly recruited personnel) and helps in their orientation.
6. Prepares manuals for personnel and job descriptions for approval by the administration.
7. Plans and conducts in-service training programs and advises on outside programs.
8. Promotes employee stabilization.
9. Informs employees of the activities of the hospital.
10. Develops procedures for job performance appraisals and sees to it that the appraisals are carried out regularly by all supervisory staff.
11. Supervises the work in the personnel department and ensures the proper maintenance of personnel files and records.
12. Sends periodical reviews to the Hospital Administrator.
13. Acts as a liaison between employees and administration
14. Attends to employee's grievances.
15. All other activities approved by the Administrator, as are conducive for better employer-employee relations in the hospital.

CHAPTER 27

Performance Appraisal System

The Hospital Administrator has to have information regarding the performance of all the personnel working in the hospital. Except for the few top administrative officers (managers), the administrator will not have direct information of those working in a medium-sized or large hospital. There is need for a system of performance appraisal.

DEFINITION

Performance Appraisal is the evaluation of work done (quantity, quality and the manner it is carried out) during a specified period against the background of the total work situation. Formal appraisal attempts at placing on record certain personality and behavioural characteristics of the individual, effectiveness at the job and contribution to the achievement of organizational goals.

OBJECTIVES OF APPRAISAL

Administrative

(Information needed by the organization for administrative purposes)
- To provide data for management decisions concerning merit, salary, increments, incentives, rewards, promotion, transfer, demotion or discharge from service;
- To weed out low performers;
- To consider the employee's suitability for different types of assignments;
- To have on hand information required for purposes like letters of recommendation, domestic enquiry, avoidance of arbitrary on-the-spot decisions, re-employment;

- To create a desirable culture and traditions in the department;
- To meet the requirements for manpower planning and Organizational Development, like identification of employees with promotion potential and their development needs – what is expected of them, what strengths they can build on and what specific weaknesses they need to overcome.

Performance Improvement

(Information specific to employees and appraisers for self-improvement and for achieving individual and organizational goals)

Employee's Objectives

- Employee gets a feedback of his or her performance which motivates him or her to perform better. It tells a subordinate how he or she is doing, brings about awareness of the strengths and weaknesses and suggests needed changes in attitude, skills or knowledge of the job;
- Employee develops role clarity with regard to the job, especially when told what is expected of him or her;
- Employee is able to clarify his or her career plan in the organization.

Appraiser's Objectives

- Superior gets feedback on how well the institutional objectives have been communicated to the subordinates, facilities provided for their effective performance and ability to motivate them to perform;
- Review of the work situation with the employee and identification of the latter's resource requirements, and helps the appraiser in defining his or her own and department's contribution to institutional objectives.

TECHNOLOGY OF APPRAISAL

The Appraiser

"Who knows best about an individual's performance" is an important issue in appraisal. Equally important is the question whether the person who knows best about the individual's performance is the best person to record this performance in the light of the organization's objectives.

Superiors as Appraisers

The conventional approach is to have the immediate supervisor of the individual to evaluate the individual. The ratings of this immediate superior, the 'Reporting Officer', may additionally be scrutinized and modified by this superior's superior, designated the 'Reviewing Officer', in the appraisal process. There are several advantages in having the immediate supervisor rate his subordinates:
- It maintains the line of authority necessary for effective functioning of the organization;
- The superior is likely to be the best person to assess the contribution of his immediate subordinates towards achievement of his department's and the organization's objectives;
- He is able to review the output of his employees in the light of the resources provided;
- He is able to compare the performance of an individual with that of his peers, a factor important for personnel decisions and for effective organizational functioning.

Having the immediate superior rate his subordinate, however, has the following drawbacks:
- Negative appraisals often result in misunderstandings, strained work relationships, demotivation of employee, decreased productivity. Supervisors normally dislike criticising a subordinate (and perhaps having to argue about it with him).
- Appraisal interferes with the more constructive coaching relationship that ought to exist between superior and subordinate as, during appraisal, the superior's position is emphasized as an authoritarian figure.

In addition to the reporting officer a reviewing officer is often necessary so as to ensure:
- Guidance to appraisers regarding interpretation of criteria;
- Uniform standards of rating among a group of reporting officers;
- Moderation of the immediate supervisor's haloes, biases, etc;
- A second-level concurring review, that maybe required for legal purposes and also to provide a mechanism for appeal.

Hospital Administration

Self Appraisal

Appraisal of one's own job performance is advocated because:
- Each individual knows himself best, and he is aware of his strengths and weaknesses and of his efforts to achieve his personal and his organization's goals;
- Self appraisal is an important factor in Participative Management and in the achievement of individual and organizational goals. However, self appraisals are not widely used, the reasons being
- Individuals do not wish to reveal their weaknesses and shortcomings on the job, more so as this information may be used against them when administrative decisions are taken.
- In general, self-appraisals are 'inflated' as most employees have an unrealistically favourable perception of their own performance.

Other Types of Appraisers

Appraisal of performance on the job is most frequently carried out by the superior and less frequently by the individual himself. It is possible to have the individual's peers or subordinates to rate him but very seldom done in a hospital situation. In organizations which primarily render service, the consumers or beneficiaries of the service may be primary appraisers.

General Appraiser Problem

Whether the appraiser be a superior, subordinate or peer, the following general problems are evident to a greater or lesser degree in every appraisal:

- *Bias* Opportunity bias (Some employees have better working conditions, supportive supervisors, more experienced co-workers); group characteristic bias (Group cohesiveness, morale, group interpretation of a fair day's work); predictor bias (Appraiser's knowledge of the past record of an individual); individual prejudices (regarding age, sex, religion, behaviour, etc.) all do affect the evaluations.
- *Equivalence* A major aim of appraisal is to compare the performance of an individual with that of his peers. These assumptions entail that all individuals being compared were subject to similar

work environments, to similar inhibitory and facilitatory factors – assumptions that are rarely true. Consequently employees subject to less competition or to lenient appraisers receive higher appraisals than equally competent or superior associates.

- *Pressure* from power groups, unions and superiors to rate the subject favourably.

Formats for Appraisal

Several techniques exist for appraisal of employees in an organization. Each has its own combination of strengths and weaknesses. No one technique by itself is able to achieve all the purposes for which management institutes the appraisal program. The choice of a particular technology depends on three major factors:

- *Utilization Criteria* Why is performance evaluation being done? The objective may be for disciplinary action, feedback for employee development, promotion, selection or training.

- *Qualitative Criteria* Consideration of organizational constraints – assumptions of the method, relevance of evaluation criteria, data availability, practicality, potential for equivalence and interpretability.

- *Quantitative Criteria* Psychometric properties of the evaluation – reliability, discriminability, accuracy, inherent rating errors.

A technique which is potentially less subjective and more objective than another is to be preferred. 'Objectivity' is the ability of the format to bring out impartial, reliable and valid information about the individual.

There are many formats available.

Free Written Ratings

Appraisers write short essays on each employee detailing the latter's strengths, weaknesses, potentials etc. The format may not be structured. The appraiser then has the choice to determine what aspects of the employee he will elaborate on. In the structured open-ended format, the superior is requested to write short notes on each of the specified criteria. This latter type ensures a more comprehensive picture of the employee. Essay ratings can be an effective means of performance evaluation as they can be 'tailor-made' to suit the individual and the particular work situation. In fact, even where scale formats are used, space is often provided for 'comments', 'remarks' or 'overall impression' to invite information on the individual that cannot otherwise be recorded through the scale.

Though this evaluation procedure is extensively used, it is important to note its major shortcomings:
- The writing skills of the reporting officer can mask the true performance of the individual;
- The method is time-consuming;
- Since the evaluations are in a descriptive form, they lack uniformity and hence comparison between individuals cannot be easily made.

Forced Distribution Technique

This technique is essentially a group-order making where the appraiser assigns each employee to one of the five groups in such a manner as to force a somewhat normal distribution, i.e., the supervisor allocates approximately 10 percent of his men to the best end of the scale, 20 percent in the next category, 40 percent in the middle bracket, 20percent in the region next to the low end and 10 percent in the lowest level.

The main advantage of this technique is that all employees cannot be given average or good ratings, some must be rated better than others. Though it is the best format when a supervisor has to evaluate a large number of subordinates, the scale is not frequently used.
- It is 'too gross' and does not discriminate between individuals in a group.
- Problems occur with 'borderline' cases.
- The scale does not explain the reasons for a certain performance gradation and the employee does not know what specifically he must do to improve his performance.

The Ranking Methods

Ranking aims at establishing a rank-order of employees based on their relative merit. In the method of Alternation Ranking the names of employees are listed in random order. The supervisor is asked to choose the 'most valuable' employee, cross his name off, and note it at the top of a list. He next selects the 'least valuable' employee, crosses him off and notes the name at the bottom of the list. The supervisor continues this procedure on the remaining list of employees till all the rates have been ranked. *Paired Comparison Ranking* entails that each employee is compared with each other employee. This method is much simpler than Alternation Ranking, requiring the appraiser to judge which of the two workers being compared is superior. The appraiser puts a tick mark on each slip against the individual whom he considers the better of the two, and the final ranking is determined by the number of tally marks against each name.

Ranking methods have the following drawbacks:

It is too cumbersome to rank individuals when their number is 20 or more.

Comparisons involve an overall subjective judgement.

It is difficult to rank employees apart from and between the top and bottom extremes.

Ranking methods however have a significant advantage in that they can be used even by untrained appraisers.

The Graphic Rating Scale

In the Graphic Rating Scale (also known as the Merit Rating Scale or the Method of Summated Ratings) an attempt is made to ascertain the degree of presence in the employee of certain characteristics. These characteristics – personality traits, knowledge, abilities, skills, quantity and quality of work turned out are listed with or without definitions or descriptions.

The responses, which can vary from three points to several points on a horizontal scale may be just enumerated numerically (e.g. 5,4,3,2,1) or the scale points may be defined to indicate the degree of applicability of the criterion as: 'excellent, good, average, poor, very poor' or 'always, often, sometimes, seldom, never'.

The Graphic Rating Scale is widely used.

It is easy and inexpensive to develop and administer;

It provides information about the employee on a number of characteristics and the degree of their applicability;

A composite score of each individual can be obtained. This enables study of an individual's performance over time as also comparison of the performance of two or more individuals at varying points of time.

The Graphic Rating Scale has however several pitfalls:
- Composite scores are deceptive. An identical total score may be obtained by two employees having significantly different specific traits.
- The Graphic Rating Scale is invariably associated with a great deal of subjectivity because personality traits are generally focussed upon.
- The Graphic Rating Scale is subject to a number of errors: Halo, Leniency, Central Tendency, Logical, Contrast, Similar-to-me and Proximity.

The Critical Incident Method

The Critical Incident approach to performance appraisal requires the appraiser to record factual incidents involving the employee which have been critical to the latter's effective or non-effective performance. The usual procedure is to have the supervisor record (in a 'little black book') actual incidents of positive or negative 'critical job behaviours' concerning the subordinate as and when they occur and to transcribe these on to the subordinate's appraisal form when required. A modification of the above method entails preparation of an extensive checklist (about 80-150 behavioural incidents) of behaviours critical to the job, the supervisor having to review the same and recollect particular behaviours observed in the employee during the relevant period.

Advantages

- Evaluation of the individual is less subjective as the supervisor is forced to focus on behaviours specific to the job rather than on vaguely defined traits.
- Appraisal interviews and counselling become easier when factual incidents can be cited to the employee.
- This technique is effective when objective work standards or quantitative goals are not available.

Drawbacks

- The idea of the 'man with the little black book' hovering in the background and taking notes on conduct is hardly consistent with a mature attitude.

- This method requires that supervisors jot down incidents on a daily or at least a weekly basis. This can become a chore.
- Appraisers are often seen to differ in their understanding of what behaviours are critical and hence have to be reported. This is partly overcome by having the behavioural checklist.
- Critical or outstanding incidents happen relatively infrequently. This may result in the supervisor not having enough critical incidents to report for a large number of employees.
- The technique tends to push the observer-recorder towards picking up things to criticise.

Forced Choice Rating Method (Mixed Standard Scale)

This is essentially a scale containing a number of statements. The appraiser is required to indicate those statements which best fit the employee and those which least describe the individual. The appraiser does not know which statements are indicative of high performance and which represent low and undesired behaviours or traits. Each statement carries a weight or score, but these scores are not revealed to the appraiser. After the evaluator completes the ratings, the personnel department arrives at an index of performance of the employee using the scoring key.

Advantages

- Performance evaluation is made more objective;
- The scale reduces halo effect and leniency error and improves reliability of ratings;
- The scale can be used for self-appraisals.

Drawbacks

- The construction of the scale takes a great deal of time and effort;
- The rating procedure tends to irritate appraisers who feel that they are not being trusted;
- A clever appraiser knows how to beat the system;
- The method is not useful for appraisal interviews.

The Behaviourally Anchored Rating Scale

First developed by Smith and Kendall for staff nurses in 1963, the BARS assumes the following:

- A person's effectiveness on the job can be best inferred from the behaviour on the job rather than on personality traits. Evaluation of behaviours is more objective than judging personality traits;
- The employee's performance is complex and results from several dimensions. The amount or degree of each dimension can be effectively recorded through statements rather than by mere numerical gradation; and
- During the evaluation process, BARS forces appraisers to focus on an employee's actual behaviour. The instrument is less subjective and shows higher validity and reliability and less halo effect.

Limitations

- The process of BARS construction is time consuming.
- With a situation of high turnover amongst appraisers, the new appraisers no longer feel they have been involved in BARS construction.
- BARS developed for one situation cannot be easily used in another situation as the job requirements may be different in another situation.

Appraisal by Objectives

In this appraisal format the employee and his superior review the achievement of the former's objectives which had been previously set up and agreed upon. The focus is on analysis of actual performance rather than on appraisal of traits or behaviours. It concentrates on what an employee does rather than what his superior thinks of him.

Appraisal by Objectives involves the following process

- The top management should formulate the goals for a definite period;
- Departmental heads next translate the organization's objectives into specific departmental objectives and lay down priority in terms of key-result areas;
- Staff of a department review the key-result areas and evolve a Results Involvement-Matrix showing the major contribution, minor contribution or advisory involvement of the person;
- Each individual then lists out specific time-bound action plans to achieve the key task. The supervisor coordinates this process;

- At the end of a specified period (six months to one year) the individual and his superior meet again to review the former's performance in the light of objectives set up earlier.

Appraisal by Objectives has much to recommend:
- The focus is on analysis of performance and not on a judgement of personality or of behaviour;
- The subordinate is no longer a 'passive' object being evaluated. He is an active agent responsible for his own career, growth and development and striving to achieve individual and organizational goals;
- The employee develops clarity regarding his work and the contribution required from him. He is involved in decision making, thus contributing towards increase work motivation.
- The method is suited for application at managerial levels and has limited applicability for lower categories of employees;
- It is possible only with the participative style of management and is not favourable in an authoritarian type of organization;
- The method is not favourable if the data generated from appraisals are to be used primarily for administrative and control purposes.

The Appraisal Interview

The appraisal interview is held periodically, between the superior (appraisor) and subordinate (appraisee). The latter is given a feedback on how his work performance during the period under review has been perceived by the superior. Depending on the nature of the interview, the discussion may include reactions the subordinate may have to the appraisal, analysis of the factors facilitating or inhibiting his performance, additional resources that may be required by the subordinate for effective performance, setting up of specific performance objectives for the future, discussion of the individual's career in the organization, identification of his training needs, superior-subordinate interaction, etc. The appraisal interview, though desirable, is not an essential part of the appraisal process.

Appraisal interviews may follow:
- The tell and sell method, where the supervisor informs the subordinate in the best manner possible of his ratings and advises him on how to improve;

- The tell and listen method, where the appraiser communicates his evaluation to the employee and allows the subordinate to react to the appraisal; and
- The problem solving approach, the focus being on 'analysis' rather than on 'appraisal' and what needs to be done to improve performance.

Objectives of Performance Appraisal Interviews

- Providing legitimate feedback to the individual on how his performance is perceived by his superior;
- Information communicated through such interviews may be a source of satisfaction and motivation to the employee, especially if feedback is positive;
- The employee can, at such a discussion, achieve role clarity with regard to his job;
- The subordinate, while coming to know of his weaknesses, can focus on corrective action. The superior can also plan training programs, continuing education, etc;
- The employee obtains greater knowledge of the organization, his superior's expectations, clarifications of his career plan in the organization, etc.

However, appraisal interviews are not often held because:

- The discussion of rating with employee often results in traumatic experiences for the subordinate and in superior-subordinate conflicts which affect the work situation;
- Negative ratings can result in demotivation and decreased performance, especially when the individual considers himself better than the superior's assessment of him;
- Appraisal is often associated with salary decisions, promotions, transfer, dismissals, etc. The employee is, thus, defensive during appraisal discussions when negative appraisals are likely to have an untoward effect on him;
- The superior feels inadequate about justifying the rating to his subordinate by citing relevant critical incidents;
- Many supervisors shun progress interviews as they fear opening a situation which they will not be able to cope with such as if the employee asked for a raise, he questions the manner of running the department, etc.

It is important to ensure that appraisal interviews do not cause ill-will. This can be ensured by having the supervisor ask himself at every stage, 'Will what I am about to say, help this man'? Appraisal interviews are effective if the employee participates actively in the discussion, is involved in setting specific performance goals for himself, and if the interview is designed primarily to improve an employee's performance rather than be connected to his salary or promotion.

Periodicity of Appraisal

Performance appraisal is most often conducted as an annual activity, though for trainees and new recruits, quarterly frequency is usually the norm. Thus employees may be rated at the same time during the year or on the anniversary date of employment of the respective individual.

CONFLICTS IN APPRAISAL

General Problems

Choice of Appraisal Objectives

Most appraisals attempt at gathering information for administrative purposes and also for self improvement and growth of the individual. Simultaneous attainment of both these objectives is not practicable as the moment data are required for control purposes, critical information pertaining to weaknesses of the person is not revealed in the appraisal process. The organization should therefore be clear about what objectives are to be achieved through the appraisal processes.

Focus on Traits versus Behaviours

Assessment of personality traits in preference to work behaviours is associated with grave implications, in that the ratings are not reliable, they tend to focus on an individual's personality rather than on his contribution to the organization, and the interpretation of traits varies markedly with people and therefore tends to be subjective.

Multiple Criteria Scores versus a Composite Score

Composite scores are often required when comparing the performance of several individuals for selection, placement, promotion, incentives, etc. However, they have the drawback that the facts of performance are not brought out through composite scores and further such composite scores are not useful for feedback and for analysis of the individual's performance.

CONCLUSION

Despite the numerous problems associated with appraisal, most organizations continue to have the formal appraisal program. It is hence clear that the alternative to a bad appraisal program need not be no appraisal program at all, but it can and ought to be a better appraisal program.

A sound appraisal program must satisfy the following basic requirements:
- The system must be consistent with the management style and philosophy, work technology and socio-cultural characteristics of the individuals concerned.
- It should be in tune with other personnel programs, such as the system of rewards, compensation schemes, training programs, etc.
- The technology in use should have the cooperation of the appraisers. It should have the ability to assess, in as objective manner as possible, the performance and effectiveness of an individual as related to his job.

Section 9: Materials Management

CHAPTER 28

Materials Management

...Expenditure on materials approximates 30-35 percent of the annual operating budget of most hospitals. Consequently, set on a task of cost containment, a Hospital Administrator's attention is drawn first to reduction of material costs... Efforts in this direction usually bring quick results, as all that is required is application of certain basic concepts, which are generally well accepted, because they also promote efficiency. Thus the importance of materials management in hospitals...

OBJECTIVES OF MATERIALS MANAGEMENT

The purpose of materials management is to bring about control over the acquisition, storage, retrievability, distribution, use and disposal of supplies and equipment in order to carry out the primary responsibilities of the organization in an efficient, effective and economical manner. Materials management seeks to ensure availability of the right materials, at the right time, to the right place, at the least cost.

THE MATERIALS MANAGEMENT ORGANIZATION

Materials management entails two basic functions: purchasing and storage/supply. These two functions may be carried out independently through separate stores and purchase departments, or they may be integrated into a single stores-purchase department.

Separate departments for purchase and for stores minimise the possibility of collusion, achieve formalization of data necessary for making effective purchases, and promote specialization (hence greater efficiency) of each of the two functions, which intrinsically are different in nature.

An integrated stores-purchase department however has the following advantages:
- A single authority can be held responsible for the availability, control and supply of materials. There is thus less scope for shifting blame from one department to another when lapses take place. Better co-ordination between the purchasing and storage promotes timely purchases *(resulting in reduction of inventory level)*, better knowledge about materials required in terms of their quality, annual quantity, variation in demand, use and standardization *(resulting in better purchases, lower safety stock and reorder levels)*. Further, unutilized materials (dead stock) can also be disposed off more easily. Besides, a single authority can handle queries from users and others more effectively.
- With an integrated department, there is less paper work as common records can be maintained *(e.g.: stock control cards can also serve for purchase history, purchase and receipt registers can be combined, etc.)* and there will be a reduction in internal correspondence between the stores and purchase staff.
- The speed of transactions can be expedited as common information can be shared easily and informally between purchase and stores personnel. This will result in decreased procurement/lead time.

THE PROCESS OF MATERIALS MANAGEMENT

The process of materials management involves planning, review and control of:
- Budgeting and materials planning
- Demand forecasting
- Procurement
- Receipt, inspection and payment
- Storage
- Inventory control
- Issue and distribution
- Usage

- Maintenance
- Disposal
- Pilferage.

Budgeting and Materials Planning

Based on data on past levels of performance and on anticipated activity/plans, capital equipment, consumables and supplies to be procured during the year ahead can be projected department-wise. Such a listing of materials in terms of units required and their cost estimates would constitute the *materials budget*, which should be prepared annually. Once this is done, it is possible at periodic intervals to carry out budget appraisal and determine the variance between the actual expenditure and the budget. Variances may result from differences in unit cost of materials and/or deviations in their usage. The former is the responsibility of the materials manager and the latter is the users'. Intensive monitoring and cost-reduction reports become necessary where actual costs grossly exceed budgeted costs.

Important in budgetary control and reduction of material costs is the concept of *standardization*. This involves grouping together similar items depending on their specifications or use so as to choose one (or a few) of those more universally acceptable for the purpose. It does not imply just cutting down on the number of sizes *(which is generally termed as 'simplification')*, but adoption of standards leading to specification of quality, reduction in sizes and varieties, facilitating interchangeability of components, etc. Standardization ensures greater relative use of the standard item in relation to similar items available in the market, non-duplication of inventories, lower purchase costs and more efficient use of materials. In a hospital, standardization is possible through preference of ISO/BIS approved items, limitation in the brands of a drug to be stocked (based on generic name, potency, company reputation, user acceptability and cost), choice of equipment and furniture built with standard and easily available components, etc. The responsibility for standardization rests not only with the stores-purchase department but also with the user departments and the management.

Related to standardization is the concept of *value analysis*. This attempts to examine all facets of the function and cost of a product/item in use in order to determine whether the cost can be reduced

or altogether eliminated, while retaining all the features of performance and/or quality of the product/item. It entails studying each item/component in use with a view to introducing lower-priced and more durable substitutes of equivalent quality, which fulfil the same objective. Value analysis attempts at addressing the following issues:
- What is the item/component?
- What is it intended to do?
- What does it cost?
- What else can do the same job?
- What does the suggested alternative cost?

Value engineering, though often used interchangeably with value analysis, specifically refers to what the user/engineering department is doing to develop a cheaper alternative.

So that standard items only are indented and also to ensure that items purchased are fully in conformity with the requisitioner's need, it is necessary for the hospital to make available to user departments a manual detailing the name, code number, description, specifications, unit and pack size of each item in regular use. For the Pharmacy this is in the nature of an approved *formulary* for the hospital, while for the Stores a *manual of indents* may be prepared.

Demand Forecasting

The greater the crisis situation and exigency for an item and the smaller the quantity required, the greater will be the procurement price and the incidental costs of purchase. It is therefore necessary to anticipate the need for the item ensuring that bulk purchases can be effected with maximum price discounts. Anticipation of future need is done through demand forecasting, which involves application of statistical techniques to predict future requirements based on past consumption patterns.

Several techniques of forecasting exist: trend line, semi-average method, moving average method, least-square method, weighting through exponential smoothing, application of trend and seasonality indices, etc.

The *moving average method* is the one used most widely. It involves summating past consumption values for a defined period of time, dividing this sum by the number of values used so as to obtain a forecast of the next period, dropping the first actual value and adding the next in the series and dividing the new sum by the number of values used so as to obtain a forecast for the second next period, and so on. A moving average, which uses a large time span, effectively neutralises the sudden temporary surges in demand and also decreases the standard deviation of the error. However, the greater the time span, the greater will be the time lag resulting in a greater error of forecasts. Hospitals typically find it convenient to work with a one year moving average.

Procurement

An effective purchasing system aims at procurement of items of acceptable quality, in appropriate quantities, at the minimum price, and within the available time.

It is not advisable for large purchases to be made by the individual departments of the hospital (decentralized purchasing). *Centralized purchasing* (by the General Stores-Purchase, Pharmacy, and Dietary departments) has certain advantages:
- Quantity discounts are possible through standardization and bulk orders.
- Purchasing costs are decreased because of consolidation and non-duplication of orders.
- Lower inventory costs result because centralization makes possible a lower safety stock.
- There is better management control as all aspects of purchase can be screened by the administration.

A group of hospitals having common interest *(e.g. run by the same management, located in the same region, etc.)* may also get together and effect bulk purchases jointly. Such *group purchasing* has advantages similar to centralized purchasing, though on a much larger scale. Group purchasing also brings hospitals together and results in sharing of price and product information. With group purchases however, forecasts must be planned well in advance, it is difficult to accommodate discrete brand and supplier preferences by individual hospitals, and hospitals forming part of the group must enjoy a good deal of trust as suppliers do tend to create dissonance amongst the members.

Beyond one-time orders, hospitals may also enter into purchase contracts with firms on a one to two year basis to ensure supply of items at fixed/predetermined prices. In *committed volume or running contracts*, the buyer commits on a fixed volume of supplies and a fixed unit price irrespective of the delivery schedule that may involve 1-12 lots spread out during the year. In *rate contracts*, the vendor offers a fixed price for a defined period, though actual quantity to be supplied must be ordered as and when required.

A hospital may wish to acquire certain expensive equipment but may not have the funds immediately available for the purpose. Such equipment, however, can still be acquired through *deferred payment* schemes or through leasing. Deferred payment involves a commitment on the part of the hospital to pay a portion of the costs immediately, the balance amount being payable over a defined period of time (perhaps even through an enhanced fee for consumables). Since the supplier must set aside funds to finance such a venture, the interest and other overhead costs so incurred are included in the price of the equipment. *Leasing* enables a hospital to make use of an equipment without actually owning it, though rent is payable by the lessee to the lessor as per the contractual terms. There are several types of leases: short term, long term, straight term, and lease purchase agreements.

Purchasing entails the following *steps:*
- Maintain a vendor list for each group of items and for unusual items. Each vendor should be known for his capabilities, reputation, etc.
- Forecast requirements and plan purchases. Beyond securing quantity discounts, proper planning will avoid stock-outs and high costs associated with emergency purchases.
- Draw up product specifications to ensure clarity, and to avoid mistakes and rejections because of wrong supplies. This expedites the procurement period and ensures that both the supplier and the receiver/user are not inconvenienced.
- Invite quotations. *'Open tenders'* ensure transparency and minimise buyer-vendor collusion.
- Prepare a comparison statement of offers based on basic price, freight and insurance charges, taxes and levies, quantity and payment discounts, payment terms, delivery period, guarantee, vendor reputation. Calculating the total value of each offer helps identifying hidden costs that are sometimes not so obvious. Further, the order value ensures reconsideration of order size and cash availability. (When dealing with out-station suppliers,

a local agent is preferable, particularly to expedite transactions and sort out disputes. Presence of a 'middle-man', however, increases the purchase cost. Further, agents are known to disown responsibility when things go wrong. Hence, even with a local agent, contact with the primary supplier should be maintained.)
- In evaluating offers for equipment, it is important to note that the basic equipment price can be quite misleading. One has also to consider the CIF value, installation costs, manpower-training costs, annual cost of consumables, spares, warranty and post-warranty service terms and cost, etc. over the 5-7 year life of the equipment. By adding all these costs, it is possible to calculate the *'life-cycle cost'* of various offers and make a more rational choice.
- Short-list offers. The final selection should preferably be by the purchase committee/authority, possibly after negotiating the price and terms of the first offer of choice. (As far as feasible, refuse advance payment, settlement through bank documents, VPP, etc. With such forms of payments, purchasers practically lose their right to reject incorrect supplies. Further, it is preferable to insist on delivery and inspection at the hospital premises even if there is an additional cost involved).
- Issue purchase orders taking care to list all requirements of the institution.
- Seek an order acknowledgement. Beyond ensuring receipt of the order, it binds the supplier to honour the terms of the order.
- Follow-up for early supply.
  A purchase order should attempt to incorporate as much of the below-cited particulars as may be relevant and justifiable. This will ensure that the order is clear to the supplier and to the receiver, and is legally valid in case of a dispute at a later stage:
    i. Order reference number and date;
    ii. Purchaser's name and address;
    iii. Consignee's name and date (especially when the purchaser is not the consignee);
    iv. Supplier's name and address;
    v. Quotation reference and date (where repeat order is placed, the previous order reference to be given);
    vi. Description of goods (specifications, brand name, catalogue number, features as per sample);
    vii. Quantity (units, pack size, weight, each/pair, quantity per pack);

viii. Price (unit price, quantity discount, payment discount, handling charges, sales tax, excise duty, surcharge);
ix. Freight and insurance charges (FOB/FOR/CIF, freight paid/to pay, insurance by supplier/buyer);
x. Packing (free/extra, special packing to be used, case markings);
xi. Shipping instructions (by air/rail/road/sea/post, name of port/railway station/post office);
xii. Delivery date (definite date to be specified; vague terms like ex-stock/immediate/urgent should not be used; for bulk orders specify quantity to be supplied at predefined intervals);
xiii. Order acknowledgement (ensures receipt of order, binds supplier legally);
xiv. General terms and conditions (specify if printed on reverse);
xv. Inspection (at hospital preferred instead of at supplier's site);
xvi. Invoicing instructions (number of invoice copies, purchase order copy to be attached, to whom to be submitted);
xvii. Mode of payment (through draft, cheque, VPP, cash);
xviii. Part supply (permissible or prohibited);
xix. Warranty (time period, what does warranty cover, replacement or just repair);
xx. Signature of authorized purchaser and designation.

The following purchase procedures additionally apply with regard to *import* of equipment, medical supplies and drugs from abroad:

- Obtain the product literature and proforma invoice listing the FOB and CIF price, mode of shipment, payment terms, etc.
- If not covered under Open General Licence, a specific import licence may be required.
- Import of drugs requires a test licence from the Drugs Controller of India. Certain drugs can be imported only through specified ports of entry as notified.
- Customs notifications are published annually and could be amended periodically, and so it is important to verify if the item is listed for duty free import. Customs duty exemption (free/rebate) is applicable to hospitals with respect to:
  —life saving drugs and equipment;
  —sight saving equipment;
  —specified medicines;

- equipment for Government and approved research institutions;
- gifts from abroad to charitable organizations for free distribution to the poor;
- aids for physically handicapped and blind;
- re-import of equipment after repairs.
* If the item or institution is not listed for duty free import, a NMI (not manufactured in India) certificate and a CDE (customs duty exemption) certificate may have to be sought. Else customs duty will be payable in accordance with the customs duty tariff.
* In the case of minor imports, the foreign supplier may seek an advance bank draft. For major imports, a letter of credit will be required.
* On receiving notification of arrival of the goods at the port of entry, prompt clearance is required to avoid demurrage.

Receipt, Inspection, Acceptance, Payment

Supplies should be received at a common Receiving Section of the Stores and should be kept aside till the receiving formalities are complete and goods cleared for issue. Receiving clerks should attempt to detect mistakes of the vendor, the supplier and/or the purchasing department. Once supplies pass this stage, the cost of remedying mistakes are much higher.

The procedure for receipt, inspection and acceptance of supplies includes the following:
* While taking delivery from the transporter/railway/customs, check container/s for deficiency and damage. If packing is damaged, insist on 'open delivery', checking quantity of packages, individual items, weights, etc. against packing slip. Any damage or loss should be registered immediately through a claims statement preferably through an insurance surveyor.
* On receipt at the hospital, check supplies for discrepancies in quantity, quality, product specification, etc. Record shortages, incorrect or damaged material, and out-dated supply and take action accordingly.
* All supplies should be inspected and certified by the receiving clerk/committee. In the case of technical items, the requisitioner/user should also certify. In the case of bulk supplies, random sampling may suffice. Samples of drugs should also be analyzed and certified by the Drugs Analytical Laboratory.

- The necessary documentation should be carried out: daybook of receipts, goods inward note, stock ledger, purchase register, bin card.
- Indentors of items purchased on specific request should be notified regarding arrival of materials.

On accepting the goods and certifying correctness, the bills should be forwarded for payment. However, before releasing payment, the Accounts Department should ensure that the bill bears proof of receipt of goods, certification of acceptance, and completion of purchase documentation. Early payment enables the hospital to avail of payment discount and establishes the credibility of the hospital for better terms from vendors.

Storage

The object of storage is to ensure that, till the time of issue for usage, the supplies are adequately preserved to prevent loss or damage.

The Stores Department should be conveniently located to facilitate easy receipt of materials from suppliers and easy despatch of supplies to the wards and departments. It should be of sufficient size to accommodate all the supplies and must provide for separate areas for receipt of materials till acceptance, storage, accumulation for issue, as well as office space for stores personnel. Special storage facilities include a fire-proof room for inflammable materials, air-conditioned rooms for materials and drugs sensitive to heat, cold rooms or refrigerators for items which deteriorate at room temperature, safe cabinets for narcotics, slotted angle racks, pallets and material handling equipment. The materials should be adequately protected from fire, pests, water seepage, etc.

Stores management entails adherence to the following 'common sense' principles and concepts:
- The Stores should be divided into homogenous sections and separate areas earmarked for different groups of items - tablets and capsules, syrups, injections and intravenous fluids, surgical disposables, dressings, minor hospital equipment, maintenance spares, stationery, furniture.
- Items in a group should be categorized based on their generic name or application, and similar items must be stored contiguously.
- The available floor and vertical space must be used as judiciously as possible while at the same time leaving sufficiently spacious aisles for material handling equipment.

- Heavy items should be kept as low and as near to the aisle as possible for easy retrieval. Bulky but light items may be placed on top shelves. Items frequently required must be as near the aisle/counter as possible for easy access.
- To minimise obsolescence, items due to expire earlier should be stored in front of batches due to expire later. The *first in first out* (FIFO) rule should be adhered to.

Each item stored in a permanent location should be given a location number for facilitating placement and retrieval of items. This location number should identify the room, rack, shelf and bin where the particular item is stored.

Each item should have a unique code-identifying number. The code numbers should be assigned in a systematic manner and should take into account the type of item, (pharmacological) group and sub-group, application, size, etc.

Every item should have a bin-card documenting the name of the item, description, code number, location number, stock control levels, as also transactions relating to receipts (invoice reference and date, supplier's name, quantity purchased, unit rate, total value), issues (indent reference and date, requisitioning department, quantity supplied, value) and stock balance (quantity and value). Such bin-cards are ideally computerized.

Beyond the main stores, each ward/department will have a sub-store. It is necessary to keep down this 'unofficial inventory' to the bare minimum to minimise inventory costs, obsolescence and pilferage. Thus maximum stock levels need to be fixed at department/ward levels taking into consideration the periodicity of issues and rate of consumption. Issues should be related to usage/replenishment and periodic physical checks should be carried out to prevent hoarding of materials in sub-stores.

Inventory Control

Inventory control principles seek to minimise investment on materials so that sufficient working capital is available for other more important activities of the organization. The primary purpose of inventory control is therefore to decrease material costs by preventing over-stocking of materials (which results in locking up of capital, possible pilferage and obsolescence) while at the same time minimising stock-out costs. In controlling inventory costs, the most crucial question to be asked is: "Is it more economical to maintain an item in inventory than to purchase it on demand?"

The following concepts are relevant in controlling inventory costs:

Periodic/Cyclic System

This system involves review of stock status at periodic/fixed intervals and placement of orders depending on the stock on hand and rate of consumption. The ordering interval is thus fixed, but the quantity to be ordered varies each time. The time interval (cycle/review time) to be chosen depends on the lead time for procurement, criticality, stock-out costs, degree of control required, etc. Where bulk orders are placed, as in committed volume (running) contracts, the time interval between scheduled deliveries is treated as the cycle time.

Two-bin System

This is a perpetual inventory system where, conceptually, the stock of each item is held in two bins, one larger bin containing sufficient stock to meet the demands during the interval between arrival of an order quantity and placing of the next order, and the other bin containing stocks large enough to satisfy probable demands during the period of replenishment. When the first bin is empty, an order for replenishment is placed, and the stock in the second bin is utilized until the ordered material is received. There is thus a maximum stock level, a predetermined point for placing an order, a minimum stock level by which time replenishments should arrive, and a zero (stock-out) level. In contrast to the cyclic system, in the two-bin system the order quantity is fixed, but the time for placing orders is not at predetermined periods during the year. Since the quantity to reorder is fixed in advance, initiation of replenishment action can be delegated to lower-level staff. The system is thus useful for low consumption value items where close monitoring and control is not required.

Lead-Time

This is the period required to obtain the supply once the need is determined. It is, therefore the average number of days between placing an indent and receiving the material. Lead-time is composed of two elements: *administrative* or *buyer's lead time* (i.e. time required for raising purchase requisitions, obtaining quotations, preparing

Materials Management 259

comparative schedules, raising purchase order, order to reach supplier, transit and clearing time when goods are sent from outstation, checking and inspection formalities when materials arrive, sending materials to the appropriate store); and *delivery* or *supplier's lead time* (i.e. time required for manufacture, packing and forwarding, shipment, delays in transit, etc.)

Lead-time is specific for each item and for each supplier and is dependent upon factors such as availability in the market, form of availability, location of the manufacturer/supplier, importation formalities, vendor response time, etc. Lead-time is important in determining the average inventory need - the longer the lead-time the higher the inventory level. Attempts should, therefore,be made to cut down the lead-time, especially for high consumption value items.

Minimum/Safety/Buffer Stock

This is the amount of stock that should be kept in reserve to avoid a stock-out in case consumption increases unexpectedly or in case the lead time turns out to be longer than normal. It is also the level at which fresh supply should normally arrive, failing which action should be taken on an emergency basis to expedite supply and replenish the stock.

Where data are maintained of the maximum demand at various points in time with frequency of such occurrences, it is possible to specify the quantum of risk to be protected against, depending on the criticality of the item, and then:

Safety stock (SS) = $(D_{max} - D_{avj}) \times L$
where: L is the lead-time in days
D_{max} is maximum demand on any day at the specified risk level
D_{avj} is average daily demand.

If this calculation is too tedious, a simple manner of determining the safety stock level is to estimate the time it normally takes to procure supplies on an emergency basis and multiply the same by the average daily demand.

Reorder Level: This is the predetermined stock level at which action should be taken to replenish the stock. It is equivalent to minimum stock plus requirements during lead time, and is calculated as follows:

Reorder level (ROL) = $(D_{avj} \times L)$ + SS

If this formula is also found too cumbersome, a simple manner of designating the reorder level is to specify 'n' months of supplies. Such an arbitrary fixation in fact takes into account the stock on hand, average consumption rate and time involved in procurement.

Maximum Stock

This is the predetermined limit beyond which the stock of an item should not be allowed to exceed in the normal course. It is equivalent to the minimum stock level plus the quantity of supplies received at any point of time.

Conceptually, maximum level is useful in minimising investment on materials. It is therefore, applied to materials whose value is comparatively high and where bulk orders are placed with staggered deliveries. Once the maximum stock level is fixed, it is possible, at periodic intervals (as in the periodic inventory system) to review the actual stock on hand and reschedule deliveries whenever the maximum level is about to be exceeded. Maximum level also helps in avoiding excess stock, which could lead to obsolescence, deterioration in storage and pilferage.

Economic Order Quantity (EOQ)

EOQ is the most economical quantity that should be ordered at any point of time. It seeks to strike a balance between the mutually conflicting ordering costs and inventory holding costs, and attempts to minimise both.

Ordering cost is the overhead cost associated with buying an item and includes those incidental costs involved in obtaining quotations, clerical work of making comparative statements, placing an order, follow-up, personnel costs, etc. The total of ordering cost per year divided by the number of orders gives the average cost per order. If 'R' is the annual requirement of an item, 'Q' the quantity of each order, and C_p the overhead costs per order, then the total annual ordering cost for that item is $R/Q \times C_p$. For a given annual requirement, the greater the quantity ordered at a time, the lesser will be the number of orders placed in a year, and lesser will be the ordering costs for that item.

Inventory carrying or holding cost is the cost incurred in connection with physical storage of inventory plus the opportunity cost of money locked up in inventory. It includes interest on investment, interest foregone because of unnecessary inventory, warehouse and personnel costs, obsolescence, insurance, pilferage, etc. Holding cost (C_H) is expressed as follows: unit purchase cost/ 100 x percentage rate. The total holding cost is equivalent to average inventory x C_H. If Q is the quantity ordered each time, then Q/2 is the average inventory. Total holding cost then is Q/2 x C_H. As can be seen from the formula, the greater the quantity ordered at a time, higher will be the holding cost.

Economic Order Quantity attempts to determine the optimum quantity that should be ordered such that both the ordering cost and holding cost are minimized.

Thus Minimum $Q° = \dfrac{R C_p}{Q} + \dfrac{Q C_H}{2}$

Hence $Q^2 = \dfrac{2 R C_p}{C_H}$ and EOQ is square root of it.

Fixation of order quantity through EOQ is, however, subject to availability of cash, storage space, variation in consumption pattern, likelihood of obsolescence, economic manufacturing quantity, lead time for delivery, government regulations, convenience possible through reduction of work, seasonal availability, etc. Further, modifications of this formula provide for quantity discounts. EOQ automatically ensures that items of high consumption value are ordered in smaller quantities at frequent intervals, thus minimising investment on materials.

ABC Analysis

This technique involves *analysing* all items in inventory on the *basis* of annual usage times *cost*. It is an aid to *always better control*. ABC analysis is one of the most effective tools in materials management. It helps in economising one's efforts to achieve greater results. Rather than 'wasting' one's time in trying to manage simultaneously all consumables in regular use, it helps in segregating those items which ought to be given priority to maximize results. Identification of such items is based not only on the unit cost of the item or on its relative quantity consumed, but on its annual consumption value, which is a combination of both.

ABC analysis tells us that 5-10 percent of all items (called 'A' category) account for 70 percent of the annual consumption costs, another 10-20 percent of the items (termed 'B' category) account for 20-30 percent of the costs, while the balance 70 percent of items ('C' category) account for about 5-10 percent of the costs. The usefulness of this management tool is that, by focussing on the 'A' category items, 70 percent results can be achieved with just 5 percent effort. And with attention to another 10-20 percent of items ('B' category), 90 percent control is achieved with 15 percent input.

Once 'A' category items are identified, it is possible to devote more attention to these items to minimise purchase costs and exercise control over consumption in a more effective manner. Other strategies in materials management such as purchase planning, forecasting, negotiating prices, minimising inventory carrying costs, minimising unofficial inventory, restricting usage, controlling wastage, managing closing stock, audit, etc. show greatest results when applied with emphasis on 'A' category items.

Similar categorization of items based on the closing stock value instead of annual consumption value is termed as XYZ analysis. Once 'X' items are identified, it is possible to further segregate the 'non-moving' items of the 'desirable' category and expedite their use, exchange or disposal to bring down the closing stock value.

VED Analysis: Items may also be classified as vital, essential or desirable based on their criticality, stock-out costs and inconvenience caused due to their absence. 'V' items require a large safety stock, whereas 'D' items can do with little or no reserve.

If the results of ABC and VED analyses are integrated into a matrix, the following groups of items can be identified for better monitoring and control by senior managers:

	V	E	D
A	1	1	1
B	1	2	2
C	1	2	3

1 = 17 percent of items
2 = 45 percent of items
3 = 38 percent of items

Group one items are the vital and/or 'A' category items which require to be monitored very closely for stock availability, overstocking and usage. Group two items require less intensive monitoring, while Group three items hardly require to be watched.

FSN Analysis

Items in stock may also be classified on the basis of their frequency of issue/consumption. Though relative and subjective in definition, fast moving items are those which are used at a rapid rate, slow moving items are used in lesser frequency, while non moving items may remain in stock for several months without being issued. These latter items should be identified and reviewed periodically to prevent date-expiry, obsolescence, damage in storage, etc.

Turnover of Inventory

This ratio is a quantitative measure of the number of times that the total inventory value is issued and replaced. The turnover rate is calculated by dividing the total money value of supplies issued during the period by the value of closing stock. A turnover rate of 12 is considered ideal, though 8-10 turns per year is more realistic. Turnover rate may be increased by eliminating surplus stock, reducing non-moving items, increasing turnover of 'A' items, reducing safety stock levels, and reducing the lead-time involved in stock replenishment.

Physical Inventory

A physical verification of inventory should be undertaken at least once a year to compare the actual stock on hand versus the number expected as per records. The variance may then be expressed in terms of money value. Other than the most urgent and vital items, regular issues should be suspended during stock checking, which should therefore take as little time as possible.

Physical inventory is the best means of evaluating the efficiency of stores personnel in material handling and record keeping. It also provides an opportunity for identification of damage, shrinkage, stock obsolescence, and pilferage. Verification of physical assets and the department stock of consumables should also be carried out at periodical intervals to prevent build up of unofficial inventory, control pilferage, and follow up on long standing repairs.

Issue/Distribution:

Items held in inventory by the stores may be issued through indents to user departments on a periodical basis (example, once a week/fortnight) or as and when necessary on a replacement basis. The latter is preferable for expensive drugs and consumables, especially if the costs are to be debited to patients.

Systems of stock replenishment to wards/departments are of the following modes:

Requisition or Drug-basket System

At defined intervals or as and when the departmental stock level gets low, a requisition, perhaps countersigned by a higher official, is submitted for replenishing the stock. The 'drug basket' involves sending an empty container/trolley with the requisition.

Par-level or Top-up System

The maximum stock level for each ward/department is predetermined on the basis of usage rate and frequency of replenishment. This departmental stock is stored in an assigned location. At periodic intervals, stores personnel visit the ward/department, carry out a physical inventory of what is available and arrange to replenish the stock to the predetermined maximum level.

Exchange-cart System

This is similar to the par-level system in that there are predetermined maximum stock levels and defined intervals for stock replenishment. The departmental stock however is stored in a cart/trolley and a similar / duplicate cart is kept by the Stores. At regular intervals, the full cart from the stores is taken to the user area and exchanged with the ward cart.

Whatever the system of stock replenishment, it is necessary that adequate controls be established for issue of consumables. Nursing supervisors, having intimate knowledge of departmental workload and supplies required, should monitor and regulate the supplies to be replenished by the stores. Special emphasis should be laid on control of 'A' category items. While sanctioning indents, nursing supervisors should also ensure that wards are not allowed to hoard supplies. Such unofficial inventory, beyond locking up capital, is more prone to obsolescence, damage and pilferage.

When issuing capital items such as equipment and furniture to the departments, wherever possible, the item code number should be painted or embossed on the article to facilitate easy identification. The Stores should also be held responsible for immediate documentation of items issued in the department's asset-register – something that is easily and effectively carried out through computerization of issues.

Usage

Inventory control techniques can bring about substantial savings in material costs, but these savings are relatively small when compared to the savings that can accrue through economical and efficient use of materials. Every effort must, therefore be made at all levels in the organization to utilise supplies in the most conscientious manner avoiding any form of wastage. Particular care should be taken to ensure that there is no over-preparation of items which have a limited shelf life. Monitoring of consumption, especially for 'A' category item, should be done through monthly 'supply-usage reports' which summarise department-wise consumption, both in stock-keeping units and money value. By relating these reports to workload and past consumption norms, it is possible to identify major variances and take needful action to restrict usage and/or purchase of higher quantities in advance.

Material costs can also be decreased by appropriate selection of materials (durables, reusable items), cheaper substitutes that meet the technical requirements and standardization of supplies.

Maintenance

Proper maintenance of equipment, furniture and fixtures not only ensures their almost continuous availability for use but also an extended life and productivity for the items, thus resulting in lower material costs.

Time and costs of maintenance can be reduced by consideration of the following factors during purchase of capital assets:

Durability

Since instruments, equipment and furniture in a hospital set-up are handled by multiple users and are subjected to varying forms of abuse and rough use, it is necessary to provide for an element of 'over-specification' so that the item is more sturdy than that available for single person use.

Periodical Disinfection

Equipment and furniture become contaminated during use and hence must be subjected to periodical cleaning and disinfection. The external surface of such items should therefore be washable and at times sterilizable.

Repairability

Care must be taken to select items which are easily repairable (e.g. steel versus wooden furniture). Decisions should be taken regarding future maintenance: planned preventive maintenance, in-house versus external maintenance, training on fault detection and trouble shooting, etc.

Spare Parts Availability

Standardization of items and opting for those easily available in the market ensures easy availability of spare parts. In the case of non-standard items and imports, it is necessary to procure certain critical spares and ensure their availability for the whole life of the equipment.

Operations and Service Manuals

It is essential to obtain the operating manual when sophisticated equipment is procured. This must be duplicated and made available to the users, the original being filed in the stores. It is also necessary to insist on the detailed service manual. This will ensure that repairs can be attended to by the hospital maintenance department without relying perpetually and solely on the supplier.

Service Contracts

Better terms for service are possible by negotiating service contracts for maintenance prior to purchase of the equipment. Such contracts should specify the minimum number of preventive overhaul schedules, unlimited breakdown calls, service charges for service with or without spares, bank guarantee and downtime payment to ensure better performance.

Materials Management 267

Standby units

Since hospital work must carry on even when the equipment is down, wherever possible, it is necessary to provide for replacements to tide over the period of repair.

Disposal/Condemnation

Indents are often improperly scrutinized and unofficial inventory builds up at the user area. Further, capital equipment, instruments and furniture are occasionally issued to departments in excess of their requirements. It is therefore necessary for nursing supervisors to periodically inspect the sub-stores attached to each ward and arrange for return of excess stock/equipment. The stores should provide for a 'stores-return' process for documenting receipt of such items.

The hospital should also have a *condemnation committee* to review used materials that are to be disposed off. At times it is possible to recycle or reuse materials or find some other use for the item. In the case of equipment, cannibalization may be possible. If no further use exists, there should be a procedure laid out for condemnation/disposal by incineration or sale as scrap.

Pilferage

Frauds involving buyer-vendor collusion are not uncommon in purchase transactions and can account for a significant percentage of avoidable material costs. For a commission or kickback, either in cash or kind, purchase personnel at times compromise the interests of the hospital. The vendor finances such payment by inflating the price, overstating the quantity, supplying substandard goods or through fraudulent payments. Such frauds can be prevented by intensive internal audit and by involving two or more departments or persons in purchase transactions. Safeguards should also be taken to ensure that bills are not paid unless all purchase transactions have been verified and goods properly certified by responsible persons.

Theft of materials is also not uncommon. Items may be pilfered by the shipper, receiver, stores personnel and/or users. Pilferage from the store shelves can be made good by 'short order filling' of requisitions as items are rarely physically counted when received by users. 'Unofficial inventory' which has accumulated in sub-stores of wards is very susceptible to theft. Maintenance personnel are also notorious for theft of hospital fittings. Control of hospital theft is possible only with intensive vigilance, though the ultimate solution is the honest hospital employee!

CONCLUSION

This chapter discusses the concepts of hospital materials management and material cost containment techniques. However, every hospital would like to evaluate the effectiveness of its materials management effort to ascertain how well it is doing in this regard.

Charles E. Housley, in his article, "Evaluating the Effectiveness of the Material Management Efforts" (Hospital Material Management Quarterly, August 1979) proposes four methods of carrying out such appraisal:

Supply-Performance Review

This appraisal reflects how well materials management is meeting the needs of the individual hospital departments in terms of availability of materials, quality of materials supplied and stock-outs. Specific performance standards need to be set up in advance. Review of actuals versus standards should be carried out at least once a year.

Supply-Price Comparison

Prices for the same product vary from hospital to hospital, from region to region and from dealer to dealer. Such price variation may occur because of greater volume of purchases by a hospital, distance of the hospital from the supplier, pricing policies of the manufacturer and dealer, negotiation skill of the purchaser, mode of supply, reputation of the hospital, promotional offers, etc. If a supply-price comparison is carried out across hospitals, it is possible to identify purchasers who have paid varying prices, thus reflecting their effectiveness in price control and cost containment.

Management Audit

The stores-purchase department can set up objectives for itself in terms of recommended materials management practices, plan of action and persons responsible for the action. These objectives may relate to material administration, purchasing, receiving, storage and issue of materials. Through the process of appraisal by objectives, it is possible to evaluate the performance of the department/staff.

The administration should also ensure that the hospital's interests are adequately safeguarded. This can be done by instituting a continuous internal audit system, the scope of which includes:
- Review of purchase documents including tenders, quotations, comparative statements, purchase decisions.
- Spot checks of card balances and actual stock in hand.
- Random checks of postings.
- Control over excess stock, date expired materials.
- Verification of balance quantity stated in indents versus that actually available at the stores and at the user areas.
- Comparative analysis of material costs in relation to patient visits, inpatient days, operative procedures, investigations carried out, etc. to detect inappropriate or excessive use of materials and wastage.
- Obtaining feedback from users and departments regarding quality and quantity of materials supplied, stock-outs, problems encountered, etc.

Material-cost-per-patient day Formula

The MCPPD formula involves dividing total material costs per day by total hospital patient cost per day and projecting a ratio of material costs to hospital costs. Such a formula compares uniformly across hospitals irrespective of size, location, age, etc. as the factors that increase material costs also increase patient per diem costs and vice versa. The MCPPD formula is probably the most objective and reliable method of evaluating the effectiveness of material management techniques.

A CASE STUDY FOR DISCUSSION
The Case

Mr. Bung, Administrator of Nice City Hospital, sent for the Purchase Superintendent, Mr. Bymore and instructed him to tender for a modern intercom system. Quotations were immediately invited telephonically for an intercom system suitable for a 300-bed hospital. Five of the eight firms contacted sent their offers; 4 other firms also heard of the hospital's interest, met the Medical Superintendent, and sent in their offers. Mr. Bymore prepared a comparative statement and forwarded the same to Mr. Bung suggesting that the lowest offer of Hira Associates be accepted. Mr. Lye, Accounts Officer, heard about the comparative statement and cautioned that only Rs. 1.9 lakhs, which had been budgeted for medical equipment, was remaining. Mr. Bung sent for the firm's representative and asked that the offer of Rs. 2.25 lakhs be reduced to Rs. 1.8 lakhs. Mr. Bung was invited to attend a series of discussions at the firm's office to witness how the system worked and to meet the local representatives. Finally the Managing Director of Hira Associates telephoned to say that the price would be reduced to Rs. 2 lakhs provided that 40 extensions instead of 50 were acceptable to the hospital. He also communicated that the firm had decided to donate a TV and VCR system since the hospital was a charitable institution, provided the order was despatched within one week along with a draft for 25 percent of the order value. Mr. Bung, on leave, telephonically advised Mr. Bymore to release the order and to negotiate the terms and conditions for maintenance of the system, which he would ratify on his return. Mr. Bymore placed the order for the communication system immediately as otherwise, in view of the year ending, the budget would expire. He further wrote to the Hospital Engineer to ascertain what terms should be insisted upon to ensure high performance and uninterrupted service of the system.

For Discussion

Were there any purchase irregularities in this transaction?

What steps should have been taken to ensure an effective purchase?

What terms and conditions should Mr. Bymore have insisted upon for supply and maintenance of the system?

Section 10: Finances

CHAPTER

29

Finances

INTRODUCTION

One of the biggest headaches for a hospital administrator is finance. Health services used to be labour intensive. Now it has become both capital and labour intensive. With escalating costs, the act of balancing income and expenditure had become difficult. The demand for expenses always seems to be far higher than the income generated. The professionals and the public demand newer costly tests and equipment. The real importance of finance is often not understood till there is a serious breakdown in the financial operation, just as the importance of health is not thought of till the person becomes ill.

Methods of Financing

These vary depending on the type of ownership. In Government hospitals, the income is derived almost wholly from taxes. The same is true for hospitals run by municipal or local bodies; grants are the main sources. Very little is received by way of patient charges. In the private sector, it is usually fee for service. The fees are relatively less in the non-profit, voluntary hospitals, whereas they tend to be high in the corporate and for-profit hospitals and nursing homes. There may be varying amounts of donations from philanthropic persons or organizations, often for capital expenditure and sometimes for the treatment of the poor and the needy. Though still very small, insurance schemes are building up, whether it be social insurance or voluntary insurance.

As a hospital administrator, you have the responsibility to see that sufficient income is generated and that the income is used wisely to provide the best possible care at the lowest possible cost. Cost consciousness is a must for all health care operations.

Health care institutions, irrespective of ownership, need an adequate system of financial planning and control for better utilization of the scarce resources and to curb the rising cost of medical care. Better trained and experienced finance officers and accountants are required. Continuous support from the top administration is a pre-requisite.

Financial Objectives

In financial planning process, the foremost task is to define the financial objectives:
1. Provide financial resources for all essential services and then for other desirable activities.
2. Maintain the service charges within the reach of the people served by your hospital, including free and concessional care for the poor and needy.
3. Improve employee satisfaction by increasing benefits such as salaries, provident fund, gratuity, pension, housing, training, loans, etc.
4. Reduce dependence on grants, donations or contributed service.
5. Provide for community health development work in the neighbourhood, if that is an institutional objective.

Funds Required

1. Regular operating income, to meet salaries and wages, maintenance, materials and labour cost and other routine expenses.
2. Reserve (emergency or sinking fund)
3. Funds for training personnel. If research is an objective of the institution, funds for research.

In order to have financial stability and to maintain the basic character of the hospital, you would do well to have a fairly large endowment fund. The above do not include capital (non-recurring) funds for building, equipment, etc.

Financial Planning

Hospitals need both short-term and long-term planning. Majority of the hospitals do not have long-term (5 years or more) plans. A few may have; often they are done as a formality rather than based on analysis of trend, projection of data and evaluation of past performance and future requirements. Financial planning must be based on analysis of hospital activities, both in terms of quantity and quality of services. The most important (and difficult) factor is to find a reasonable basis of projection of future activities. The short term plan (annual) should fall in line with the objectives of the long-term plan.

Policies Influencing Financial Plan

1. Service mix and decisions regarding specialization.
2. Pricing.
3. Free and concessional care.
4. Community health and involvement in social development activities.
5. Training and research.
6. Growth, expansion and modernization.

Implementation of the Financial Plan

Many persons play important roles in an effective planning system.

Administrator

   i. Assumes responsibility for implementing the plans and policies approved by the Governing Board/Government/Higher Authority.
  ii. Meets with the heads of departments and others concerned to discuss the plans, policies and strategies.
 iii. Appoints a budget committee or designates a budget officer (generally the Finance Officer).
  iv. Assumes responsibility for the development, applying corrections needed, control and execution of the plan within a time frame.

Finance Officer (Finance Controller/Treasurer)

i. Provides information about past experience and historical trend.
ii. Translates the effect of change in hospital activities – addition or modification of facilities and services.
iii. Provides data on environment –population changes in the hospital service area, price trend, changes in regulations such as taxes, provident fund contributions and gratuity.
iv. Translates the effect of changes in policy, such as pay scales, allowances and perquisites.
v. Compiles and collates data generated by departmental heads.
vi. Provides information about financial performance variances.
vii. Advises on investments and endowments.
viii. Co-ordinates annual budget; does cash flow budgeting; monitors budgetary – actuals variances.

Department Head

i. Accepts responsibility for the departmental portion of the budget.
ii. Analyses the financial and statistical data generated by the department or supplied to him/her.
iii. Studies critically the departmental operations and performance.
iv. Develops indices for planning and control.
v. Assesses the operation of the department in relation to the total plan and co-operates with the total plan of the hospital.
vi. Monitors and controls income and expenditure related to the departments.

Budgeting

Budgeting is an important financial procedure, which must receive full attention by the Administrator. Many administrators do not like budgets; to them budgeting represents restrictions. But well-thought out budgets bring about guidance, stability, balance and direction. The administrator should not only understand fully the budgeting process but also give wholehearted support to it.

A budget expresses the plan of the hospital to provide optimum care at reasonable cost in financial terms. A budget is a financial plan. It is usually a short-term (annual) plan.

In order to be an effective tool to (i) provide for a quantitative expression of the plans of the hospital, (ii) evaluate financial performance in accordance with the plans, and (iii) control costs

The budget must be planned and prepared well. Often, the tendency is to take the financial performance for the previous 8 or 9 months for which accounts are available, add pro-rata for the succeeding 4 or 3 months and an adhoc percentage (say 10-20%) to the total to offset inflation and make a forecast. Another method suggested is zero-based budgeting; this has not caught on.

Budgeting is an opportunity to consider better performance by the hospital. While planning a budget, we must apply our minds to think in terms of improved quality and quantity of care.

All departments and sections must co-operate in the preparation of the budget. The individual plans of the departments and sections must fit into the overall plan of the hospital. The plans must be realistic so that they can be implemented.

There can be different kinds of budgets:
1. Appropriation,
2. Forecast, and
3. Flexible.

Government hospitals usually have appropriation budgets. They provide for a certain level of spending. Normally, this level cannot be exceeded. If it becomes essential, a supplementary appropriation has to be made available. Forecast budgets are more flexible, which is seen fully in the flexible budgets. It provides for variations in the level of activity. Flexibility presupposes realistic standards to measure activity.

Budgets can be divided into:
1. The operating budget, and
2. The capital budget.

Operating Revenue Budget

In order to have a proper revenue budget, we must have full statistical data. The prediction of revenues is somewhat speculative even with good quality data. It is related to the volume of work anticipated. Any change in workload will affect revenues. It also depends on the rate or schedule of charges.

The revenues come from the activities of the hospital:
1. Patient services,
2. Activities incidental to patient services,

3. Income from investments, and
4. Other income – donation, grant, etc.

The income from patient services represents the largest part of revenue for voluntary and private hospitals. It consist of two parts:
1. Daily service charges (room, nursing care, diet, etc.). This varies with the daily census, mix of accommodation and type of service. There may be fees for outpatient registration and/or consultations.
2. Special services (operative procedures, investigations, etc.). There may be some deduction, such as free and concessional care.

Operating Expenditure Forecast

Recurrent (operating) costs are required for the operation or maintenance of facilities and services. The more important costs are for salaries and wages, supplies like drugs, dressings, reagents, fuel, etc., utilities including electricity, water, telephone, etc., and equipment maintenance and purchase of spare parts. An often neglected item is the budgetting for on-the job training.

Salaries and Wages

Once we know the work load for each service unit, the staff requirement could be easily projected. From the analysis of past year's data we know:
- Doctor : Patient Ratio
- Nurse : Patient Ratio
- Lab. Technician : Test Ratio
- X-ray Technician : Examination Ratio.

In this manner detailed indices could be developed. The trend could be analyzed; over-staffing could be avoided. The salaries have to be fixed for all the personnel. In fixing the salaries, consideration must be given to the requirements of qualification, experience and skills, nature of work, fatigue, prevailing salaries in similar, nearby hospitals, etc. For certain categories, the minimum wages have been fixed statutorily; these have to be implemented. In addition to salaries (pay and allowances, as per scale), provision has to be made for provident fund contributions, gratuity and other benefits.

Supplies

Supply indices could be developed for various services, working out per OPD visit, I.P. day, normal and abnormal delivery, various types of operation, laboratory test, radiograph, meals, housekeeping, etc.

Utilities

There is need to know the expenditure on utilities of high consuming areas like X-ray, Central AC, C.S.S.D., laundry, kitchen, and others.

Maintenance Expenditure

To a considerable extent it could be projected in advance.

Capital Budget

Funds should be available for expenditure on capital (non-recurring) items. These are required for:
1. Growth, with new facilities being provided, and
2. Replacement of obsolete, worn-out equipment, furniture and machinery.

The new facilities may be by way of buildings, plant and machinery or equipment.

There will be many competing requirements. Funds are never available to meet all the demands. Choice has to be made. The needs may be classified as essential and desirable. Some of the demands like those for replacement of inefficient life-saving equipment have to be met. Others may be cost-saving proposals. Yet others may improve conveniences and comforts.

Hospital T had a number of proposals: (1) a communication system, replacing the old inefficient telephone system, (2) new building for the casualty, and (3) image intensifier. The hospital decided to install the new communication system, which was given top priority. The hospital also decided to put up the building for casualty because a philanthropist offered to meet one-half of the cost. The purchase of image intensifier was postponed.

Cash Budget

Enough cash must be available to meet the obligations as and when they arise. There is need to maintain the right flow of cash. Yet unnecessary cash in hand must be avoided; it must be invested to yield optimum returns. This is done by cash planning.

Cash receipts and disbursements must be estimated: amounts and time. Among the receipts will be revenue for patient services. Some of these will be paid when the bills are presented. Other bills may take time. This is so for credit bills, especially those for services rendered to employees of companies and firms, who have arrangements for payment. It is also true for payment from insurance organizations. Estimates should be made of other revenues. Interest on investments will fall due at certain times of the year. Investments can be so made that the flow of returns is smooth and spread over, as thought best to meet the demands.

The major item among disbursements is pay roll. Salaries have to be paid on pay day. Along with salaries, other items like contributions to provident fund have to be met. Payments have to be made for electricity and water so also insurance (like fidelity) premiums, taxes on vehicles and property, and service contracts. Payments have to be made for supplies and expenses. Most of these payments are usually made at the beginning of the month. Good planning will help in an even flow of cash as required.

Categories of Expenditure

The hospital expenditures can be classified into following three categories:

Capital vs Recurring (Revenue)

Capital costs are initial one time expenses to make available a particular service. These include expenses on building, equipment, instruments, fixtures and furniture.

Recurring costs are incurred on a continuing/periodical annual basis. They include salaries, consumables and supplies, water, electricity, maintenance and contingent expenditures.

Fixed vs Variable

Fixed costs are expenditures incurred irrespective of the quantum of workload. When fixed costs are high, average cost per procedure can be brought down by increasing the number of procedures. Overheads are then shared output base, resulting in lower unit costs. Variable costs include the portion of operating costs which vary in proportion to the volume of work (number of patients served; type and number of services provided).

Direct vs Indirect

Direct costs can be apportioned directly to the particular activity or procedure.

Indirect costs include those miscellaneous costs which are incurred but which cannot be wholly or conveniently linked to one particular procedure.

Factors Affecting Hospital Expenditures

Size of the Hospital

There is an optimum size of each type of hospital and the area it serves. As the size of the hospital increases, the range and comprehensiveness of services increase, resulting usually in a higher cost per patient day.

Volume of Activity

Higher the patient turnover, higher the number of staff required and greater the total number of procedures carried out. This leads to higher total operating costs; the unit cost may be lower.

Competition

Competition between hospitals usually does not lower charges to the patient. It often results in higher costs but more facilities and conveniences are provided by the more competitive hospitals.

Service Intensity

Specialization leads to higher cost per patient day. High technology care warrants sophisticated, costly equipment, expensive procedures, greater use of consumables and supplies and more skilled staff.

Degree of Investment

Higher operating costs result when capital and fixed costs are high. Availability of costly equipments and facilities lead to greater use and higher costs to the patient.

Efficiency

With an efficient management system, manpower and material resources are deployed economically, resulting in a better output to input ratio.

Design of the Hospital

The age, location, architecture, layout, type of building material and facilities provided have a bearing on maintenance costs, number of staff employed, work flow etc., and thus affect hospital expenditures.

Reimbursement Pattern

Payment of hospitalization bills by third parties often results in rising hospital costs. Beneficiaries want to be hospitalized, even where ambulant treatment might have been sufficient or tend to remain longer in the hospital. Not feeling the pinch, they demand more services than what is necessary. Hospitals too, to play safe or to increase their revenue, might administer more procedures than necessary.

Expenditure Containment

There are many elements in an expenditure containment program:

Cost Awareness

Intensify awareness of all hospital personnel what the costs (direct and indirect) are, how they can be managed and the processes available to contain them.

Cost Monitoring

Provide a mechanism to identify, report and analyse actual expenditures, against budgets and standards. What are the reasons for major variations? Contrast against workload for the period. Focus on where, how much and why excess money is spent.

Cost Management

Establish a responsibility system for communicating and controlling the attainment of plans, strategies, and programs involving

expenditure containment. Focus on what can be done to contain costs and by whom.
Motivate all personnel to contain expenditures.

Strategies for Expenditure Control

Decrease the Cost of Inputs Relative to Outputs

a. *Materials*: All suggestions given under "materials management" must be followed. These include standardization, demand forecasts, inventory control, centralized and group purchases, purchase contract, periodical and preventive maintenance and avoiding pilferage.
Carry out a value analysis to use lower priced and more durable substitutes of equivalent quality, which fulfil the same objective. Every effort must be made at all levels to utilize supplies in the most conscientious manner; avoid any form of wastage. Monitor consumption. Relate monthly supply – usage reports with the workload.

b. *Manpower*: Periodical appraisals of job positions should review the need for existing posts, their contribution to overall objectives and possibility of amalgamation of jobs currently assigned to different individuals. Identify which category of staff can perform the tasks at an optimum of quality and cost. Allot the work to the personnel at the lower skill level, satisfying the requirements.
Sometimes personnel may not be kept fully occupied but it is necessary to have them on hand. Identify ways and means of sharing the services of such an individual across departments and tasks.
Leave should be planned to coincide with periods when the patient census is low.

Increase Output Relative to Input

a. *Scheduling*: Ensure proper scheduling of procedures. Remove bottlenecks at service areas. Smooth flow of services can lead to higher turnover without altering the inputs.

b. *Automation*: Higher output can result from the use of automated equipment. This involves initial capital expenditure but the costs can more than be offset by savings.

c. *Sharing*: Expensive equipment and facilities can be shared between departments of a hospital and between hospitals. This results in decreased capital investment and lower operational costs.

Alter the Technology

a. Focus on promotive and preventive care, in preference to curative services.
b. Preference for ambulant care instead of hospitalization. An extension of this would be the provision of a day-care centre.
c. Narrow the service mix to increase efficiency and reduce cost per patient.

Other Economy Measures

Depending on the situation, there will be many ways of increasing output and reducing costs.

With good management, the Hospital Administrator can control expenditure, without compromising quality.

Rate Setting

An important administrative function is to determine the schedule of charges for the services to be rendered. The charges must be reasonable; yet sufficient income must be generated. The first requirement is to find the actual total cost for providing each of the services. The fixing of rates would depend on

Cost Factors

There are direct and indirect costs. The direct costs include salaries, and wages (including employee benefits) and cost of supplies. The indirect costs are many and have to be apportioned equitably – electricity and water, housekeeping and maintenance, depreciation and overheads.

Non-cost Factors

They include the philosophy of the hospitals in general and with respect to a particular service (e.g., rehabilitation), and comparision with rates in vogue in other similar hospitals in the neighbourhood.

Cost finding is complex. Determining the cost to the hospital of any test or procedure is important though not done usually. Most often, the charges are fixed comparing the charges levied by neighbouring hospitals or diagnostic centres. Not ascertaining the real cost to the hospital can lead to loss.

Dr. Narendra, Clinical Pathologist, wanted to introduce a new test: Serum iron and total iron-binding capacity. Kits (for 20 tests) were available at Rs. 185/-. Dr. Narendra suggested charging Rs. 10/- per test. He had overlooked many other forces in costing:
- Standardization, Calibration, Wastage
- Other reagents, cleaning glassware with acid and distilled water
- Use of colorimeter
- Time of technologist
- Overheads, including reporting.

The charges were ultimately fixed at Rs. 30.00 per test, even this was less than the prevailing rate in nearby laboratories.

The cost of a laboratory test can vary greatly, e.g., with the time of the day. If the test is done along with many others during the routine working hours, the cost of each test will be much less than if the test is done singly as an emergency at night. It is usual to determine the average cost.

Determining Rates

There are many methods of affixing rates.

Relative Values

The rates may be fixed on the basis of time and skills involved as also considering the cost of supplies. This procedure is usually adopted in fixing rates for operative and other procedures. The total cost for laboratory tests can be determined and then, the rate fixed.

Cost plus a Percentage

This is usually done in the Pharmacy. The rate fixed must be within the maximum retail price determined by the Government.

Hourly Rates

This method is often used to determine charges for use of operating rooms, anaesthesia and use of ventilators. Costing operating room charges by the hour is often criticized. Different surgeons operate at different speeds.

Routine Services

Room charges (including nursing care) are fixed based on the type of accommodation and facilities provided – general wards and semi-private and private rooms. Often the charges are fixed on a differential/graded basis, depending on whether the patient is in the general ward or special ward. Philosophical, moral and economical issues stem from such differential charges. Is it right to charge different rates for the same service provided? For example, the charge for estimating blood urea may be fixed at Rs. 10/- per test for a patient in general ward and Rs. 15/- per test for a special ward patient. Is it ethical to charge higher rates, just because it is presumed that the person in the special ward can afford to pay more to offset the inability of the person in the general ward, who cannot afford to pay the actual cost? The general consensus is, given the conditions in the country, it is perfectly valid to charge the richer client a little more to offset the inability of the poorer patient to pay the full charge.

Rate setting is important for many purposes, including budgeting. It should be such as to ensure adequate income for the operating and capital budgets. Rates must be refixed periodically, based on changes in the cost and other factors.

Depreciation

Buildings, machinery, equipments, furniture and fittings, vehicles and other assets are acquired by making sizable investment. Each of these assets have a limited life span and shall be unusable and obsolete after varying periods. Depreciation accounts for that part of value of capital assets which are considered "used up" during the accounting year. It has a number of important implications. Although it is considered as an expenditure, there is no 'cash outflow'. For taxable institutions, depreciation works as a 'tax shield'. As such, while analysing the sources and uses of funds or cash flow it adds up to the flow of cash till such time the amount is invested as depreciation fund.

Depreciation was considered as a provision to replace the assets which become unusable over a period of time. For this to occur, the amount has to be funded. The more modern view is that the assets can be imagined as a "bundle of future services", to be used over a period of their usefulness. Accordingly, the process of charging depreciation is the mode of recovering the cost of expiration of the assets over a period.

Depreciation is the allocation of the depreciable amount of an asset over its estimated useful life. Depreciable assets are assets which
- Are expected to be used during more than one accounting period;
- have a limited useful life; and
- Are held for use in the production or supply of goods and services.

Depreciated amount of a depreciable asset is its historical cost less the residual value.

There are many ways of calculating depreciation.

Straight Line Method

The asset value is depreciated by a fixed equal annual amount for the entire life span of the asset. This method has two distinct disadvantages. First, the cost of repair and maintenance of an asset is negligible during the initial years and keeps on increasing during the later years. By following the straight line method, for the same equipment and same use, the expenditure is low in the initial years and grows gradually during the later years. Secondly, the replacement cost of the equipment will always be higher than the initial cost due to inflation as well as technological changes.

Hospital 'H' bought an Ultrasound Machine for Rs. 9lakhs. The estimated life span is six years. The depreciation expense shall be Rs. 1,50,000/- per year by straight line method. But by the end of six years, the equipment cannot be replaced with Rs. 9lakhs accumulated through depreciation. Let us assume that it will cost Rs. 15 lakhs after six years. In that case, the hospital is required to have in hand Rs. 15 lakhs at the end of the sixth year to replace this equipment.

Accelerated Rate of Depreciation

A higher rate of depreciation is charged in the initial year. The amount of depreciation gradually goes down, usually on a percentage basis. Once larger amounts are invested in the earlier years, they could generate additional returns to meet the replacement cost of the machine at a later date. For taxable and profit-making institutions, it provides a larger 'tax shield'.

Generally, for assets like building, plant and machinery, furniture and fittings, etc., depreciation is charged on straight line method. But the high value medical and surgical equipments which have higher rate of obsolescence due to change in technology, accelerated rate of depreciation is preferable. The Administrator should draw up a policy, with the approval of the management, for application of the method of depreciation as well as fixing the rate of depreciation. The rate of depreciation should be within the limits fixed by Government.

Internal Control

It is mandatory for the Administrator to have a control over the finances of the hospital. Unfortunately, this is an area which many Administrators skim over leaving it to the Finance Manager/Accounts officer to deal with. The Administrator must be conversant with what is the financial status, day today, month to month, year to year and in the long perspective. Adequate accounting system should be instituted for all income, expenditure, assets and liabilities. The Finance Manager/Accounts Officer will not be discharging his duties fully, if he does not explain the situation and provide reports in a manner understandable by the Administrator and the Governing Body. They have a right to know how the money is received and used.

Organizational structure should provide appropriate segregation of functional responsibilities, and a system of authorization and recording, adequate to provide accounting control on assets, liabilities, revenue and expenses.

Financial Information System

Financial Information System is designed to economically collect, carefully organize, properly process and selectively transmit financial data to designated points in the organization. The focus is on the flow of information. It presents a network of information required for management decisions.

INTERNAL CONTROL

Assets	Liabilities	Revenue	Expenditure
Land & Building	Accounts payable	Patient Revenue	Salaries & Wages
Accounts Receivable	Major Fixed Supplies and Equipment	Long term Loan	Expenses
Minor Equipment Fund	Specific Purpose	Grants & Donations	Repair & Maintenance
Cash	Capital	Income from Property	Plant Operation
Investment		Other Income	Utilities Admn.
Inventory			Exps. Research Training Development

Reports and Statements for Effective Management

Daily Reports

1. Daily Cash Collection and Cash Disbursement
2. Daily Census Report
3. Daily Bank / Cash position

Monthly Reports

1. Monthly Financial Report (income and expenditure statement), with departmental break-up in budget format.
2. Free and concessional care.

Quarterly Reports

Budget Performance—Comparative statement of all major departments.

Half-Yearly Reports

1. Revenue/Expense summary with comparative analysis.
2. Balance Sheet (if possible). If Balance Sheet is drawn, following ratios also could be calculated
   a. Current Ratio
   b. Working Capital
   c. Inventory Turnover

d. Collection Period
   e. Payables Outstanding.

Yearly Reports
1. Comparative Balance Sheet
2. Analysis of departmental income and expenses and balance sheet
3. Cost analysis—broken down by departments and further broken down to give unit costs of service.
4. How much does it cost to a patient, General/Semi-private / Private, servicewise?
5. Salary and Wages Content (includes pay and allowances, wages and all employee benefits like provident fund, gratuity, pension, uniform, etc.)

Requirements of a Control System

a. A functional chart of account with detailed explanatory note on each account head.
b. A well drafted "Accounting Manual" containing detailed system and procedure for cash handling; payment; purchase, storage and issue of items of supply (medical, surgical and others); inventory control; asset accounting; condemnation and replacement.
c. Detailed procedure for preparation of long term plan, annual operating budget, cash budget, capital budget and budgetary control.
d. Procedure for cost analysis: segregation, accumulation, grouping and analysis of required financial and service data for identification of direct cost and allocation of indirect cost; basis of allocation of indirect cost and use of cost data for decision making and control.
e. A detailed procedure for internal audit and internal control.
f. System and procedure for periodical review, evaluation and corrective action.
g. Financial reporting system for internal control, external reporting, evaluation of financial performance by the governing body/ council or other authorities.

PREPARATION OF INCOME & EXPENDITURE ACCOUNT AND BALANCE SHEET

Hospital accounting is a special branch of accounting. The majority of the finance managers and auditors, responsible for preparation of financial statements, are not familiar with the special requirements of hospitals. It is high time for the management and the administrator to discuss and decide their own format and ask the auditor to follow the format.

Separate O.P.D. income and expenditure from inpatient income and expenditure. Depending on the size of the hospital, the income and expenditure of various departments are required to be worked out and shown departmentwise. Departmentalized income and expenditure help in evaluating the financial performance of each department, allocation of resources and also in the determination of cost of providing each of these services.

Income

Routine Services

- Room, medical care, nursing care, food, etc.
- OPD Services like registration, consultation, dressing, injection, minor operation, and other procedures.
- Casualty services
- Nursery / Neonatal care services.

Special Professional Services

- Operation theatre
- Delivery room
- Intensive Care Unit
- Medical and Surgical units – wards
- Clinical Pathology
- Radiology
- Pharmacy
- Physiotherapy

OPD Income and IP income should be separated

Free Care and Concessional Services

These should be shown as a deduction from the operating income

Other Income

- Fees for training programs—school of nursing, laboratory training, radiographers training, others.

- Recoveries from staff for accommodation, food, electricity, water, etc.
- Income from ambulance, canteen, parking lot, etc.

Non-operating Income

- Donation
- Grants
- Bank interest
- Property income
- Investment returns
- Sale of assets.

Expenditure

Operating Expenditure

- Salaries and Wages including employee benefits like provident fund and gratuity,
- Supplies and expenses
- Utilities
- Maintenance
- Administrative expenses

Other Expenses

- Training Programs – School of Nursing, laboratory training
- Community health and community development.

Non-operating expenses

- Depreciation
- Fund raising –internal and external
- Property management / upkeep

If there is departmentalized income and expenses, the income and expenditure summary shall include the heads mentioned above and a complete department break-up needs to be shown in the attached schedule.

Balance Sheet

Balance sheet is a snap shot picture of the assets and liabilities of an institution on a particular date. It is very important to use a proper format for preparation of balance sheet without which financial analysis becomes very difficult.

Preparing A Balance Sheet

Assets (what the Hospital Owns)

Fixed Assets

These are intended for use over a long period.
- Land and improvements to land.
- Buildings—value of hospital building, residential building, nursing school and other buildings should be available separately in the schedule together with accumulated depreciation.
- Plants and Equipments—Laundry equipments, large sterilizers, central airconditioning, boilers, piped oxygen, suction, lifts, etc.
- Furniture and Fittings—general furniture could be separated from special hospital furniture.
- Medical and surgical equipments
- Vehicles.

Current Assets

These vary from day to day.
- Cash in hand and at bank
- Investment
- Accounts and notes receivable
- Prepaid expenses
- Other receivables
- Inventories

Specific Purpose Fund Cash and Investment

- Cash in hand
- Cash in bank
- Investment

Other Assets

- Properties
- Farms

- Buildings on rent which are not normally located within the same premises/campus.

Liabilities (What the Hospital Owes)

Current Liabilities

- Salary and wages payable
- Accounts and notes payable
- Accrued expenses
- Taxes payable
- Secured liabilities

Long-term liabilities

- Bank loans
- Long term notes
- Mortgages
- Bonds

Specific Purpose Fund

Emergency Fund, Contingency Fund, Scholarship Fund, Training Fund, Endowment Fund for free care.

Capital

Capital shall be divided into two parts:
a. Original capital plus additions by capital, grants and donations
b. Summary of Income and Expenditure.

Each year's excess of income over expenditure or excess of expenditure over income is required to be adjusted in the summary account and the net capital or net worth worked out. This will help to find out the original amount that was invested as capital (fund investment) and subsequent additions to it.

CHAPTER
30

Activity Based Costing in Hospitals

DEFINITION

Activity Based Costing (ABC) is a technique developed for strategic management. It analyses the cost of all activities involved in the production processes. This technique is very well suited to calculate cost in a service institution like hospital. It is also useful to determine the costs in each department or activity center in the hospital and for each activity—test, procedure or intervention.

Improved financial management is a must if hospitals are to survive and flourish providing quality health care.

"...the Indian hospital industry is a sinking one. Government hospitals are in a pathetic state; private hospitals are closing down".

—*Studying health care: Business India, December 28, 1998 to January 10, 1999.*

Hospital Bed capacity in India

Even as it is, the installed capacity of beds per 1000 population is least in India compared to other regions of the world (Source: Organization for Economic Co-operation and Development, 1990, WHO data). China has nearly four times the number of beds per 1000 population as India. Even Sub-Saharan Africa has about double the number of beds. The established market economies have about 12 times the number of beds per 1000 population. A major reason for the small number of beds in India is the absence of awareness of cost factors relative to the revenue and action taken based on cost and revenue.

Cost determination and analysis are not carried out satisfactorily in most hospitals. Cost finding is complex. There are direct and indirect costs. Examination of how resources have been utilized to perform an activity is necessary for many purposes:

Objectives of activity based costing

1. Rate setting (pricing the service)
2. Better management
    - Cost consciousness; cost control; cost effectiveness.
    - Eliminating waste
    - Bench marking
3. User fee and cost recovery
4. Insurance; Medical aid plan
5. Fund allocation (esp., in government sector)
6. Regulation by government
7. Transparency

Rate setting

The main purpose of this chapter is to determine how pricing may be done equitably to meet the true costs.

"The present system of pricing seems to be ad-hoc. Fee levels are set without reference to cost....Service charges are set on the basis of an initial market survey of comparable services in the private sector. A fee for a chemical pathology test, for example, is set after checking the prices charged by closely located competitors."

The costs and financing of health care,
VHS, Madras, Ford Foundation, 1990.

Cost Consciousness and Cost Control

Once we know the actual costs (direct and indirect), we can create cost awareness among all hospital staff. This can lead to better cost monitoring and cost management. Various strategies can be adopted like
- Decreasing cost of inputs relative to outputs;
- Better utilization of personnel; and
- Changing the technology.

"The cost control systems are weak in almost all institutions. Most institutions did not have information on the costs for different services, such as X-rays and diagnostic investigations ... An analysis of the costs of various hospital services will not only help to rationalize the fee structure

but will also point out avenues for cost reduction .... The economies so achieved can be passed on to the patients."
"High technology services .... are not charged at their full cost,, which would be prohibitive as relatively smaller number of patients require them. Such services are therefore cross-subsidized by other users".
—**Peter Berman and M.E. Khan** *(1993): Paying for India's Health Care, New Delhi, Sage Publications.*

If we know the elements of cost for various services, we can manage them better, minimising waste and controlling costs.

Needlessly expensive inputs and technologies can be avoided by:
- Substitution by less expensive, but no less efficient, cadres of health personnel;
- Questioning the need for the number and extent of diagnostic services requested;
- Using less costly, but equally effective technology for investigations and treatment; and
- Use of less costly, but no less efficacious, drug regimes.

Hospitals must always be conscious of cost-efficiency and cost-effectiveness.

More efficient : carrying out the service cheaper; less costly with less resources—staff, materials, money, time.

More effective : concern for the results (outcomes) and achievement of the objectives.

Clinical Budgeting

Sharing data of costs with doctors can have a salutary effect on reduction of costs. The UK National Health Service observed that doctors had little consideration of cost, leading to
- Inappropriate use of resources, and
- High health care costs.

Attempts by administrators to control costs were not successful. It led to cutting services, either in quantity or quality. Clinicians are:
- Suppliers of health care, and
- Demanders of health service resources.

Doctors take decisions on behalf of the patients.

By cost awareness doctors learn to cut down unnecessary hospitalization, over- investigation and irrational prescribing.

Advantages of Clinical Budgeting

There are a number of advantages in getting doctors fully involved in the budgeting of hospital services.
- Heads of clinical units are involved in planning, allocation of resources and achievement of objectives.
- Head of the clinical unit seeks specific resources, personnel, and equipment to perform optimally the services.
- Each clinical unit is responsible for expenditure including referrals, investigations, drugs and materials, and services from other departments.

Clinical budgeting leads to cost containment and control over wastage.

User fee and Cost Recovery

There is clamour to introduce user fee everywhere, including government run health facilities. User fee has been in vogue in the voluntary and private hospitals. To do this rationally, we need to know the true costs of the services.

There are many arguments against user fee. The most important is "equity". Health care services must be accessible and affordable. When charges are made, the very poor will be excluded. Health care services are too important to be left to market mechanisms.

Cost recovery raises many questions:
- What to charge for?
- Whom to charge and whom not charge?
- How to charge?
- How much to charge?

When exemptions are proposed, it is seen that many more people become exempted and exemption fails to reach all those it is intended to reach.

Insurance

There is increasing demand to cover health care services by insurance, which is being opened up to the private sector and even transnationals. For fixing the premium for the coverage being provided, it is necessary to know the cost.

Many hospitals have arrangements with industries and business firms to provide health care and health check-ups. These plans can be executed beneficially for both parties if the costs are known.

Allocation of Funds

To have cost-effective allocation of funds, we need reliable information on alternative interventions.

"Cost-information alone can promote allocative efficiency, as the experience of a Brazilian non-profit maternal and child hospital demonstrates. By estimating costs for 'cost centers' and relating them to outputs, the hospital discovered that its pediatric intensive care unit would drain resources from other departments....The decision was made to limit the intensive care unit to newborns"

- World Development Report, 1993.

Regulation by Government

Many states have introduced or are considering regulation of hospitals, including fixing ceilings for various services. Because the health profession and health care facilities have not fixed the criteria for charges being levied (lack of information) of costs, politicians and bureaucrats are fixing the charges. They (and their advisors) have no or little idea of the costs involved and are least competent to fix the charges.

Factors Influencing Hospital Costs

- *Case mix*: The more severe or complex cases increase the cost per patient.
- *Choice of technology:* Sophisticated technologies are usually very expensive.
- *Volume of services:* Higher volumes mean that the fixed costs are spread out over a large number of units of output, leading to lower average costs.
- *Activity and Occupancy levels :* Number of patients treated; bed occupancy; length of stay.
- *Medical practice style:* Differences in response to particular medical conditions affect cost, choice of drugs, etc.
- *Quality of care provided*
- *Efficiency*: Inputs versus output (and outcome); wastage; higher productivity. With an efficient management system, human and material resources are deployed economically.
- *Training programmes;* research; health and patient education.

- *Competition:* Competition between hospitals leads to more facilities and conveniences but does not usually lead to lower costs.

Cost Centers

A cost center is a functional unit which provides "services" and incurs "costs". Many activities are incorporated in each cost center (which is also a revenue center).

There are various ways of classifying cost centers:

Direct Patient Care Cost Centers

- Outpatients
- Emergency services
- Inpatient wards
  —male medical; male surgical
  —female medical; female surgical
  —pediatric (medical; surgical)
  —maternity; gynecology.
  —post-operative
  —intensive care; coronary care
  —special (private; semi-private; speciality)
- Special clinics (diabetic, allergy, cardiology, well-baby, antenatal, postnatal, etc.)
- Operation theatre (?)

Ancillary Services

- Clinical laboratory
- Radiology; ultrasonography; CT scanning
- Pharmacy

These centers are often called "cash cows", because they usually generate larger revenues, compared to the cost. They often offset deficits elsewhere. Hospitals charge "what the market allows". Sometimes, the number of investigations done are not medically "necessary" but may be medically "justifiable".

Overhead cost Centers

These centers do not produce patient services directly but give inputs into patient services. Among them are

- Administration
  —general
  —plant and machinery; building; housekeeping; premises
  —personnel and materials management
- Accounting
- Dietary
- Laundry
- Mortuary
- Transport
- Security

The overheads are allocated to the other cost centers on a proportionate basis. Even the ancillary service centers costs are allocated to the patient care centers, which are then called the final cost centers.

Training

Many hospitals have training programmes
- Nursing
- Laboratory technicians
- Radiographers
- Dieticians
- Others

The costs of these programmes are calculated and then apportioned.

Costs Can Be

Direct costs Costs of inputs which can be traced clearly to a particular cost center, e.g., laboratory reagents; X-ray films; staff who spend their whole time working in a single cost center.

Shared costs Costs of items that are shared among more than one cost center, e.g., electricity; housekeeping materials; staff who contribute to the output of a number of cost centers.

Allocation of shared costs can be done, though not exactly. Do not expect 100 percent accuracy.

Administration All cost centers require the support of administration. Work out the share based on proportion of staff time, direct costs or other criteria. Use the same criteria for all cost centers.

Staff When staff are involved in different activities, the amount of time spent on each activity can be considered. Draw a schedule of their activities during a typical week. (What really happened and not what was expected).

Supplies Volume of different items used for each activity (including wastage, if any).

Housekeeping Share can be worked out based on amount of space (including corridors and waiting area) used.

Costing Steps

- Identify the resources (direct and shared) used to produce the service being costed
- Estimate the quantity of each input used
- Assign monetary values to each input (including shared inputs and overheads)
- Calculate the total cost of the input.
- Allocate the costs to activities in which they are used.

Capital (development) Cost

Establishing productive capacity. These costs are necessarily incurred irrespective of scale of activity. The capital costs should be apportioned between the life years of the asset and between the cost centers. Apportioning between the life years is usually done by the straight line depreciation method (spread evenly over the useful life span of the item : total cost ÷ expected years of life).

Buildings   :   20-25 years (depending on type of building)
Equipment: 5-10 years (depending on the nature of equipment)
Furniture   :   10-15 years (wooden; steel)
Vehicles   :   5 years.

Building

Measure the area of each room, including corridors and waiting areas and apportion cost.

Equipment

Make an inventory of all equipment, according to the main activities for which the equipment is used or shared.

Equipment are of various kinds
Imaging : X-ray, ultrasound; CT scanner, etc.
Surgical : Operation tables, lights; anesthesia apparatus, diathermy, etc.
Intensive Care : monitors, defibrillators, ventilators, etc.
Laboratory : auto-analysers, centrifuges; microscopes; cell counters, etc.

Equipment cost includes initial purchase cost, post-warranty costs, upgradation, support contracts, repairs and maintenance. The cost of 'supplies' would be additional. In the case of sophisticated equipment, the cost of training personnel has to be included, unless it is borne by the manufacturer / supplier.

Furniture

Make an inventory of the furniture present in each room in the facility.

If land has been obtained on lease the cost of the lease also has to be considered.

There can be investment in "human capital", where training is given to the staff. But this is not often taken as "capital" but included in recurring (operating) costs.

Recurring (operating) Costs

1. *Personnel :* Make list of all personnel and calculate the cost for each staff member.

Full cost   :   take home pay + fringe benefits (gross emoluments)
+ employer's contribution
Salaries and allowances

Calculate staff allocation on a 'typical shift'. How much time do they spend on each activity? Calculate unit cost per minute / hour.
2. *Drugs and Medical supplies*
Full financial cost of drugs and supplies consumed by each cost center. Include drugs and supplies lost or wasted.
3. *Vehicle operating and maintenance*
Fuel, lubricants, insurance, registration, tyres, batteries, spare parts and personnel.
4. *Building recurrent costs*
Lighting, water, insurance, materials for cleaning, painting, maintenance and repairs, plumbing

5. *Equipment recurring costs*
   Refrigeration, sterilization, maintenance, upgradation.
6. *In-service training and staff development*
   Actual expenditure : average of 3 years.
7. *Administration*, accounting, house-keeping, etc.
   One of three methods can be used for allocation:
   i. Patients contacts in the cost center
   ii. Space occupied by the cost center
   iii. Number of staff (full-time equivalent) working in the cost center.

Some Examples of ABC

The method of activity based cost management is to link up all activities that need to be performed to provide a service. The cost of each input (direct and indirect) is calculated and then totalled up to give the total cost.

Pharmacy

(costing a drug dispensed)
When drugs are dispensed in hospitals, pricing can be done by adding a certain margin to the cost. A useful formula would be
Purchase cost x 140 percent (a suggestion only): price at which the medicine is made available to the patient.

Notes   Hospitals are offered "discounts" and "incentives". The actual cost will be less than the cost shown in the bill, eg., 3 bottles of IV fluids are given free when 10 bottles are purchased. The benefits must be shared between the patient and the hospital.
The ultimate price should not exceed the maximum retail price. The extra 40 percent should cover all overheads and losses due to 'spoiling' of drugs, breakages and expiry date.

Operation

(for a single operation)
In a study on cost-effectiveness of extraperitoneal laparoscopic inguinal hernia, conducted in University Hospital, Utrecht, The Netherlands, Mike S.L. Liem et al listed the following costs of main resources:

- Pre-operative screening (including ECG and X-ray chest)
- Anesthesia : type of anesthesia and anesthetics used.
- Operating room
- Operation time
- Personnel during operation (medical, nursing, others)
- Sterilization and maintenance
- Drugs and supplies
- Hospital days
- Post-operative medical care
  —follow-up visits
  —pain medication
- Outpatient visits
  To the above must be added proportionate cost of overheads.

Clinical Laboratory

(costing a single test)

Staff Time

- Technician; helper
- Supervisor/specialist – Pathologist, Microbiologist, Biochemist.

Laboratory Time

Training (in-service or external)
Equipment, eg., autoanalyser – apportion
Reagents (include calibration, wastage, etc)
Other chemicals, washing, etc.
Glassware, pipettes, etc (apportion)
Sample collection
Overheads : housekeeping; utilities
Forms/requisitions/registers/computer time
Administration – apportion
Reporting.

Inpatient Ward

(for a single patient)

Admitting Service

Staff time: Consultations; procedures
 Doctor, nurse, aide, other staff
 Supervision
Supplies: Drugs, oxygen, ventilator, etc.
 Dressing; health accessories

By costing each activity, we can determine the real cost of each activity, test, procedure or service of any kind, which can be used for rate setting and other decision making. We will need that information; the public will demand it.

Section 11: Quality Assurance

CHAPTER

31

Quality Management in Our Hospitals

...This chapter reviews the need for quality assurance in hospitals, the benefits of an active system for quality management and the implications of a non-existent program...

OBJECTIVES OF QUALITY MANAGEMENT IN HOSPITALS

Ensuring Quality is a general function of Management

Though relevant in every sector, quality is vitally important in the field of Hospital Management for it determines what, when and how much will be the sum effort of care. Unlike the manufacturing industry where output is easily definable, the input-output relationship well known, and quality of output measurable in absolute and relative terms, the same is not true of the service industry. Quality in service establishments has to be ensured more by emphasis on 'processes' rather than on the final 'output'. This is all the more true of hospitals since Medicine is not only a science but also an art, heavily dependent on human judgement and labor. The most effective means of ensuring quality care—and thereby outcome of service—is thus to guarantee that particular processes, shown to deliver good outcomes, are *always* used. Monitoring and improving the process factors of care and Quality Management

(QM) therefore, assume importance as a means of regulating the outcome of hospitalization.

Mandatory Requirement

Quality Management is a mandatory requirement in certain countries.

Globally, maximum work with regard to establishing quality standards for hospitals and enforcing adherence to these standards through the process of accreditation has been in the United States. Consequent to the foresight and efforts of Dr. Ernest Codman, Dr. Edward Martin and Dr. John Bowman, in December 1919, the American College of Surgeons adopted five criteria, which became known as the 'minimum standard'. When first announced, only 89 of 692 US hospitals surveyed had met these standards, but though voluntary in character, by 1950 they had become a national norm met by 3290 hospitals which represented over half of the hospitals in the United States.

Formation of the US Joint Commission on Accreditation of Hospitals in December 1951, and the need in the mid-1960s for hospitals to be accredited to participate in Medicare and Medicaid, gave greater impetus to improvising these standards. In August 1966, the Joint Commission undertook a complete revision of the standards to reflect an 'optimal achievable' rather than a minimal essential level of care. Publication of the 152-page 1970 Accreditation Manual for Hospitals was a landmark in that it set out the state-of-the-art standards that were to be achieved at that time, given the prevailing medical / hospital routines and legal and other concerns. Almost all American (and Canadian) hospitals now have well structured quality assurance programs and undergo inspection for continued accreditation once in two years. Though JCAHO accreditation is voluntary, over the years it has assumed a mandatory character for routine functioning and growth of the hospital.

France also has a well-defined, though somewhat bureaucratic, inspection system. Costly procedures and prolonged stays in hospital have to be scrutinized and authorized by Physicians employed by the social security administration. Hospitals are also inspected periodically by civil servants.

In the UK, the 1991 'Patient's Charter' set out seven rights for patients: to receive health care on the basis of clinical need; to be registered with a GP; to receive emergency medical care at any time; to be referred to a consultant if thought necessary by a GP; to be given a clear explanation of any treatment proposed; to have access to health records; to choose whether or not to take part in medical research. Three further rights were added in 1992: the right to detailed information about available local services, quality standards and maximum waiting times; guaranteed admission to hospital no later than two years from the day a patient joined a waiting-list (subsequently reduced to 18 months and then a target of 1 year); the right to have any complaint investigated and to receive a full and prompt written reply from the chief executive of a trust or district or family health service authority. The UK also has a well established system for investigating patient complaints: the Hospital Complaints Procedure Act, 1985 requires all health authorities to establish a designated complaints officer; the Wilson Report of 1994 suggested further streamlining of the complaints procedure in the NHS; serious professional misconduct and medical negligence remain within the domain of the General Medical Council and Courts. The system for Confidential Enquiry into Perioperative Deaths (CEPOD), the limited use of the quality standard BS 5750 by providers, and monitoring of waiting times are other attempts in the UK at promoting quality as a minimum norm.

In India, quality management is not as yet a mandatory requirement mainly because there is no statutory body that lays down standards for hospitals, inspects adherence to these standards and accredits hospitals that fulfil these standards in terms of infrastructural requirements, process factors and final outcome of care. Government hospitals are assured of their annual revenue and so there is no compulsion to meet targets in terms of quantity and quality of services provided. Private hospitals, however, have to compete for clientele, which makes quality management a mandatory requirement, for as Casurella avers in his article "Managing a Total Quality Program" (Federation of American Health Systems Review, 1989, 7/8, pp 31-33), "... in a truly competitive market, quality is the most important competitive strategy an organization can adopt."

Efficiency and Effectiveness through Quality Management

Quality Management is a means of ensuring Efficiency and Effectiveness:

Abundant literature now exists to show that QA projects in hospitals do indeed result in higher administrative efficiency and significant cost savings. Hospitals with top management commitment and active quality assurance programs have reported higher patient satisfaction, lesser waiting time, shorter length of stay, lower incidence of nosocomial infection, better risk management and overall improvement in cost-efficiency and cost-effectiveness.

Shortell et. al., in a review article "Assessing the Evidence on CQI (Continuous Quality Improvement): is the Glass Half Empty or Half Full?" (Hospital & Health Services Administration, 40:1, 1995, pp 4-24), reports on the US national survey of 3303 community hospitals which showed that CQI (Continuous Quality Improvement) hospitals were significantly more satisfied with their quality improvement efforts, had board members that took a significantly greater number of quality improvement actions, had a greater perceived impact on human resource development (e.g. improved hospital-physician relationship and greater employee empowerment), had greater perceived impact on productivity and profitability, and reported more statistically significant measurable cost savings than did non-CQI hospitals.

Improved Clinical Outcome

Quality Management ensures improved Clinical Outcome.

With regard to the traditional tools of QA, there is no question that techniques such as setting and monitoring of clear standards, systematic statistical review of quality linked data, retrospective medical audit, peer review, credentialing and accreditation, mortality and morbidity audits, risk management, nursing audit, utilization review, monitoring of nosocomial infection, appraisal of provider profiles, etc. have indeed resulted in improved patient care processes, higher standards, and improvement in the final outcome of care. Shortell's review also reveals the abundant testimony by health care executives and providers that, beyond cost savings, individual QA projects have indeed resulted in improved clinical outcomes.

Higher Patient Satisfaction

Quality Management programs result in higher Patient Satisfaction:

Although it is possible to have a dissatisfied patient who may have actually received a high standard of care and vice versa, in most cases, the index of patient satisfaction correlates fairly well with the end results of care. Further, patient satisfaction assumes importance because it is probably the best indicator of quality of art-of-care and quality of amenities-of-care. It is for this reason that most developed countries insist on proper patient complaint mechanisms and on patient surveys to document delay in attendance by providers, patient waiting times, discourtesy shown to the patients, lack of physical amenities, and incidents of incorrect treatment and iatrogenic complications.

Further, as advanced by O'Connor et. al. in the article "Service Quality Revisited: Striving for a New Orientation" (Hospital & Health Services Administration, 40:4, 1995, pp 535-552), service quality has been shown to directly influence patient satisfaction that, in turn, improves patient retention, financial performance and productivity and reduces staff turnover and malpractice suits. He thus reiterates that, "...even if clinical outcomes are satisfactory, the long waits, the impersonal treatment, the cost and just about everything else about the experience can be and often is negative."

Patient satisfaction is all the more important in a private enterprise, for it is the perception of quality by regular clients that determines the continued patronage of managed care programs and becomes the determining factor for market share, profitability, return on investment - in fact the basis for survival of the hospital.

Job Satisfaction

Quality Management activities promote Employee Job Satisfaction:

Quality management programs, particularly CQI and TQM, indirectly result in participative management, which in turn results in increased employee involvement and commitment, higher job satisfaction and lower staff turnover.

A JCAHO study (Striving Toward Improvement: Six Hospitals in Search of Quality, Chicago, 1992) highlighted the importance of the chief executive officer becoming the champion, mentor and coach rather than 'director', and the need for greater employee empowerment and decentralized decision making as a means of quality improvement.

Counte *et. al.*, in an article "Total Quality Management in a Health Care Organization: How Are Employees Affected?" (Hospital & Health Services Administration, 37, 1992, pp 503-18), examined 5174 employees in an academic medical center in which one-half had been exposed to TQM principles, practices and values, and one-half had not. Among those exposed to TQM, significant associations were found between increased job satisfaction, more favourable opinions of the organization, and more favourable opinions of their work than those not exposed.

Shortell's review (1995) also reports on a 1994 study of 8 hospitals, ranging from 125 to 850 beds, where a positive relationship was found between integrative cultures emphasizing commitment and the effectiveness of and longer job tenure for both professional and non-professional employees. The study also brought out the significant relationship between leadership, innovation and patient focus and the perceived quality of care provided. Hospitals scoring high on group developmentally oriented cultures (emphasizing teamwork, consensus building, adaptability, flexibility and growth) were significantly higher in employee-reported quality improvement implementation activity than hospitals with cultures emphasizing hierarchy and bureaucracy.

Constraints in Rendering Quality Care

Hospitals and doctors, especially in less developed countries, often encounter constraints which result in poor quality of care:

Lack of Resources

Insufficient or improper infrastructure, equipment, money for recurring expenditures, salary, manpower make it impossible for output of the desired quality to be turned out given the prevailing circumstances.

Drugs and Medical Supplies

Non-availability of essential drugs and supplies, spurious, adulterated and sub-standard drug preparations and medical consumables, improperly sterilized or pyrogenic materials, etc. have a deleterious effect on the course of hospitalization and final prognosis.

Improper Maintenance

Building and equipment require proper maintenance for efficient use. To minimize equipment downtime, it is necessary to ensure adequate after-sales service, availability of spare parts, service manuals, etc.

Personnel Problems

Lack of trained, skilled and motivated employees, staff indiscipline, irresponsible union activity, etc. compromise on the quality of care.

Unreasonable Patients and Attendants

Illness, anxiety, absence of immediate response to treatment, ignorance about prognosis, late attendance, etc. cause patients, their families and friends to adopt unreasonable and uncooperative attitudes.

Impetus for Quality Management

A Well-informed Populace

Because of the high level of illiteracy, the ready willingness of patients to accept their fate or *karma*, and particularly since, in less developed countries, the demand for healthcare services grossly exceeds supply, it is unlikely that patients and lay organizations can exert sufficient pressure on the medical establishment to demand a better standard of care. To improve care, it is necessary that people become knowledgeable and assert their rights to quality care. However, in India, with increased literacy and awareness, and because of certain pronouncements by Consumer Courts, the situation is fast changing, though one hopes that this will not lead merely to practice of 'defensive medicine', which is to the detriment of the patient.

Hospital Accreditation Laws:

Unlike most developed countries where there are statutory organizations empowered by Government to lay down standards for hospitals, in India there is no such body empowered by legislature to accredit hospitals and thereby enforce compliance of a minimum standard of care. The Medical Council of India looks into the requirements of medical education and for this purpose it inspects facilities available in medical college hospitals. The quality of care rendered is however not appraised and there is no regulatory/supervisory body for granting recognition to non-teaching hospitals and nursing homes. The State Medical Council does look into complaints from aggrieved patients regarding negligence and

unethical practices against doctors, but it is largely ineffective in regulating the standard of care. India requires a law that provides for setting up a hospital accreditation authority in each State to:
- Lay down at least minimum standards to be complied with by hospitals;
- Inspect hospitals and ensure that basic requirements are met;
- Enquire into major incidents of negligence, and
- Take action against hospitals and health professionals who are guilty of malpractice consequent to breach of these standards.

Third-party Payers

In many countries, bills relating to hospitalization are met by third-party payers—Government agencies, insurance firms, employers – and beyond payment of premiums, patients are not involved in settlement of the major portion of the hospital bill. It was therefore, customary for patients to demand the 'best' and hospitals and practitioners, to play safe and to increase their revenue, administered more diagnostic and treatment procedures than necessary, claiming the full charge from the same third-party payers. All this resulted in spiralling costs of medical care. With the introduction of diagnosis related (DRG) reimbursement, a way has been found of curtailing hospital costs while at the same time ensuring quality and increasing efficiency. The US Government Health Care Financing Administration now reimburses hospitals involved in Medicare and Medicaid predetermined amounts based on the diagnosis reported and not on the basis of the actual procedures carried out, length of hospitalization, etc. This practice is spreading to other countries—Australia, United Kingdom, Germany, Nordic countries. Efficient hospitals can profit through this system by retaining the difference between the amount reimbursed for the particular disease treated and the actual costs of treatment, whereas inefficient hospitals must absorb the difference. In India, there is an increasing trend toward third-party payments. They, along with the Government, can exert sufficient pressure to demand a better quality of service at a reasonable cost.

Legal Redress

The Law of Torts makes it possible for aggrieved patients or their families to file malpractice claims against doctors for compensation for damage arising out of negligence. Further, under the doctrine of *'respondeat superior'* (let the master be responsible), hospital management too can be held responsible for vicarious liability, i.e. the conduct of its employees, including doctors, and can be held liable for payment of malpractice claims.

The duties of a hospital/doctor to a patient, the ambit of medical negligence, and the factors necessary to establish liability in India have been detailed extensively in AIR 1969 Supreme Court 128-135, AIR 1975 Bombay 306-324, and AIR 1985 Madhya Pradesh 150-171 as below:

"The duties which a doctor owes to his patient are clear. A person who holds himself out ready to give medical advice and treatment impliedly undertakes that he is possessed of skill and knowledge for the purpose. Such a person when consulted by a patient owes him certain duties, viz.: a duty of care in deciding whether to undertake the case, a duty of care in deciding what treatment to give or a duty of care in administration of that treatment. A breach of any of those duties gives a right of action for negligence to the patient. The practitioner must bring to this task a reasonable degree of skill and knowledge and must exercise a reasonable degree of care. Neither the very highest nor a very low degree of care and competence judged in the light of the particular circumstances of each case is what the law requires." (Halsbury's laws of England, 3rd edition, vol. 26, p 17)

"Mistaken diagnosis is not necessarily a negligent diagnosis. No human being is infallible. A practitioner can only be held liable if his diagnosis is so palpably wrong as to prove negligence."

"A person is not liable in negligence because someone else of greater skill and knowledge would have prescribed different treatment or operated in a different way nor is he guilty of negligence if he has acted in accordance with a practice accepted as proper by a responsible body of medical men skilled in that particular art, even though a body of adverse opinion also existed among medical men."

"A doctor cannot be held negligent simply because something went wrong. It would be wrong and indeed bad law to say that simply because a misadventure or mishap occurred, the hospital and doctors are thereby liable." (Lord Denning in Hatcher v Black and others, 1954)

"We must not condemn as negligence that which is only a misadventure. The doctor is liable when he falls below the standard of a reasonably competent practitioner in his field so much that his conduct might be deserving of censure or inexcusable."

"To establish liability, it must be shown: (i) that there is a usual and normal practice, (ii) that the defendant has not adopted it, and (iii) that the course in fact adopted is one no professional man of ordinary skill would have taken had he been acting with ordinary care."

Despite the above clear pronouncements by the courts in U.K. and the major Courts in India, with the prolonged delay in fighting legal battles in the country, only the rich, the well informed and the persevering will seek the necessary legal help. Besides, the traditional reverence that doctors enjoy (for when the patient is sick, the doctor is God!) precludes a patient from seeking compensation for damages caused, more so since the patient may have further need of the same doctor. Legal redress is therefore not an effective impetus at present to quality assurance of health care. But, as stated earlier, with the ready access to Consumer Courts, the situation is changing.

Forums of Medical Administrators

There is an understandable reluctance on the part of doctors in defining parameters and standards within which they will render care and, traditionally, no doctor likes to sit in judgement over his colleagues. If health care providers have to play a role in ensuring a higher quality of care, the responsibility rests on the hospital administrators. It is the administrators who generally have to face the consequences of malpractice in terms of poor reputation of the hospital, loss of clientele, legal expenses, compensation for iatrogenic damages and higher hospital cost. Hospital administrators and their professional forums must strive towards bringing about the needed changes: adoption of quality assurance programs, laying down minimum standards for hospitals and professionals, instituting an accrediting process and regulating the quality of hospital care in India.

CHAPTER

32

Quality Management Programs: Techniques and Tools

...Since the early part of the twentieth century, quality assurance concepts have undergone development, trial and change in emphasis. Starting with the 1919 five-point 'minimum standard' of the American College of Surgeons, which developed in 1966 into 'optimal achievable standards' of the US JCAHO, the 1990s have witnessed further change: from the traditional model of medical audit, utilization review and monitoring standards, to application of CQI/TQM and managed care. Though future will tell, the years ahead are likely to witness increasing use of clinical pathways, clinical indicators, benchmarking and adoption of 'best practices'......

Elements of a Comprehensive Quality Management Program

Quality control is not a one-time retrospective audit. Nor is it a periodical enquiry system into incidents of negligence. A comprehensive hospital based QM program ought to include the following features:
- It should be a *systematic* on-going activity.
- The emphasis should be on *monitoring for improvement* rather than on a faultfinding punitive approach. That is:
  — the focus should be system oriented rather than on picking up individual inefficiencies;
  — it should be kept separate from negligence related enquiries;
  — the current emphasis is on identifying and adopting 'best practices'.

- It must focus on **efficiency, effectiveness** and **economy,** i.e. not the 'best care at any cost' but 'reasonable standard of care at a reasonable cost'. That is:
  — quality assurance is not synonymous with use of sophisticated procedures, super-specialization and superfluous invasive technology;
  — it does not advocate excellence at all costs;
  — efficiency addresses the degree of professional competence and smooth flow of hospital services;
  — effectiveness aims at achieving maximum productivity or optimum results given the cost and other constraints
  — economy relates to eliminating wasteful and unproven practices.
- All three variables associated with provision and outcome of care need to be documented and appraised: *input, process, output:*
  — medical professionals must agree on the optimum input/ structural infrastructure required for a particular service: building requirements, type and number of equipment needed, availability of consumables and drugs, number and competence level of various categories of staff, inter- and intra-departmental organization, clinical privileges, budget;
  — emphasis on process factors aims at guaranteeing that particular processes, shown to deliver good outcomes, are *always* used: there must be therefore clarity regarding protocols for routine patient care, nursing regimen, relationship of ancillary and supporting services, patient trail, manner of patient care documentation, review of tissue and blood utilization, rational prescribing practices, antibiotics policy, control of nosocomial infection.
  — appraisal of quality through outcome measure involves review of patients' final outcome and productivity of the hospital. Since these are difficult to define, the following surrogates are often used for inter/intra hospital/departmental comparison: mortality rates, managed care defined outcomes, length of stay, index of patient satisfaction, incidence of iatrogenic complications, provider profiles, DRG/HRG costs, hospital turnover statistics.
- QM looks at all aspects of care, i.e. the *quality of technical care,* the *quality of art-of-care,* the *quality of amenities-of-care:*

Quality Management Programs: Techniques and Tools

— technical care involves correctness of diagnostic and therapeutic procedures applied to the patient which assures a defined outcome given the clinical presentation.
— art-of-care relates to the quality of provider interactions with the patient/family, and includes attitude, courtesy, communication, professional conduct.
— amenities-of-care include the essential and assured hospital environment which promotes rest and recovery, such as cleanliness, privacy, lack of noise, appetising food, conveniences of daily living.

Prerequisites for Success of Quality Management Programs

- It is important to have a written vision statement that clearly outlines the hospital's quality improvement goals and strategies.
- There should be strong commitment from the top management.
- QM should have a mandatory element, in that it should be an essential activity for every department.
- The QM program must be synchronous with the organizational culture and management style.
- The organization must set aside sufficient resources to demonstrate its commitment to QM in terms of:
  — a QM co-ordinator/advisor/department;
  — a Quality Council;
  — an agreed upon plan of activities;
  — a computerized hospital information system which facilitates review of performance related statistics.

Policy Issues in Choosing the Best Quality Management Technology

- Quality management concepts and techniques have witnessed changing emphasis over time, as below:
  — *statistics and Audit*—the focus here was retrospective review (of medical records, utilization, statistical data) aimed at identifying unacceptable levels of performance so as to focus on areas for improvement;
  — *QA* – the emphasis was on inspection to improve quality, i.e. measuring the level of care provided at some point of time, identification of outlier statistics far enough from the

acceptable standard, reviewing causative factors, effecting improvements;
— *TQM* – this novel approach aims at creating an organizational culture with devolution of powers and employee empowerment so that the responsibility for problem identification, analysis and resolution is transferred as far down the organizational hierarchy as possible;
— *CQI* – the premise here is that organizations need to continually seek opportunities to enhance the quality of their products or services, and that application of statistical analysis and control techniques commonly found in industry will facilitate the assessment and enhancement processes; in contrast to the older theories of quality improvement which aimed at identifying and eliminating the 'bad apples', CQI attempts at identifying 'best practices' so that overall quality of care improves;
— *QIP*—current thinking suggests that problems in quality are more the result of poor job design, failure of leadership or unclear purpose, than because of poor employee motivation and effort; therefore real improvements in quality depend on understanding and revising the processes themselves; the focus is thus on continuous improvement throughout the organization, through constant effort to reduce waste, repetition of tasks and task complexity; quality improvement occurs when those involved in the processes stop being observers of problems and begin to become problem-solvers;
— *TQT*—quality management is still an evolving concept and there is no single agreed upon approach to 'this quality thing'!
- Choice of appropriate technology:
  — The traditional QA approach is more successful in organizations that emphasize control, stability, rules, accreditation, credentialing;
  — CQI/TQM is possible only with flexible organizational cultures that emphasize member participation, employee empowerment in decision making, teamwork, adaptability, flexibility, growth. Suggestions for improvement should essentially come from those who actually provide the service.
- Disadvantages of the traditional QA approach:
  — in order to identify outliers, QA becomes heavily dependent on measurement tools for inspection; most measurement

tools, however, eventually become controlled by those being studied because workers, forced to prove that their work complies with the established acceptable standard, become focused on how they can make the measurement acceptable;
— employees become defensive when considerable variance exists between actual performance and accepted norms; in attempting to justify the inadequacies, a negative approach develops—denial of data validity and reliability, counter-accusations against management, peers and systems, demands for unreasonable conditions which are difficult to comply with;
— management promotes what it measures with regard to emphasis it lays on volume, cost, quality.

- Heidi Boerstler *et al*, in the article "Implementation of Total Quality Management: Conventional Wisdom versus Reality" (Hospital & Health Services Administration, 41:2 1996, pp 143-159), stresses five basic requirements for implementation of CQI/TQM/QIP:
    — a philosophy of continuous improvement of quality through improvement of organizational processes;
    — use of structured problem-solving processes incorporating statistical methods and measurement to diagnose problems and monitor progress;
    — use of teams including employees from multiple departments and from different organizational levels as a major mechanism for introducing improvements in organizational processes;
    — empowering employees to identify quality problems and improvement opportunities and to take action on these problems and opportunities;
    — an explicit focus on 'customers' - both external and internal.

Techniques for Managing Quality

As elaborated upon by P.E. Plsek in his article on "Techniques for Managing Quality" (Hospital & Health Services Administration, 40:1, 1995, pp 50-76), Juran's trilogy sets out 3 basic sets of techniques:
- Quality improvement
- Quality planning
- Quality measurement or control.

Techniques for Quality Improvement

Quality Improvement Projects and Teams

A quality improvement project is a 'focused effort' at solving a particular problem or achieving a specific objective - e.g.: decreasing outpatient waiting time at a clinic, expediting reporting time of emergency investigations, etc. On agreeing that the problem must be tackled, the senior management commissions a team of 3-9 people from various disciplines involved, with a clear mandate to investigate all aspects of the issue and propose specific solutions. Their proposals are reviewed by the respective line managers and implemented where feasible.

Models for Improvement

Quality improvement models aid the work of quality improvement teams and strive towards two modes of thinking:
- Divergent thinking: thinking broadly, exploring various options, avoiding being restricted to traditional approaches;
- Convergent thinking: focusing efforts, making choices, getting down to business.

Such models set out a methodology for understanding the work processes, involvement of staff, and use of scientific method.

Methods of Collaborative Work

- *Brainstorming* is a form of unrestricted, divergent thinking usually held amongst interdisciplinary groups. The topic/subject and its scope should be well defined (e.g. a service, a process, a problem, viable solutions). Ideas and suggestions related to the topic are generated in a set time period. There is no detailed discussion on any idea advanced so as to encourage a positive approach and free flow of ideas and suggestions.
- *Boarding* is a visual display of information on flip charts or other media that all group members can see.
- *Multivoting* is a form of convergent thinking. Following brainstorming or discussion of various ideas, the group members review the long list of options, problems, theories or suggestions and select the one-third they feel are most significant. Assigning points to each item can further help to prioritize options for improvement or for activities.

- *Decision matrices* help the group to prefer the best option given the advantages and drawbacks of each option in terms of feasibility, moderate in terms of effectiveness, and high in terms of cost.

Tools in Quality Assurance

- *Statistical tools* utilized in Quality Assurance studies include tools for process description, for data collection, and for data analysis.

Tools for Process Description

- *Flowchart or Patient Trail* The flowchart graphically depicts the sequence of steps in the work process, chronologically describes the process, and describes flow of patients, information, materials, thought. As teams document sequence of activities, they uncover redundant steps, wasted effort and unnecessary complexity.
- *_Cause-Effect Diagram:* This pictorially describes the process in terms of its causative relationships. Instead of blaming people for not doing work properly, the premise is that work processes are complex causal systems consisting of 4Ms and a P - machines, materials, methods, measurements, people. Divergent thinking helps to list hypothesized theories of cause on lines extending from the main categorical spines. A completed good diagram is balanced, with theories associated with each category. Such diagrams are also called fishbone or Ishikawa diagrams.
- *Pareto Principle* The basic premise here is that in any collection of factors that contribute to a common effect, a few of those factors will account for the majority of the effect. However, despite the many steps in the process and many theories about the causes of problems, focus on the 'vital few' steps or theories will yield the greatest improvement.

Tools for Data Collection

- *_Checksheet* is a form for gathering data that enables analysis directly from the form. The simple tick marks go to make up a stratified bar chart and help to immediately identify the problem. However, with the simplicity, there is less ability to explore the situation further.
- *_Data sheets* are forms for recording data for which additional processing is required. They provide the means to dig deeper. The choice between a checksheet and data sheet depends on trade-off

between desired ease of collection and ease of analysis. Hence, teams often use checksheets earlier on to determine if there is an opportunity for improvement, then switch on to data sheet for more detailed analysis and later switch back to checksheet to monitor performance after improvements are implemented.
- *Interviews* can be one-on-one or in focus groups of multiple participants. They are helpful initially before launching on an in-depth survey. Interviews are also helpful as one can ask open-ended or follow-up questions to deepen understanding.
- *Surveys* summarise perceptions of a large sample of people. However, the questions must be carefully selected and phrased since responses cannot be probed further.

Tools for Data Analysis

These include several graphical methods of presenting data such as pie chart, bar graph, pareto diagram, histograms, line graph, scatter diagram, and control chart. A pareto diagram is a special type of bar graph where categories are arranged on the horizontal axis in the order of decreasing frequency of occurrence, while bars indicate the number of occurrences in each category as read on the vertical axis. The first few tallest bars account for the majority of the occurrences (the 'vital few'), while the remainder of the categories have only a little effect (the 'useful many').

Techniques for Quality Planning

Models for Process Design

In designing or redesigning new processes, the following aspects merit clear thought:
- The aim of the new process should relate to needs of the external and internal customers;
- The processes should not be designed by staff or managers who will not finally work with the process;
- Involvement of multidisciplinary teams ensures a holistic approach across the whole spectrum of activities;
- It is easier to design control and feedback systems before the new process is implemented than to retrofit them later in the climate of defensiveness that occurs after problems crop up.

Quality Management Programs: Techniques and Tools

Planning Tools used in Quality Management:

- *Affinity Diagram or Kawakita Jiro (K-J) Method* is a group brainstorming and organising technique where team members brainstorm on a defined topic. The ideas are written on individual cards or adhesive note papers and arrayed on a surface for all to see. After a period of brainstorming, team groups ideas into sensible categories. In this way, all cards are placed into 6-10 groups. Each group is examined to identify the central theme that ties the ideas together and this theme is written on a header card and individual items arranged under it.
- *Relations Diagram or Interrelationship Diagraph or ID* documents complex cause-effect relationships among items. The items are written on individual cards and displayed on a flip chart. Considering one card at a time, the group determines which other items are driven by or influenced by the respective factor. Thus arrows are drawn from the factor of interest or 'driver' to the items it influences. Identifying drivers gives a sense of priorities; items with many incoming arrows are key effects. The completed diagram gives a greater appreciation of the system as a whole.
- *Tree Diagram or Systematic Diagram* Here the team starts with the end result (driver, problem, objective) to be achieved, and, by going down various levels of the tree, splits in increasing detail. The final level is reached where the tasks can be assigned to a particular person. This exercise ensures that all tasks are taken into consideration, and that, in the end the people working on individual tasks will see how what they are doing fits into the whole scheme of related activities.
- *Process Decision Program Chart (PDPC)* Here the activity focuses on pre-empting conceivable but undesirable events and on planning contingencies. At the first level, the team begins with a tree diagram and sets out the goal. At the second level, the major activities that contribute to the goal are listed out. Instead of further dissection, at the third level, the team lists what could go wrong with each of the second-level activities. At the fourth level, the team plans preventive or countermeasures to avoid failure. At the fifth and final level, the team evaluates these contingency plans and marks out the impractical ones with 'X', and those to be implemented with 'O';
- *Activity Network Diagram or Arrow Diagram* shows the sequence of tasks required to accomplish the objective, along with time

estimates for each task. The team defines the start and completion dates, identifies the critical path of activities that dictate the minimum total time required to accomplish the objective, manages the slack time in parallel tasks, and monitors progress.

Managed Care Technique

- *Critical paths or Care paths or clinical paths* A pathway attempts to describe the care experienced by a patient undergoing an uncomplicated course of treatment. Pathways describe the continuum of care, including preoperative planning, hospital stay and postoperative care. For patients of a specified diagnostic category, it specifies key milestones in the care process to be achieved within clearly set time schedules. Involvement of multidisciplinary teams is essential. Managed care achieves co-ordination of care, reduction in length of stay, improvement in quality of care, higher patient and family involvement, and higher inter-departmental co-operation.

Techniques for Quality Measurement

Traditional Approaches to Quality Assessment

Standards developed by the US Joint Commission for Accreditation of Healthcare Organizations and the Donabedian's approach of monitoring input, process and output factors have resulted in the application of the following techniques:
- *Accreditation*
- *Credentialing and Clinical Privileges:* A doctor's credentials (licensure, specific training, experience, current competence) need to be verified prior to granting clinical privileges to function independently and perform selected high risk and invasive (diagnostic or surgical) procedures independently, while others can do so only under their supervision.
- *Enquiry into patient complaints.*
- *Risk Management—Incident Review*: During a patient's hospitalization several incidents can occur which have a bearing on the treatment and the patient's final recovery (e.g.: delayed attendance by a physician/nurse, incorrect medication, improper nursing care, procedure on a wrong patient, iatrogenic complication, patient fall, unexpected death, etc.). Risk management

involves maintaining a record of such critical incidents and analyzing them for their nature, frequency, time and place of occurrence, personnel involved, and listing of their causative factors. Corrective action can then be taken to reduce the frequency and seriousness of such incidents that cause risk to the patient's well being.
- *Committees* Quality assurance activities are effectively carried out through standing committees for infection control, surgical case review, blood bank, and pharmacy and therapeutics. These report to the medical staff committee.
- *Medical Audit—Peer Review* It should be the responsibility of various clinical departments to conduct Medical Audit, Mortality Audit and Utilization Review. Specifically, the following matters require monthly/periodical review:
  — medical records documentation to ensure that case notes are legible, complete and factual and that they accurately summarize the events which have occurred during hospitalization,
  — retrospective analysis of outpatient and inpatient case notes to ascertain accuracy of diagnosis and treatment regimen;
  — screening of all deaths and, in more detail, unexpected deaths;
  — length of stay grossly in excess of the norm for that ailment/speciality/DRG, factors contributing in general to increased length of stay, bottlenecks in the system;
  — unnecessary admissions;
  — inappropriate use of investigations;
  — therapeutics review (non-ethical prescribing practices, irrational use of antibiotics, use of irrational drug combinations, unindicated transfusions, blood and IV transfusion reactions);
  — review of nosocomial infection statistics;
  — tissue utilization (unindicated surgeries, normal tissues removed/amputated, correlation of pre and postoperative diagnosis, surgical complications, deaths arising out of or during surgery/anesthesia).

It is important that minutes of such meetings be forwarded to the QA Department regularly so that the Administration is kept informed of quality assurance initiatives being carried out at the departmental level.
- *Nursing Audit:* The Nursing Department is required to carry out nursing audit on a monthly basis. The following areas need to be specifically reviewed:

- non-conformance to recommended nursing regimens;
- inappropriate/excessive use of consumables and ward supplies;
- incidents arising out of poor nursing care (e.g.: fall from cot, bedsores, patient burns, etc.).
- *Patient Satisfaction Surveys* The QA Department should carry out periodical and on-going surveys to ascertain index of patient satisfaction. By administering questionnaires and conducting interviews of patients chosen by random sampling, it is possible to obtain the following feedback on the hospital / particular services:
  - delay in attendance (by doctors, nurses, paramedical staff, others);
  - staff discourtesy, inefficiency, dereliction of duty;
  - lack of amenities, quality of meals, cleanliness, pest control;
  - perception of incorrect treatment.
- *Statistics* The QA Department should compile data which reflect the quantity and quality of care and enable inferences to be drawn on hospital and staff productivity. These statistics include comparative analysis of:
  - number of admissions, bed occupancy, surgical procedures, length of stay, inpatient turnover, outpatient visits, mortality rates;
  - practitioner profiles (outpatient load, admissions, surgeries, complications/deaths, patient satisfaction);
  - activity audit (use of surgical time, delayed/ cancelled surgeries, incidents regarding non-availability of blood/drugs/ medical supplies, equipment out of order, etc.).

Clinical Indicators and Benchmarking

- *Clinical indicators* are valid and reliable quantitative measure of process or outcome, which are related to one or more dimensions of quality (defined in terms of accessibility, appropriateness, effectiveness, satisfaction, outcomes, and/or cost). The JCAHO, as part of its Indicator Measurement System, is currently field-testing around 75 indicators and it is expected that monitoring of certain indicators will become mandatory for accreditation. There are 2 types of indicators: An *event-based indicator* is used to produce a quantitative value of performance to identify cases, situations or circumstances which should be subject to more intense peer-based evaluation. (e.g.: A patient with myocardial infarction for whom thrombolytic therapy was not contraindicated but who did not receive the therapy within the time limit specified.) Here, the purpose of peer review is to determine why the event occurred, and the action to be taken to prevent recurrences of similar unacceptable situations. A *rate-based indicator* is a proportion or ratio of events across an aggregate of cases which could be subjected to peer review when the actual rate of events differs significantly from the accepted norm. (e.g.: Mortality rate at one year following infarction significantly exceeds 10%; or intra-hospital mortality of patients undergoing isolated CABG, PTCA or MI expressed as a percentage of all patients undergoing isolated CABG, PTCA or acute MI.) Here, the purpose of peer review is educational, i.e. to determine whether the standard is valid, and if so, what treatment protocols need to be modified to achieve the target.

- *Benchmarking* is the process of comparing an institution's performance to that of the best. It involves a process by which valid and reliable indicators or benchmarks are developed at various levels: institutional, departmental, clinical processes, clinical outcomes, patient satisfaction, waiting time, work turnover, cost-efficiency, cost-effectiveness, etc. The organization's performance with regard to these benchmarks are then measured and documented. Comparison is next made within the institution and with other institutions to highlight differences and to identify 'best practices'. Site visits are made to these 'best practice organizations' institutions to compare and contrast one's own policies with theirs, and thereby understand why, despite seemingly similar processes, they have a better performance level. One's own practices are then modified by assimilating relevant best practices and continued monitoring of benchmarks is undertaken to review and improve performance.

There are 4 types of benchmarking: Internal-benchmarking compares similar processes and services within the organization. Competitive benchmarking compares an institution with its competitors. Functional (or group) benchmarking compares performance against those who are the best in the industry. Generic benchmarking involves comparison of similar processes across industries to imbibe key practices responsible for success achieved by those innovative centers of excellence.

Comprehensive Measurement System

The hospital's MIS should be so designed as to provide appropriate quality related information relevant to various hierarchy levels. This ensures proper data utilization and avoids information overload. Thus, basic 'dashboard' indicators suffice for top management to monitor overall organization performance in terms of outcome, customer satisfaction, productivity, cost. Departmental managers will need more detailed information for operational control, while still lower down, more indicators of performance may need to be tracked.

Section 12: Infection Control

CHAPTER

33

Control of Hospital Acquired Infection

INTRODUCTION

There is constant danger of patients admitted into the hospital getting infection while in the hospital. Such infections are known as nosocomial infections. They invariably prolong the length of hospital stay (on an average seven days). The incidence of nosocomial infection varies
1. From one hospital to another,
2. With the primary disease condition of the patient, and
3. With the nature of treatment.

Causes

The *causes* of such infections are:

Endogenous

When the infection (microorganisms) is derived from the patient's own body. It is also termed 'opportunistic infection'. It occurs as a consequence of
- Debiliated condition of the patient
- Extremes of age—very young and old

- Compromizing the person's immune system (genetically, by disease, or following immunosuppressive therapy)
- Breach of the individual's skin/mucous membrane barrier (following severe burns, widespread dermatoses, surgical wounds, catheterization, intubation
- Following diagnostic/treatment procedure (e.g., pulmonary infection developing in a patient on respirator)
- Secondary to malignant disorders, diabetes mellitus
- Prolonged broad-spectrum antibiotic therapy.

Exogenous

When the source of infection is external. Also referred as 'cross-infection'. This occurs as a result of:
- Improper asepsis of environment, equipment, instruments
- Poor sterilization/disinfection techniques
- Invasive monitoring and therapeutic procedures
- Transmission of infection by staff carriers
- Consumption of infected food/water
- An epidemic arising in the community and spreading to the hospital.

The highest incidence of nosocomial infection occurs amongst patients subjected to invasive technology in vulnerable areas such as critical care and premature nurseries. Urinary tract infections constitute about 40 percent of all nosocomial infections. Next in frequency comes respiratory, surgical wound and blood stream (bacteremia) infections.

Bacteria are the commonest microorganisms involved; less often fungi, parasites and viruses may cause cross-infection. Seventy percent of nosocomial infections are caused by gram-negative bacteria, with Escherichia coli, the most frequently encountered. Twenty five percent of hospital-acquired infections are caused by gram-positive organisms, with Staphylococcus aureus by far the most troublesome. The remaining five percent are due to fungi, with Candida albicans heading the list. Viral nosocomial infections are rarely included in statistics because the technology for identifying viral agents is still primitive.

Common Nosocomial Infections and their Causative Agents

Type of Infection Commonly encountered	Infectious Agent
Urinary tract	E.coli
	Klebsiella
	Enterobacter
	Proteus sp.
	Ps. aeruginosa
	Staph. Aureus (Coag. +ve)
	Strep.faecalis
Respiratory tract	Respiratory viruses
	P-haemolytic streptococci, group A
	Klebsiella pneumoniae
	Other coliform bacilli
	Ps. aeruginosa
	Candida
	Pneumocystis carinii
Wound/Burns	*Staph, aureus* (Coag.+ve)
	Ps.aeruginosa
	Coliform bacilli
	Proteus sp.
	P-haemolytic streptococci
	Strep. faecalis
	Clostrida (may lead on to tetanus
and gas gangrene)	
Gastro-enteritis/dysentery	Enteropathogenic E.coli
	Salmonella, esp. *S. typhimurium*
	Shigella
	Rota virus
Bacteraemia, Septicaemia	Ps.aeruginosa
	Enterobacter
	Non-fermenting Gram negative
bacilli	
	S.*typhimurium*
Others	Hepatitis B Virus

Although the hospital, by its very nature, is densely populated with infectious organisms, it is the people in *hospitals rather than the physical environment which generally constitute the reservoirs*. It has been found that significantly reducing environmental bacteria rarely alters the rate of nosocomial infection, while studies repeatedly confirm hospital personnel as significant carriers.

The routes of transmission of exogenous infection:
- Airborne: dust particles, droplet nuclei are common modes of transmission of respiratory infections, and at times, wound infection.
- Contact with cases or carriers, especially applicable for wound infection
- Through contaminated food, water, etc.; enteric infections.
- Instrumentation: use of contaminated/unsterile instruments cause wound infection, urinary and respiratory tract infections.

Prevention of Hospital Acquired Infections

1. The greatest single factor in the spread of nosocomial infections is the failure of health care workers to wash their hands often enough. *Conscientious washing of hands between patient contacts* effectively prevents most of the cross-infections which tend to occur between patients.
2. Adequate *disinfection of the environment and provision of properly sterilized materials* for all diagnostic and treatment procedures is a necessity. Sterilization of instruments and consumables is more effective when carried out in a Central Sterile Supply Department (CSSD). Use of pre-sterilized packs, disposables, and routine disinfection of ward, equipment, furniture, linen, etc. is important in preventing nosocomial infection. The use of a large number of disinfectants, especially without knowing the proper concentration and antimicrobial spectrum, should, however, be discouraged. In situations when the use of disinfectant is indicated, *it is important to ensure that:*
   - The choice of the disinfectant is appropriate
   - The concentration used must be adequate
   - The contact time should be enough.
3. Adhere strictly to *aseptic techniques* while performing various surgical and instrumentation procedures. These include:
   - A strict 'no touch' technique while changing surgical dressings, insertions or removal of a drain, catheterization, etc.
   - Use of adequately sterilized packs
   - Periodical removal and reinsertion of sterilized catheters, drains, etc.

- Proper handling of catheter and suction tubings and related equipment.
4. *Segregate contaminated instruments*: keep them aside for disinfection, cleaning, repacking and resterilization. Infected materials should be discarded and incinerated wherever possible. Soiled infected linen should be sluiced, washed separately using steam and sterilized. Sputum cups to be incinerated (if disposable) or disinfected and autoclaved. Bedpans and urinals to be washed and disinfected between uses.
5. *Isolation facilities and procedures* must exist in critical care areas (intensive care unit, newborn nursery, burns unit, etc.), both for patients with communicable infections (*source isolation*) and for those who are particularly vulnerable to infection (*protective isolation*). Source isolation should ensure that the patient should be isolated. The transmission mode of a given infection determines the necessary precautions; single room cubicle, wearing of gowns and/or masks and/or gloves by anyone entering the room, hand washing by everyone upon entering and leaving the room, special attention to articles taken into and out of the patient's room. Isolation ward facilities should be available for admitting patients with communicable diseases.
6. *Indiscriminate and inappropriate use of antibiotics* should be thoroughly discouraged as this leads to spread of drug-resistant strains of bacteria. The following guidelines may be considered in determining an *antibiotic policy*:
    - Use of antibiotics only when clearly indicated
    - Use of antibiotics in adequate dosage, for sufficient period of time.
7. *Precautions with Staff*: Immunise staff periodically against typhoid, and, if possible, against other common infections such as hepatitis-B. Screening of staff working in dietary and canteen is essential to rule out carriers of organisms causing amoebiasis, typhoid and diarrhoeas. Personnel harbouring significant number of Coagulase staphylococcus aureus in nose and throat should not be employed in a newborn nursery. Staff with overt infections should be discouraged from operating on a patient. Monitor personnel employed in high-risk areas bacteriologically.
8. *Surveillance* of nosocomial infection entails an ongoing scrutiny of hospital patients and procedures to determine the types of nosocomial infections occurring, and why and how they are

occurring. It requires the active follow-up of specific infections in terms of morbidity and mortality in time and place, keeping track of the sources and spread of the infecting agent, and the study of conditions that may favour or inhibit the spread of infection in the hospital. *Outcome surveillance* focuses on results of practices and procedures, provides a profile of endemic infection rates and pinpoints increases. Process *surveillance* involves on-the-spot checks to see whether or not these infection control policies and procedures are being carried out. Surveillance of either type must be actively pursued to be fully effective in recognition as well as prevention of nosocomial infection. Give special attention to critical areas in terms of opportunities for patients to become colonized or contaminated by organisms from the environment or instruments. These include the operation theatres, delivery room, various nurseries, intensive care units, dialysis unit, transplantation unit, isolation units/wards, CSSD, IV manufacturing unit and source of water supply. Beyond taking *swabs* for *culture* on a monthly basis from the environment, equipment, instruments and consumables in these areas for checking the bacterial load, type and antibiotic-resistance, it is also important to check the sterility of fluids prepared or used in these areas. Statistics of cross-infection involving patients in these areas should be reviewed periodically, as also adherence to recommended procedures and routines.

Role of the Central Sterile Supply Department

The Central Sterile Supply Department (CSSD) is now an accepted feature of hospital planning. With a CSSD set-up, *nursing time is saved, sterilization processes are more effectively controlled, aseptic techniques are safer* and can be *standardized* throughout the hospital. These contribute to reduction in incidence of hospital infection.

Functions of CSSD

- Supply of sterile instruments and materials for dressings and procedures carried out in wards and departments.
- Sterilization of instruments and linen for use in the operation theatre.
  The CSSD may also look after:

- Disinfection and sterilization of medical and nursing equipment such as ventilators, baby incubators, oxygen tents, etc.
- Selection and distribution of single-use (disposable) sterile supplies such as catheters, suction tubing and syringes.

Working Principles of CSSD

The salient working principles of the CSSD to ensure adequate control of cross-infection are responsibility for the supervision of sterilizing tasks should be clearly defined, clearly understood, undivided and vested in the CSSD in-charge, who is invariably a trained nurse. She may report to the Microbiologist, Infection Control Officer, Nursing Superintendent, and/or Medical Superintendent.

- There are three categories of articles to be dealt with in CSSD– contaminated, clean and sterile. Contaminated and potentially *contaminated* articles are those instruments and reusables which are used for a procedure and which may be contaminated by bacteria. Such articles require to be kept aside, washed and thoroughly cleansed. Clean articles include those items which have been cleansed as also those reusables which have been exposed though not used for a procedure, date-expired packs and new items that have not yet been sterilized. Sterile items are those that have undergone the steriization process through autoclaving, gas sterilization, gamma irradiation, etc., and which are free of vegetative forms and spores. There should be *no scope for these three types of articles to get mixed* together. Contaminated articles should always be kept separate from clean goods and sterile supplies. Sterile supplies and contaminated articles should not be carried on the same trolley at the same time.
- Pay attention to the proper direction of work flow and economy of labour. Articles should move only in one direction through receipt, washing, drying, sorting, checking, reassembly and packing, sterilization, and storage for reuse. Careful and logical work flow should ensure that clean packs awaiting sterilization can at no time become confused with sterile supplies.
- The CSSD should deliver all sterile supplies to users, and should also undertake collection of contaminated articles.
- Machines often provide more satisfactory and economical solutions in CSSD than manual work. It is necessary to address the following issues:

- Can the task be more efficiently done by hand or by a machine?
- Is the task an unpleasant one?
- Is the volume of the task great enough to justify the cost of mechanical equipment?

In *Planning* a CSSD, the following concepts may be kept in mind:
Space: about 4 sq.feet per bed.
The rooms in the CSSD are as follows:

Sl.	Room	Nature of work	Proportion of space percent
1.	Wash room in which everything is washed up	Dirty	10
2.	Work room in which all packaging is undertaken	Clean	26
3.	Syringe and Instrument processing room	Clean	9
4.	Unsterile Pack Store	Clean	4
5.	Bulk Store	Clean	11
6.	Sterile Store	Sterile	16
7.	Miscellaneous rooms, including glove room, office, rest room, lavatories, etc.	Clean	19
8.	Autoclaves	Clean	5/100

Location: preferably sited close to the operation theatre and wards. CSSD may be located in the basement under the ward blocks it serves. This enables delivery and receipt of materials through hoists or dumb-waiters.

The colours chosen for the department should contribute to its quiet efficiency. White background is suggested for ceilings and walls, white for woodwork, grey for bench surfaces and floorings. Doors should have the following strong colours to signify the different zones to which they give access; red denotes a contaminated zone, yellow a clean zone, green sterile zone. These colours brighten the department and act as continual reminders to the staff, when they enter a room, of the type of work on which they will be engaged.

Major *equipment, furniture and fixtures*
- Work benches: 35" height, 24" width, water proof surface, top of stainless steel covered with loose sheets of thin polyfoam material to deafen noise, reduce breakage and absorb wetness.

- Work chairs with back rest and footrail, seat 25" from the floor.
- Storage cupboards, unsterile pack cupboards, sterile bins, trays.
- Glove processing bench with central pile-up and packaging area and accommodation for sorted gloves.
- Linen folding table: acid-etched glass-topped, 60" x 36", lit internally by two 80-watt tube lights so as to reveal holes in linen when the same is placed on the table for inspection and folding.
- Soaking sinks
- Washing machines, high pressure water jet type of machine, needles holder flushing device, ultrasonic washer.
- Drying chamber, hot air incubator/oven
- Autoclaves, gas sterilizer.

Salient features in the cleaning, drying, packaging and sterilization processes

- Rinse reusable catheters and tubings immediately after use to prevent lumen blockage by exudates, blood, pus, etc., which encrust with heat because of protein getting baked.
- Immerse visibly contaminated instruments in a disinfectant solution after use.
- Surgeons should rinse their gloves in the theatre before removing them.
- Soak instruments for at least four hours before loading into a machine (ensures better cleaning).
- Washing may be done mechanically using ultrasonic waves, spin wash or with high-pressure water jets.
- Drying may be carried out naturally or in hot-air oven.
- Examine instruments and needles for their sharpness, impairment of performance, etc.
- Packing should be done using two layers of *linen or kraft paper*. Paper acts as a better filter against bacterial penetration as compared to linen. The kraft paper used should
  — allow efficient penetration of steam,
  — have adequate wet strength to withstand the sterilizing process,
  — provide an efficient bacterial barrier between the atmosphere and the sterile material it encloses,
  — be conformable and act as good a drape as cloth, and
  — have sufficient water-repellency to prevent liquid from passing through.

If paper is used, it may be finally wrapped with linen or placed in a cardboard box for autoclaving, transport and storage. Sealing of packs should not be done with staples but by use of heat sealing or heat-sensitive tape after the paper/linen is folded on itself and corners mitred.

The sterilization process must be adequately monitored through use of heat-sensitive Bowie-Dick autoclave tapes, temperature charts, ethylene oxide indicators, etc.

If sterile articles are packed in two layers of linen/paper and the storage conditions are of good standard, a *shelf life of 28 days* is safe. Thus each pack should carry an expiry date of 28 days from that of sterilization.

Infection Control Committee

1. The hospital infection control committee plays a vital role in laying down policies for the control of nosocomial infection.
   Inspection Control Committee: Members
   - Medical Superintendent : Chairperson
   - Representatives from major clinical departments (Medicine, Surgery, etc.)
   - Representative from Nursing Service
   - C.S.S.D. –in-charge
   - O.T. – in-charge
   - Microbiologist.

   A doctor/nurse/microbiologist may be designated as Infection Control Officer and serve as the Convenor of the Committee. He or she follows up action on the recommendations of the Committee.

2. The committee formulates *policies* and *procedures* to be followed in relation to
   - General cleanliness, termite and pest control
   - Surveillance
   - Maintenance of proper aseptic techniques
   - Disinfection procedures, including use of chemical disinfectants
   - Antibiotic use; control of indiscriminate use
   - Periodical immunization of personnel
   - Notifiable diseases.

   The committee will:
   - Conduct periodical review of statistics on nosocomial infections,

- Carry out evaluation of routine surveillance activities including reports on bacteriological swab counts of critical areas surveyed,
- Supervise epidemiological investigations,
- Review current policies, and
- Convey infection control information to hospital staff.

Monitoring and Control of Cross Infection

1. It is necessary to monitor the prevalence of cross infection and initiate eradication and control measures whenever an outbreak or epidemic of nosocomial infection is threatened or is evident.
2. Monitoring is done by:
   - Periodical *review* of statistics of hospital-acquired infections as reported in the medical records of patients and as compiled by the Medical Records Department or by the Infection Control Officer.
   - Ensuring that all cases of suspected cross-infection *are reported to the Medical Superintendent* by the attending physician/nurse.
   - Such intimations serve to alert the hospital administration regarding the increased incidence of cross-infection in any particular area of the hospital, to trace the source of such infection, and to take suitable measures to control it.
   - The *Microbiology Department* plays a major role in collection and analysis of laboratory data on nosocomial infection. Through review of bacteriological counts and culture and sensitivity *studies of routine swabs* taken of the environment and appliances in critical areas of the hospital, it is possible to obtain a clear picture of the endemic prevalence of microorganisms responsible for hospital-acquired infections. Further, the Microbiology Department, through review of culture and sensitivity *reports of specimens sent from patients in a particular ward,* can identify the existence of such infection. The hospital administration and the relevant doctors/ward incharge can be alerted and further studies undertaken to determine the source of infection, identification of the organism, antibiotic sensitivity, phage or serotype, etc.
3. Depending on the nature of the microorganism, the source of infection, mode of transmission, and severity of the infection, it may be necessary to:

- Modify the manner of carrying out a certain procedure, e.g., type of sterile pack used, preference for disposable material versus reusuable, choice of a different chemical disinfectant or mode of sterilization, use of gloves or other aseptic techniques, adequate disposal of contaminated materials, etc.,
- Isolate patients with the particular infection to limit the spread of such infection and use barrier nursing techniques, and
- Disinfect the environment by fumigation/formalin aerosol.

Staff Health

Disease transmission can occur from and to persons who have direct contact with patients—doctors, nurses, paramedical workers and others. Infection control objectives should focus on
- Maintenance of sound habits of personal hygiene and individual responsibility in infection control;
- Monitoring and investigating infections, diseases and potentially harmful exposures; and
- Instituting appropriate preventive measures.

Section 13: Ethics and Law

CHAPTER

34

Ethics

A Hospital Administrator has to face many ethical problems and dilemmas. It is not easy to arrive at a decision on problems in health which have scientific, clinical and ethical components. The issues in medical ethics often involve life and death. Life saving and sustaining technologies are expensive. They give rise to issues of access and distributive justice. Serious ethical issues are raised over patients rights, informed consent, confidentiality, competence, advance directives, negligence and many others.

We face different choices of conduct, uncertainty and dilemma when dealing with patients. We have to make a choice. Ethics deals with the right choice, considering all the circumstances. It deals with the distinction between what is considered right or wrong at a given time, in a given culture. It is based on values.

Medical Ethics is derived from values in health care. It is concerned with the obligations of the doctors and the hospital to the patient, other health professionals and the society.

All of us have a set of personal ethics, so also each profession. The health profession has a set of ethics, applicable to different groups of health professionals and health care institutions. Ethics is not static, applicable for all times. What was considered good ethics a hundred years ago may not be considered so today. It varies with the values held by the Society and its culture. Ethics for the health professions in India is influenced by ancient Ayurvedic teachings.

Charaka Samhita has elaborate code of conduct; the medical profession has to be motivated by compassion for living being (*bhuta-daya*). Charaka's humanistic ideal becomes evident in the advice to the physicians. "He who practises not for money nor for caprice but out of compassion for living beings (*bhuta-daya*), is the best among all physicians. Hard is it to find a conferor of religious blessings comparable to the physician who snaps the snares of death for his patients. The physician who regards compassion for living beings as the highest religion fulfils his mission (*siddharthah*) and obtains the highest happiness".

Medical Ethics in India today is in a flux because of the impact of newer developments in the West on the ancient concepts as also the socio-economic situation. The problems are:

1. Those concerning the professional activities of the doctors and related ones eg., informed consent and rights of patients,
2. Those connected with social justice and equity, including the use of sophisticated technology, experiments on human beings and right to health (unmet needs of many), and
3. Those related mainly to the beginning and end of life, including right to life.

Commercialisation of health care services is producing greater erosion of medical ethics.

Heirarchy of Values

Medicine places emphasis on certain values:
- Preservation of life.
- Relief of suffering.
- Cure of disease.
- Care of the person.
- Prevention of disease.
- Promotion of health.

Such a heirarchy is sometimes questioned as greater benefit may accrue to the people in general by placing greater emphasis on promotion of health. Hospital doctors have a wide ranging role in the maintenance of the health of the people. Hospital doctors have access to large numbers of patients, their families and friends. They have great opportunities to advise on diet, life style and smoking, which could prove more valuable than the drugs prescribed. Minor changes in lifestyle can substantially reduce death and disease.

In earlier days, the people had unbounded trust in doctor, the nurse and co-workers, as also in the hospital. This situation is changing. Patients are questioning the action of doctors and hospitals. They have begun to assert their rights.

Many countries and associations, consumer and professional, have issued bills of rights of patients, eg., the American Hospital Association's "A Patient's Bill of Rights". The patient has the right to obtain complete information about his or her condition. The patient has the right to refuse treatment (to the extent permitted by law). Procedures can be carried out only after getting informed consent.

Informed Consent

There is a general belief among doctors in India that it is not possible to get 'informed consent' because of rampant illiteracy. They believe that the patients are unable to make a reasoned choice because they cannot appreciate the intricacies of alternative medical treatment, procedures or drug trials. Often a paternalistic view is taken: "the doctor knows best". Giving information is troublesome and time consuming. Why take all the trouble when the patient will anyway agree to what the doctor suggests? Is not consent implicit in the very fact that the patient has sought the expertise of the doctor? It is the usual practice to get patients (or other responsible persons) to sign consent forms, which are often unread by them. Practically nothing is explained to them.

Dr. Srinivasamurthy and colleagues at the National Institute of Mental Health and Neuro Sciences, Bangalore, conducted a study into the relevance of obtaining informed consent. Almost all (99%) of the subjects invited to participate in a drug trial gave a clear choice whether to participate or not. Their decision was based on adequate information being supplied. Patient's level of understanding and decision-making related to the amount of information provided. They did not depend on social, economic, educational or other background characteristics. The patient must be told enough in a language he or she can understand, to make decision.

Can the doctor withhold treatment, if there is no 'informed consent'? There seems to be conflict between the moral duty of the doctor and the legal rights of the patients. Can a man refrain from benefitting from medical treatment and forfeit saving his life? Will the doctor be assisting suicide? On the contrary, does not the patient have the right to determine what shall be done to his / her body?

What is the status of 'informed consent' when a patient is admitted to the hospital in a critical condition but in full possession of his/her senses?

An interesting case came up in the State of Kerala. A patient with acute abdominal pain was diagnosed to have perforated appendix with general peritonitis, which required an immediate operation. But the operation was not performed by the surgeon and the patient died the next day. An action was laid against the doctor personally for pecuniary damages by the patient's dependents and against the Kerala Government vicariously. The doctor's defence was that the consent of the patient was necessary before he undertook the operation and, as the patient did not give it, the operation was not done. The court rejected this plea and granted a decree against the doctor personally, absolving the Government however. The decree was confirmed by the Kerala High Court in the appeal preferred by the doctor.

Two specialist Surgeons who were called as expert witnesses stated that they would have operated on the patient without the explicit consent.

Contrasting to the above is the view that every human being has a right to determine what shall be done with his or her own body; a surgeon who performs an operation without the patient's consent commits an assault for which he is liable.

"Every human being of adult years and of sound mind has a right to determine what shall be done to his/her body".

"In the medical context, the mere fact that one puts oneself into the hands of physicians does not mean that they can proceed as they deem fit. They have a duty to explain what sort of treatment they propose and why and to point out significant risks or reasonable alternatives. They also have a legal duty to limit treatment to that to which one has consented. If they go beyond the boundaries, even for the patient's good and with good results, physicians violate the patient's right"— Angela Roddey Holder. Indian physicians who are trained abroad or have imbibed this principle find themselves in a conflicting situation.

What is the ancient teaching in such circumstances? *Charaka* advises the physician to take into confidence the close relatives, the elders in the community and even the State officials, before undertaking procedures which might end in death of the patient. The physician is then to proceed with the treatment.

In India, ethics of trust has been and continues to be in vogue. But more and more people are questioning the practice. They want to make their decision especially in the light of what is happening in the West. They are no longer willing to accept mistakes, even if inadvertent. The old idea to accept philosophically any harm done, attributing it to *karma* or fate, with ethics of trust based on 'goodness' of the doctor is slowly giving way to ethics of rights.

Confidentiality

> *"All that may come to my knowledge in the exercise of my profession or outside of my profession or in daily commerce with me which might not be spread abroad, I will keep secret and will never reveal".*
> - Hippocratic Oath.
>
> *"I will respect the secrets which are confided in me even after the patient has died".*
> - Geneva declaration

The health care personnel will come across many confidential matters regarding the people cared for. The information given should be treated as confidential. It can be shared with other members of the health care team to the extent necessary for the proper management of the person concerned or as required by law, e.g., in the matter of notifiable diseases, birth and death, and when required by the courts.

Patient records are the property of the hospital. It is the duty of the administration that access to the medical information is available only to authorized persons. Insurance companies, employers and government agencies will request for information. Confidential information can be given to them only with the consent of the patient. The Administrator should also be careful in the matter of research and publications that no harm is done, directly and indirectly, to the interests of the patient.

Sometimes, the patient and family members of the patient request for access to the medical charts and records. Discretion is to be used in allowing such records. Only the relevant portions for better understanding and future care of the patient are ordinarily given. A recent ruling of the Mumbai High Court gives the patient the right to a copy of the medical records.

The patients have the right to privacy. The administration should see that this right is not violated. Every individual must be treated with respect and human dignity.

Negligence and Incompetence

Many ethical problems arise in the hospital because of negligence and incompetence of the personnel.

A patient was operated upon for enlargement of thyroid gland. The anesthetist, under the influence of alcohol, did not take sufficient care and the vital functions failed. Though the patient was resuscitated, she never regained consciousness and later died. The hospital and the anesthetist were sued and the court gave judgements against both and awarded damages.

Kalyani, a staff nurse, used to pinch pethidine from the wards and inject the drug into herself. This was detected and, after due enquiry, she was dismissed from service. She filed a Writ Petition, which was dismissed by the High Court, who confirmed the dismissal.

Veli, a semi-conscious patient was placed in a bed without railings. She fell down from the bed and fractured her pelvic bone.

Dr. Prabhakar, a young house surgeon gave an intravenous injection. The fluid, which was irritant, went outside the vein and caused sloughing of the tissues.

There was a mix-up of two patients. Krishnan who had come to the laboratory for a blood sugar test was taken to the blood bank and bled 350 ml of blood. This occurred because the technician did not care to check the name, hospital number, fitness report or requisition.

Giving of wrong medicines, wrong dosages, charting without giving the medicines, not charting the medicines given, and many other acts of negligence and incompetence are causing havoc in hospital care. The ultimate responsibility rests on the Administrator to protect the patient and the hospital.

Unethical Advertisements

There are a few instances of unethical advertisements by doctors. These are frowned upon by their colleagues but little action follows. The Medical Council is to look into such matters but, because of technical flaws, the doctor often escapes.

Recently, with the proliferation of the mercenary health care institutions, advertisements by hospitals and diagnostic centers are coming up in a big way making all kinds of claims. This is producing ethical problems. But it is the general trend in the country in all commercial industrial advertising. Such practices are bound to affect the 'health industry' also. Professional ethics is seen only as a specialized part of general ethics.

> *"Solicitation of patients directly or indirectly by a physician, by groups of physicians or organizations is unethical"*
> *- Medical Council of India Code of Ethics.*

Diagnostic Aids

There is a growing supermarket in diagnostic equipment. Sophisticated equipment is bought by third world countries at great expense of scarce foreign exchange. Most of the imaging equipment currently in use in the various hospitals and diagnostic laboratories is excessive when related to the needs and the complexity to operate and maintain. Artificial demands are created.

Third world countries are sometimes used as dumping grounds for equipment not needed elsewhere or substandard diagnostic aids, withdrawn from the developed countries.

Yet another problem with the purchase of equipment from abroad has been the difficulty of servicing and maintenance. Doctors trained abroad in sophisticated procedures influence the Administrator to order costly equipment. The aspirations of the specialists are understandable. But should not these need to be tempered by the realities of the situation? The equipment may function for some time. When they go out of order there is no back-up service and the equipment lies idle.

Is it ethical for the doctor and the hospital to order for costly sophisticated equipment, which is not likely to function, utilising scarce funds including foreign exchange? Is it ethical for firms to supply these items without back-up service?

Drugs and Pharmaceuticals

There is a huge proliferation of drugs in the Indian market, with more than 60,000 formulations. They are manufactured by large, medium, small and tin-shed factories – multinational and national.

Many of the small and tiny factories work on the basis of 'loan licences' from the large firms. These small scale industries are not subjected to the more stringent rules and regulations. The larger firms then market the product under their brand name.

There are many drugs in the Indian market which are banned in other countries. There are drugs which are banned in India itself but continue to be marketed, after getting 'stay' orders from the courts. Legal proceedings take a long time. During this period, doctors continue to prescribe these hazardous drugs.

Many of the drugs in the market are spurious or of substandard quality. As a rule 20-25 percent of the samples tested are substandard.

These are products manufactured by firms irrespective of whether they are national or multinational.

Manufacturers are expected to give the indications, contraindications, side effects and adverse effects. They often do so but in such a way that it will not attract attention: *the greater the hazard, the smaller the print.*

"One of the most distressing aspects of the present health situation in India is the habit of doctors to over-prescribe or to prescribe glamorous and costly drugs with limited medical potential. It is also unfortunate that the drug producers try to push doctors into using their products by all means – fair or foul. These basic facts are more responsible for distortions in drug production and consumption than anything else. If the medical profession could be made to be more discriminating in its prescribing habits, there would be no market for irrational and unnecessary drugs"—ICSSR-ICMR study on health for all, 1981.

The drug firms do not generally follow the WHO ethical criteria for drug promotion. Gift giving is rampant in the country and raises many ethical issues.

Right to Health

"Everyone has the right to a standard of living adequate for the health and well-being of himself and of his family, including food, clothing, housing and medical care and necessary social services""-- Article 25 of the Universal Declaration of Human Rights. The Alma-Ata conference called for a new approach to health and health care, to close the gap between the 'haves' and have-nots', achieve more equitable distribution of health care resources and attain a level of health for all citizens of the world that will permit them to lead a socially and economically productive life.

The right to health brings on another issue of distributive justice in health care delivery: to make available an acceptable and affordable care to all. Health is included in the Directive Principles of state policy, which is considered as the 'conscience' of the Indian constitution. Article 39 of the constitution directs the State to make policy to ensure health; article 47 requires the improvement of public health to be among the primary duties of the State. What is the role of the hospital administrator in making the right to health a little more real?

Equity

Equity may mean many things to many people. It is often confused with equality:
- *Equal health*. It is practically unattainable
- *Equal access to health care*. Is it workable?
- *Equal utilization of health care services*. This is desirable.
- *Equal access to health care according to need*.
- *Equal utilization of health care services according to need*. This is probably the possible way of ensuring equity.

Health Policy

The policy of the hospital should generally fall in line with the health policy of the country, unless there are serious objections to parts of that policy. Many questions arise:
- Who shall receive what health care?
- What resources can be allocated, how and to whom?
- How do we set our priorities?
- What is an acceptable form of health care?
- Who should decide on health policy?

These and many other issues are being debated currently. There is a wave for more *equitable* distribution of the benefits of medical knowledge. But against it is the much more powerful force for the use of *sophisticated, spectacular* and *costly* technology for the benefit of the few. Newer gadgets, machinery and technology are skyrocketing the expenses for diagnostic and therapeutic procedures.

Control of Fertility

The Government of India and the people of the country are concerned with the increase in population. The Government thinks that the benefits of economic development are not seen because of the excessive growth in population. Hence, the Government wants to control population growth by any means.

One method proposed is that of incentives and disincentives - - incentives to those who subject themselves to sterilization and disincentives to those who are not willing to undergo sterilization. This leads to discrimination. Such discrimination raises an ethical issue. With limited resources, discrimination in favour of one works out to be discrimination against another, it also amounts to coercion.

The majority of leaders in the country consider that control of population is necessary. The difference in opinion is mostly with respect to the methods. There are many people against any artificial methods of control of fertility. They approve only natural family planning methods.

Right to Life

Article 3 of the Universal declaration of human rights declares: "Everyone has the right to life, liberty and security of person". Article 6 states: "Everyone has the right to recognition everywhere as a person before law". The International Covenant on Civil and Political Rights (1966), Article 6 states: "Every human being has the inherent right to life". These and other declarations and affirmations raise the question: How do we define a "person", a "human being"? Upon the answer to that question will depend the rights to life.

According to ancient Samkhya philosophy, there are two ultimate principles in the universe: *Purusha* (soul) and *Prakriti* (the body). The soul is immutable (*Kutasta*) and imperishable (*nitya*). The soul or *atman* descends into the zygote, produced from the union of the sperm and ovum, along with the mind, which carried with it the influences of major actions done in previous states of existence. "Life starts with the union of the sperm and the ovum. Individuality is reckoned from that moment. It is at the moment of the sperm-ovum union with the transmigrating *atman, purusha* (the individual) gets his material encrustation, as dictated by his previous *karma*".

But there are many other views of when the growing embroyo/foetus becomes a person.

Abortion

The Indian law allows abortion, "if the continuance of pregnancy would involve a risk to the life of the pregnant woman or grave injury to her physical or mental health".

Abortion was being practised earlier by many. Because it was illegal, it was practised in a clandestine manner. Many a time it ended in maternal death from bleeding and sepsis. The passing of the Act made medical termination of pregnancy legal, with certain conditions, for safeguarding the health of the mother.

From April 1972, Indian doctors started performing with zeal, abortions at women's request. Doctors advertised and invited women to have abortions done at their clinics. All these have raised many ethical issues.

Though abortion is legal, many find it 'immoral'. But most people including physicians in India do not see anything unethical or immoral in carrying out medical termination of pregnancy within the first trimester, for the 'greater good' of the country in the light of the expanding population. Abortion is severely condemned in the *Vedic*, *Upanishadic*, the later *puranic* (old) and *smriti* literature.

There arises a conflict of the rights of two persons, the mother and the growing foetus. Has the mother the right to destroy the life of the child she is carrying in her womb? Is the right something akin to the possession of some material good, which can be disposed off as the mother wants, without consideration of the right of the unborn child?

There is a likelihood of demand for foetal tissue, e.g., foetal brain in the treatment of Parkinson's disease. Is it ethical for the doctor or the hospital to participate in the venture of women getting pregnant and aborting the foetus for monetary considerations?

Sex Pre-selection, Sex-determination and Female Foeticide

A number of methods are available for sex determination and sex selection. Like traditional practices and mores, these methods of selection are pro-male and anti-female.

It is perhaps peculiar to India that pre-natal determination of sex is employed for rejection of a female foetus. If the test shows a female foetus, at the request of the parents, the doctor performs an abortion. Such abortion clinics thrive in the country, in spite of public opinion against it. Many doctors in the country continue the selective abortion of female foetuses, the justification often being the problem of dowry.

Infanticide

There is a tendency in some parts of the world to do away with life, if the newborn is detected with deformities, compatible with life but likely to put a great burden on the person and the family(e.g., children with spina bifida). Such practice is much less in India. The parents usually accept the children as part of their fate or karma. But there is a growing number of persons who advocate that the choice be left to the parents.

There are also instances where infanticide is resorted to because it is a female child. There was a practice in Ancient India to do away with the newborn female child, if the mother died during childbirth. But the practice no longer exists.

In the Vedic times, there is a reference to the exposure of the newborn child by unmarried women. But even then there were many against such practice. Manu advises the king to award death sentence to him who kills a woman, a child or a brahmana.

Euthanasia

"Hasn't a person the right to quit life which, according to him or her, is not worth living? Is the right to die implicit in the right to live?".

No ancient documents allowing euthanasia are seen. But there were advocates among the ancient physicians for abandoning treatment, when the disease had reached a stage from which recovery was considered unlikely.

Most people reject positive euthanasia, of bringing about death in an active manner. The exceptions are among the intellectuals at present. People, by and large, accept suffering as part of their fate, resulting from Karma. But there are many who favour the omission of heroic treatment, with the intention of not prolonging the process of dying. They also favour measures to relieve the constant agony, suffering and pain, even if these measures might have a secondary deleterious effect on the length of life.

Organ Transplants

There is a big demand for organ transplants, especially for kidneys. These demands and the means of meeting the demands often raise ethical nightmares because of unscrupulous activities.

There is a small group of transplants where close relatives of patients donate their kidney. This is possible because of the strong family ties. But the large majority of transplants are carried out on a commercial basis. Very few cadaver transplants are done in India. Most of them are kidneys "donated" by the very poor for monetary considerations.

Some doctors in India saw a potential goldmine in kidney transplants. There were unlimited number of kidney patients from the rich Middle East, in addition to the rich Indian patients. They were prepared to pay large sums. Kidney transplant became a commercial proposition. A new class of organ procurers rose up. The doctors involved were not bothered about the ethical issues of robbing a kidney from an unsuspecting person. A few doctors raised their voice: "The trafficking that is taking place in kidney is ethically unacceptable, morally wrong and sociologically degrading". But the hospitals continue to have such transplant programme.

Terminally Ill

Physicians have been brought up to preserve life to prevent death. The ancient teaching has been that knowledge of incurability of the disease should not make the physician withdraw care of treatment. As long as the patient breathes, it is the duty of the physician to provide treatment (*tatvat pratikriya karya yavae chvasiti manavah*). But there is also another view; one should know when to stop treatment. Among the qualities that brought credit to the physician is the withdrawal of treatment of one whose condition is definitely moribund *(upekshanam prakristheshu)*. The two apparently contradictory dictums may probably mean only that the heroic specific treatment was to be withdrawn and care to be given to the terminally ill, to reduce suffering.

The present thinking is also in line with the above. Prolonging life with the help of machines when there is no chance of recovery or in patients suffering with great pain and distress because of incurable illness has been questioned more and more in recent times. If restoration of health is no longer possible and death is imminent, the physician need not do anything extraordinary or heroic to prolong living (dying)but it is proper and necessary to relieve pain and suffering. These measures have to be taken, even if they may incidentally shorten life. The physician is expected to assist the patient in achieving a peaceful death.

To Tell or Not to Tell

According to Charaka and other physicians of the ancient days, the physician must be careful in telling the patient about the possibility of the incurable nature of the illness. Charaka advises that it should not be told bluntly. It may shock the patient. It is preferably made known to the patient's relatives and even to state officials (fear of punishment, should the patient die under his care!). Treatment of a heroic nature is to be undertaken only with the consent of the relatives and elders.

In modern days doctors differ in their approach about how much and when to tell the truth to the patient, while caring for the dying. There are many conflicting considerations: the patient's right to know; the benefit to the patient; possible harm. Most of the doctors favoured involvement of the family members and close relatives. In view of the family structure and the close ties among the relatives in the Indian set-up, this aspect is of obvious importance.

CONCLUSION

Ethical issues are probably among the biggest headache producers for the Hospital Administrator. They have to be tackled taking into consideration the values of the Society and the good of the patient and the people.

One way of tackling the problem is to have Hospital Ethics Committee. Many hospitals have such a committee. The major objectives of the committee would be
- Ethical care of the patient
- Ethical research.
- Education of the staff on biomedical ethics.
  The Committee should have members from various disciplines – representatives of administration, clinicians, social workers, nurses, lawyers, and priest/philosopher/ethicist.

CHAPTER
35

Laws Applicable to Hospitals

The laws applicable to hospitals directly and specifically are the various "Hospitals and Nursing Homes Acts" passed by the States and Union Territories legislatures and which have received the assent of the Heads of States / Union. The various Public Health Acts also regulate the functioning of the hospitals. But there are many other laws which are applicable to hospitals. Hospital Administrators must be conversant with them. Among them are:
- The Consumer Protection Act, 1986
- The Indian Medical Council Act, 1956
- The Indian Nursing Council Act, 1947
- The Pharmacy Act, 1948
- The Medical Termination of Pregnancy Act, 1971
- The Drugs and Cosmetics Act, 1940
- The Drugs and Magic Remedies (Objectionable Advertisements) Act, 1954
- Transplantation of Human Organs Act, 1994
- The Dangerous Drugs Act, 1930
- The Opium Act, 1978
- The Drugs (Control) Act, 1950
- The Poisons Act, 1919.

The above acts are applicable to Medical and Health Institutions. There are other Acts which are applicable to Institutions and Organizations in general and, as such, applicable to Hospitals also. They include:
- Industrial Disputes Act, 1947
- Payment of Wages Act, 1936
- Minimum Wages Act, 1984
- Maternity Benefit Act, 1961

- Employment Exchange (compulsory Notification of Vacancies) Act, 1959
- Payment of Gratuity Act, 1972
- Employees Provident Fund (and Miscellaneous Provisions) Act, 1952
- The Indian Medicine Central Council Act, 1970
- The Homeopathy Central Council Act, 1972
- The Societies Registration Act, 1860
- The Companies Act, 1956
- The Income-tax Act, 1961
- Foreign Contributions Regulations Act, 1976.

Besides the above Acts and Rules framed thereunder, there are many decisions of the Supreme Court and various High Courts which have bearing on the functioning of the hospitals.

The Public Health Laws provide for compulsory notification of certain diseases and action to be taken in such diseases. Medical evidence can play a crucial role in many civil and criminal cases. Documentary evidence provided by a hospital includes

- Medical certificate, generally referring to ill-health, disability, unsoundness of mind, etc.
- Certificate of death, giving cause of death and identity of the deceased;
- Medico-legal reports; and
- Dying declaration.

Hospitals and Nursing Homes Acts

Governments have a duty and responsibility to ensure the health of the people. Hospitals form an important component of the health care system. Hospitals function at different levels and provide varying levels of care.

The standards of care are based on what is desirable and what is feasible under the given circumstances – location (rural or urban), size (large, medium, small and tiny), services provided (primary, secondary and tertiary) and the economic and social situation of the region. Standards are based on some form of collective judgement of knowledgeable persons. Standards are also value-based. Government should set appropriate standards and the hospitals must follow the standards set for each group. Hopefully, this will ensure good quality of health care and health outcome.

The legislation aims to ensure that the hospitals follow the standards set for that group.

The objectives of the legislation should be to assure quality of health care and not mere control or regulation.

State Acts

There are a large number of state laws, regulating hospitals and nursing homes in various states. Some are at the bill stage. One of the first Acts was the Bombay Nursing Homes Regulation Act, 1949. The Act had three objectives:
1. To provide for registration of nursing homes;
2. To effect inspection of nursing homes;
3. To provide for other purposes connected with the registration and inspection of nursing homes.

Nursing Homes, as per definition, are premises used for the reception of persons suffering from any sickness, injury or infirmity and the providing of treatment and nursing for them and includes a maternity home. All hospitals are 'nursing homes'. Consultancy rooms and clinics are excluded from the purview of the Act.

The Rules framed under the Act provided for
- Application for registration or renewal of nursing home;
- Fees chargeable; and
- Form of registration certificate.

The next Act was the Delhi Nursing Homes Registration Act, 1953. It followed mostly the Bombay Nursing Homes Act. The rules framed under the Delhi Act were also similar to the Bombay (now Maharashtra) Act.

Another State Act that came into being was the Karnataka Private Nursing Homes (Regulation) Ordinance 1976 and the Rules thereunder. This Ordinance and rules did not come into force and have lapsed. A new bill is now on the anvil:

Karnataka Private Medical Institutions (Regulations) Legislation, 1998

1998 Legislative Act No.15.

The objective of any such legislation should be the improvement of the quality of care provided by the health care institutions in the state, whether they be Governmental, quasi-governmental, voluntary not-for-profit or private-for-profit. Unfortunately the focus of such bills is not quality assurance but 'regulation' and 'control'. Such regulation and control might indirectly bring on better quality.

Governments, central and state, have been asking for greater participation by non-Governmental organizations in providing health care services. This must be reflected in the legislation. Non-governmental participation must be assured in decision and policy making bodies, such as the Recognising Body and those fixing standards.

Government of Karnataka has recognized the need for grading institutions. This is a welcome step. This must be done based on specified criteria—size of the hospital, type of service provided, location, etc.

If the regulatory functions are to be carried out effectively the 'standards' must be fixed. Government must specify the mechanism for fixing standards for each grade of hospitals. Who will fix the standards? How will they be fixed? Expert committees, with adequate non-governmental representation, must be appointed to set the standards, which must be feasible.

Supervisory Authority

It is necessary to create an autonomous, statutory authority, having government officials, and representatives of hospitals as also people's representatives. In the larger states, Divisional supervisory bodies may be created on similar lines, to avoid delay.

Pro-active role

Governments should play a pro-active role to ensure that the health care of the people is of the required standard. The same must be improved continuosly. It is the duty of the government to provide adequate health care services. The people have a right to health. If other non-governmental agencies are providing health care services, they are helping the government to discharge its duties and obligations. Such agencies must be encouraged by providing financial, technical and educational support. The function of the government must be facilitatory and regulatory.

Accreditation

It will be a very good idea to encourage the process of accreditation of the hospitals by professional bodies on the lines of accreditation in USA, Canada, Australia, England, Spain, Malaysia, China and other countries. The outstanding example is the Joint Commission on Accreditation of Health Care Organizations in USA.

CHAPTER 36

Consumer Protection Act, 1986

Among the many laws affecting the practice of medicine, whether it be by the medical practitioner or the health care institution, the legislation affecting most the medical profession today is the Consumer Protection Act. It is necessary to be knowledgeable about the legal provisions under this Act, and to take appropriate action.

One of the most important subjects that have come into litigation involving doctors and hospitals is negligence. Medical negligence alleged to have caused harm has seen many persons and hospitals being taken to the courts and more recently and in a much greater measure to Consumer Redressal Fora under this Act.

Medical Negligence

Negligence is a careless act and may result in harm. A person is said to be negligent when he/she acts without due care in regard to the harmful consequences of his/her action.

When a member of the medical profession (or a health care institution) falls short of the standard of ordinary skilled person, the patient (or the heirs) has a right of action for damages.

A doctor (or health care institution), negligent in providing medical services to a patient is liable criminally as also to compensate the patient by way of pecuniary damages.

The concept of punishment when harm results from negligence is not something new.

Brihaspathi Shruti records as follows:

"A physician who, though unacquainted with drugs and their effects or is ignorant of the nature of diseases, yet takes money from the sick (for giving treatment), shall be punished like a thief".
- Sacred books of the East : Vol, 15

Manusmriti has the following to state:
> "All physicians who treat their patients wrongly
> shall be liable to pay fine".
> -Sacred books of the East, Vol. 2

Legal remedy

There are many avenues of legal remedy when negligence has occurred and it has caused harm:
- *Criminal liability:* IPC Section 304A : Grossly rash or grossly negligent act, which is proximate, direct or substantive cause of patient's death.
- *Civil liability :* Indian Contract Act sections 73 and 74 : Medical services rendered on payment of a fee.
- *Law of torts :* Breach of contract, whether patient pays or not.
- *The Indian Medical Council Act, 1956.*
- *Consumer Protection Act, 1986.*

Formulating the general principles of the law of negligence in England, Halsbury's Laws of England (4th edition) says:

"Negligence is a specific tort and in any given circumstances is the failure to exercise that care which the circumstances demand ..... it may consist in omitting to do something which ought to be done or in doing something which ought to be done either in a different manner or not at all.

"Where there is a duty to exercise care, reasonable care must be taken to avoid acts or omissions which can be reasonably foreseen to be likely to cause personal injury to persons or property".

What are the duties of a doctor?

When consulted by a person, the doctor owes the person a duty of care in
- Deciding whether to undertake the care of the person,
- Deciding what advice/treatment to give, and
- The administration of that treatment.

"The duties which a doctor owes to his patient are clear. A person who holds himself out ready to give medical advice and treatment impliedly undertakes that he is possessed of skill and knowledge for the purpose.

Such a person when consulted by a patient owes him certain duties, namely a duty of care in deciding whether to undertake the case, a duty

of care in deciding what treatment to give or duty of care in the administration of that treatment".
—*Laxman vs Trimbah, AIR 1960, p131-2*

The duty of a medical practitioner arises from the fact that he owes something to a person which is likely to cause physical damage unless it is done with proper care and skill. There is no warranty of success when treatment is given. Deviation from normal practice is not necessarily evidence of negligence. Also, mistaken diagnosis is not necessarily a negligent diagnosis. A practitioner can only be held liable if his/her diagnosis is so palpably wrong as to prove negligence (AIR 1975, Bombay 306).

There is also a duty of care in answering questions put to the doctor by the patient in circumstances in which he (the doctor) knows that the patient intends to rely on his answer.

What is the Degree of Care Required of a Doctor?

It is the law that a practitioner must bring to his/her task a reasonable degree of care. Halsbury's Laws of England, 4th edition, Vol.30, para 35 states:

"Neither the very highest nor a very low degree of care and competence, judged in the light of the particular circumstances of each case is what the law requires and a person is not liable in negligence because someone else of greater skill and knowledge would have prescribed different treatment or operated in a different way; nor is he guilty of negligence if he has acted in accordance with a practice accepted by a responsible body of medical men skilled in that particular art, even though a body of adverse opinion also existed among medical men".

Actionable negligence by a physician (doctor) in USA is connoted by the expression "medical malpractice", which is defined as a particular form of negligence that consists of not applying to the exercise of the practice of medicine that degree of care and skill which is ordinarily employed by the profession generally, under similar condition and in like circumstances. The law does not expect of the members of the medical profession utmost degree of care and skill attainable or known to the profession but they should possess and exercise reasonable degree of skill, knowledge and care ordinarily possessed and exercised by members of their profession under similar circumstances. However, the law does recognise that medicine is a progressive science and, therefore, in determining the degree of care and skills, regard will be had to the state of advancement of the profession at the time and place of treatment.

McNair, J, in Bolam vs Friern Hospital Committee (1957 (2) All E.R. 118), enunciated the law:

"A doctor is not guilty of negligence if he has acted in accordance with a practice accepted as proper by a responsible body of medical men skilled in that particular art….. At the same time, that does not mean that a medical man can obstinately and pigheadedly carry on with some old technique if it has been proved to be contrary to what is really substantially the whole of informed medical opinion. Otherwise, you might get men today saying : 'I don't believe in anaesthetic. I don't believe in antiseptics, I am going to continue to do my surgery in the way it was done in the 18th century! That clearly would be wrong".

To establish liability by a doctor where deviation from normal practice is alleged, three factors must be proved:
- There is a usual and normal practice.
- The defendant has not adopted the practice.
- The course the doctor adopted is one which no professional of ordinary skill would have taken if he / she had been acting with ordinary care.

McNair J, stated

"Counsel for the plaintiff put it this way, that in the case of a medical man, negligence means failure to act in accordance with the standards of reasonably competent man at that time. That is a perfectly accurate statement, as long as it is remembered that there may be one or more perfectly proper standards, and if a medical man conforms with one of those standards, then he is not negligent".

Negligence would not be inferred merely because there was a body of opinion which took another view.

The onus of proof of negligence rests squarely on the plaintiff. Justice Chagla and Baghwati of the Bombay High Court stated:

"The law on the subject is really not in dispute. The plaintiff has to establish that there had been a want of competent care and skill as to lead to a bad result. The plaintiff has also to establish the necessary connection between the negligence of defendant and the ultimate death of the plaintiff's son".

Failure to conform to the required standard of care resulting in material injury is actionable negligence if there is proximate connection between the defendant's conduct and the resultant injury. The standard required will be that of an average practitioner of the class to which he/she belongs or holds to belong. In the case of specialists, a higher standard is expected.

There is a classic judgment given by Justice M.N. Rao of Andhra Pradesh High Court, which is quoted often:

"Law imposes a duty on everyone to conform to certain standards of conduct for the protection of others. Persons who undertake work requiring special skill must not only exercise reasonable care but also measure up to the standard of proficiency that can be expected from persons of such profession. Failure to conform to the required standard of care resulting in material injury is actionable negligence if there is proximate connection between the defendant's conduct and the resultant injury. A surgeon or anaesthetist will be judged by the standard of an average practitioner of the class to which he belongs or holds himself out to belong. In the case of specialists a higher degree of skill is called".

The above judgment was given in the case of a brilliant boy of 17 years, whose IQ fell to that of a boy of 6 years as a result of loss of blood supply to the brain during a tonsillectomy operation. It was alleged that the anaesthetist and surgeon were negligent, causing loss of blood supply leading to the brain damage.

Error of judgment

Often a plea is made that there was no negligence but what had gone wrong was due to an error of judgment. The position has been made clear by a number of judgments.

"The true position is that an error of judgment may, or may not, be negligent; it depends on the nature of the error. If it is one that would not have been made by a reasonably competent professional man professing to have the standard and type of skill that the defendant holds himself out as having, and acting with ordinary care, then it is negligence. If on the other hand, it is an error that such a man, acting with ordinary care, might have made, then it is not negligence".

-Lord Fraser, 1981, 1 All ER, 267,
Quoted by Hon'ble S. Saghir Ahmed and G.B. Patnaik, JJ. AIR 1998 SC 1801.

A common defence put forth by a medical practitioner to a charge of medical negligence, is consent. The question can arise in two ways:
1. That the patient gave consent for the treatment and therefore, cannot on facts or in law or in equity complain about the effects of the treatment.
2. That the patient did not or was not in a position to give consent and therefore, the doctor did not act and the doctor cannot be held responsible for any result flowing out of such omission.

Both these do not absolve the doctor of charge of negligence.

Damages

If the negligence causes harm to the patient, then the patient (or his/her relatives)is entitled to damages. These damages may be for:
— pecuniary losses, called special damages, and
— non-pecuniary losses, called general damages.

The special damages include
— expenses incurred for treatment as a result of the negligence
— loss of earnings, and
— future monetary losses, because of disabilities.

The special damages must be pleaded and proved:
General damages include payment for:
— pain and suffering,
— loss of amenities of life, and
— shortened expectation of life.

The plaintiff must establish that the damage he/she suffered was caused by the negligence of the doctor.

CONSUMER PROTECTION ACT

Litigation to get redressal of grievances for negligence and claims of damages is time consuming. It is also expensive. The Consumer Protection Act was passed by the Parliament in 1986 with a view to provide for the better protection of the interests of the Consumers. It provides for the establishment of Consumer Councils to educate the public and creation of authorities for the settlement of Consumer Disputes and for matters connected therewith. The Consumer Protection Act does not confer any new right to the patient (or the relatives). The Act is designed to provide for a quicker and cheaper remedy when there is deficiency in service and claims for damages are made arising from such deficiency in service.

According to Section 2(1)(d)(ii) of the Act, Consumer means any person who hires or avails of any services for a consideration which has been paid or promised or partly paid and partly promised or under any system of deferred payment.

Section 2(1)(o) of the Act defines 'Service'. According to it, "Service" means service of any description which is made available to potential users.

Health care services will be service, within the meaning of Section 2(1)(o) of the Act, if such services are obtained for consideration.

"........ the activity of providing medical assistance for payment carried on by hospitals and members of the medical profession falls within the scope of the expression "service" as defined in Section 2(1)(o) of the Act, and that in the event of any deficiency in the performance of such service the aggrieved party can invoke the remedies provided under the Act by filing a complaint before the consumer forum having jurisdiction"—V. Balakrishna Eradi, President of the National Consumer Disputes Redressal Commission, in Cosmopolitan Hospitals Vs. Vasantha P. Nair, AIR 1992 CPJ 302, 312 (NC).

The judgement of the National Commission was appealed against in the Supreme Court by the Indian Medical Association and others.

An opposite view was taken by the Madras High Court in the Writ Petition by Dr. C.S. Subramanian. D. Raju and A.R. Lakshmanan, J.J., held that doctors and hospitals do not come under Consumer Protection Act. According to them, 'consumer' meant a consumer of service of commercial and trade oriented nature and 'service' by way of diagnosis and treatment would not come under the purview of the Act.

Transfusion was given in heart surgery. The first three bottles of blood had been tested fully. The fourth bottle was given without the full results being known, because of the urgency. The test for fourth bottle of blood came out as HIV (Human Immuno Deficiency Virus) positive. The woman became infected and passed on the infection to her child. The hospital was sued in the consumer court. No damages were awarded as it was a charitable hospital and the patient was treated free of charges.

There were a few other judgments which were appealed against.

The appeals against the decisions of the National Commission and judgments of some of the High Courts have been heard by the Supreme Court. In its judgment on November 13, 1995, the three-bench court has stated categorically that the medical profession and the hospitals come within the ambit of the Act. (Supreme Court of India, Civil Appeal No. 688 of 1993).

Salient points

- Service rendered by a medical practitioner or hospital (or other health care institutions) by way of consultation, diagnosis and treatment, when rendered on payment by all or by some and free of charge to others, falls within the purview of the Act.
- Service rendered to person, whose charges are borne by an insurance company or employer as part of the conditions of service falls within the purview of the Act.
- Service rendered where no charge whatsoever (except a token amount for registration only) is made from any person availing the service and all patients (rich and poor) are given free service, is outside the purview of the Act.

The Act provides for the constitution of the Consumer Forum for the settlement of Consumer Disputes. Under the Act, the consumer need not pay any court fees or process fees. The dispute is required to be decided in three months, if it does not involve examination by an expert or adducing expert evidence.

The fora that are formed under the Act are
- District forum
- State Commission, and
- National Commission.

District Forum

The District Forum consists of three persons:
1. a person who is or has been or is qualified to be a District Judge – President, and
2. two persons known for ability, integrity, knowledge of economics, law, commerce, accounting, industry or administration, one of whom shall be a woman.

The forum can entertain complaints where the compensation claimed does not exceed Rupees Five Lakhs.

The complaint has to be made to the district forum within whose jurisdiction the cause of action arose or the opposite party resides or carries on business at the time of the complaint.

Appeal against the order of the district forum lies with the State Commission. It has to be made within 30 days.

State Commission

The State Commission has three persons:
1. A person who is or has been a judge of the High Court – President, and
2. Two persons known for ability, integrity, knowledge of economics, law, commerce, accounting, industry or administration, one of whom shall be a woman.

The Commission entertains complaints where the compensation claimed is more than five lakh rupees and less than twenty lakhs and also appeals against the orders of the district forum in the State.

Appeals against the orders of the State Commission lies with the National Commission. It has to be made within 30 days.

National Commission

The National Commission has five members:
1. A person who is or has been a judge of the Supreme Court – President, and
2. Four persons known for ability, integrity, knowledge of economics, law, commerce, accounting, industry or administration, one of whom shall be a woman.

CONSUMER PROTECTION COUNCILS

The Consumer Protection Act provides for Consumer Protection Councils at the center and in the States. The objects of the councils are:
- Promotion and protection of the rights of consumers, and
- Consumer education.

Central Consumer Protection Council

The Central Consumer Protection Council consists of
- The Minister in charge of the Food and Civil supplies of the Government of India—Chairman

- Official and non-official members representing such interests as may be prescribed by the Government of India.

State level Consumer Protection Councils

Consumer Protection Councils are present in the States. They are constituted along the same lines as the Central Council and have similar objectives. State council consists of such members as may be specified by the State Government by notification from time to time.

Medical Profession's View of CPA

Many doctors are against the inclusion of doctors under the Consumer Protection Act.

Arguments Against CPA

1. Medical Services cannot be compared to defective household appliances. Questions of medical negligence are highly complex.
2. Medical Services are personal in nature and not the type offered by manufacturers of consumer products.
3. The State Medical Councils are the proper authorities to hear complaints of this nature.
4. Inclusion of doctors under the Act would encourage frivolous complaints, as no fees are charged. The complainant goes scot free in case of malicious intent.
5. The doctors would be harassed; corruption will seep in.
6. The patient will ultimately be the loser; doctors will not take the treatment of patients with even slightly complicated ailments.
7. Many unnecessary tests will be done as abundant precaution —defensive medicine.
8. No treatment is absolutely safe.
9. There are only non-professional people in the forum/commission; they cannot appreciate the complex issues in medical care.
10. Only the President of the forum / commission has a legal/judicial background; in case of difference of opinion, the opinion of the majority (non-medical; non-judicial) will prevail.

11. Irreparable damage will be done to the reputation of the doctor, even if the complaint is dismissed.
12. Doctors will have to spend time defending themselves.

Arguments For CPA

1. Doctors are accountable for their actions
2. Doctors are not above law
3. Speedy justice does not mean a summary trial. The procedures followed in Civil Courts are applicable to consumer forums.
4. Medical Councils cannot give compensation.
5. Malpractice suits are decided by civil courts.
6. The composition of the forum / commission is such that the decisions will be made on the basis of law, reasonableness, fairness and good faith.

Some Suggestions

1. The Court should have the power to examine a complainant on oath before issuing a notice to the defendant.
2. Consumer courts should be able to grant compensation to the defendants, if the court finds the complaint to be baseless. The Consumer Protection (Amendment) Act, 1993 gives powers to the forum / commission to require the complainant to pay such cost, not exceeding ten thousand rupees, where the complaint instituted is found to be vexatious or frivolous. This amount is too small; the amount may be stipulated as 10 percent of the damages claimed.
3. A screening committee which has a senior medical person as member of the consumer court should screen all complaints.
4. The Commission / Court should have at least one senior medical person, when complaints against hospitals, nursing homes and doctors are heard.
5. When a deficiency of service is alleged, the matter may be decided by arbitration by a board, consisting of one doctor nominated by the complainant, one doctor nominated by the defendant and the presiding judge of the appropriate forum.

The Consumer Protection (Amendment) Ordinance, 1993.

Section 26 : Where a complaint instituted before the District Forum, the State Commission or the National Commission, as the case may be, is found to be frivolous or vexatious, it shall, for reasons to be recorded in writing, dismiss the complaint and make an order that the complainant shall pay to the opposite party such cost, not exceeding ten thousand rupees, as may be specified in the order.

Will payment of rupees ten thousand be adequate to compensate for the loss of reputation, psychological trauma and harassment and damages claims of many lakhs of rupees and even crores of rupees?

What Should the Doctor or Health Care Institution Do?

- Accept a patient only if the management of the patient is within your skill and competence or if it is an emergency and first aid and life-saving measures have to be taken.
- Have genuine concern for the patient. Think and act in the best interests of the patient.
- Create an atmosphere of trust and friendship with the patient and the family.
- Inform the patient (and, where applicable, the close relatives, without breaking confidentiality) of the proposed procedures and the possible outcome and the other alternatives.
- Always obtain informed consent. Record it. Where informed consent is not given, record that also with witnesses.
- Give maximum possible care.
- Be honest.
- Update your knowledge, skills and attitude through:
  —CME programes
  —journals, books, audio and video tapes.
- Maintain detailed records:
  — history
  — findings of examination
  — investigations
  — diagnosis
  — treatment given
  — monitoring
- If a second opinion is needed, facilitate it.
- Be available, till your services are no longer required.
- Get cover under the medical indemnity scheme.

Section 14: India's Health Policy

CHAPTER

37

Hospitals in the Framework of India's Health Policy

INTRODUCTION

Hospitals play an important role in the health care services in the country. In order to do so effectively and efficiently, the hospitals must fall in line with India's Health Policy. If they work at cross purposes, the efforts will be counter productive and the health of the people will suffer.

A country's health policy is determined by the answers to three basic questions:
1. What kind of society do we want?
2. What are our goals, explicit and implicit?
3. Are we prepared to give priority for the implementation of our goals and provide the necessary human, financial, material and other resources?

Do we have clear cut ideas of the type of society that we would like to have? We had been striving for a democratic, secular, socialistic republic. Today, there seems to be a change in our thinking. This change could affect our health policy. We are also in the midst of globalization and commercialization. We are already seeing the effects of these changes.

Ancient systems

India's Health Policy has evolved over a long period of time. We had the heritage of an ancient civilization with Ayurveda and Siddha and similar philosophies. Ayurveda (the Science of Life) had its own theory and practices. It emphasized the need for personal codes of health and hygiene. It emphasized daily and seasonal rituals and cleanliness for the preservation and maintenance of health. The precepts have been codified by Charaka, Shusruta and others in their *samhitas*. Other systems such as Unani followed. These systems continue and flourish even now.

British Period

During the British rule, provision was made for the care of the defence personnel. This was slowly extended to the civilians. Hospitals and dispensaries (modern medicine) came to be established in many parts of the country. The health care institutions were few, accessible to a small population and used by still fewer people.

The civilian Government hospitals and dispensaries were almost completely free and catered for the poor. The standard was not high. The available health care institutions were overcrowded. The exceptions were the 'military' hospitals, which were well maintained. There was no particular health policy.

Later, public health departments were started. These took care of public health aspects (mainly hygiene) and functioned fairly well.

During the struggle for Independence, the leaders realized the need to plan the development (including health) of the country. The Sokhey Committee of the Indian National Congress worked out the details of the health plan.

The Planning Commission was established in 1950. This had health as one part of it. The First Five Year Plan was launched in 1951 with emphasis on Community Development, establishing Community Development Blocks. Health was an integral part of development. But the efforts at Community Development did not succeed because there was no Community Organization and participation by the people.

Health Survey and Development Committee (1943-1946)

Our health plans have stemmed largely from the report of 'Health Survey and Development Committee', under the chairmanship of

Sir Joseph Bhore. This report was a stupendous effort and has been responsible for guidance of our health policy over the years. The stated objectives could be summarized as follows:
1. No individual should fail to secure adequate medical care because of inability to pay for it.
2. The health services should provide all the consultant, laboratory and institutional facilities necessary for proper diagnosis and treatment.
3. The health programme must lay special emphasis on preventive work.
4. There is urgent need for providing medical relief and preventive health care to the vast rural population of the country.
5. The health services should be placed as close to the people as possible in order to ensure the maximum benefit to the communities to be served.
6. It is essential to secure the active co-operation of the people in the development of the health programmes by health education.
7. The health development schemes should be in the hands of the people's representatives.
8. The doctor of the future should be 'social physician protecting the people and guiding them to a healthier and happier life'.
9. The active support of the people is sought to be secured through health committees in every village and through stimulation of local effort.

The Bhore Committee had short term and long term comprehensive plans

Short term plan
The short term plan was for 15 years. It fixed targets to be achieved by the year 1971.

Personnel requirements

Type of personnel available	Number ratio (1946)	Existing ratio (1971)	Suggested (1946)
Doctors	47,500	1:6,000	1:2,000
Nurses	7,000	1:43,000	1:300
Health Visitors	750	1:400,000	1:5,000
Midwives	5,000	1:60,000	1:100 births
Pharmacists	75	1:4,000,000	1:6000
Dentists	1,000	1:300,000	1:4,000

Long term plan

The comprehensive long term plan, also called the Three Million Plan, aimed at a district with three million population. The Plan would have:
- Primary Unit for 20,000 population
- Secondary Unit for 600,000 population
- District organization for 3,000,000 population
- 30 bedded hospital for every 4 primary health units.
- 200 bedded hospital for a secondary unit.
- 500 bedded district hospital.

The number of hospital beds was to be raised progressively from the then existing (1946) 0.24 beds per 1000 population to 1.3 beds for 1000 population in 10 years, 2.0 beds for 1000 population in 20 years and finally to 5.67 beds for 1000 population (long term). These targets are never likely to be achieved. Even today (more than 50 years later), the ratio of hospital beds is less than 1 per 1000 population.

Health Survey and Planning Committee, 1961

Our progress in the implementation of the Bhore Committee Plan was very unsatisfactory. Government decided that it is necessary to reconsider the Plan and appointed another committee under the chairmanship of Sir A. Lakshmanaswamy Mudaliar in 1961. The Committee scaled down the Plan of the Bhore Committee. More importantly, it aimed at regionalization of health care with primary health centers, taluk hospitals, district hospitals and state level hospitals.
- Primary Health Centers : 1 for 40,000 population
  Beds : 10
  Medical Officers : 2
  Public Health Nurses : 4
  Midwives : 4

  Other technical and non-technical staff.
  Residential accommodation for all staff.
  Provision of residential accommodation was considered critical.
- Taluk hospitals : Referral center for primary health centers. It would ensure availability of staff at all times in the rural area.

Beds : 50 (minimum)
Specialists in Medicine, surgery and
Obstetrics & Gynaecology.
Other technical and non-technical staff.
- District Hospitals: Referral center for taluk hospitals
    Beds : 300-500
    Specialists in all major specialities
    District Tuberculosis Clinic
    Public Health Laboratory.
- State level hospitals   : One or more hospitals for
    —Children
    —Maternity
    —Cancer
    —Leprosy
    —Infectious diseases
    —Psychiatry
    —Eye.

The immediate target for hospital beds was fixed at 1 for 1000 population. Even this target could not be achieved.

Other Committees

Government appointed many other committees but there was poor implementation of the reports and recommendations. A committee which went mainly into hospitals and hospital beds was the Study Group on Medical Care Services, under the Chairmanship of Sri. Ajit Prasad Jain (1966). They recommended certain norms to be attained by 1971.

Hospital		Number of beds
Teaching	:	500 (to be increased based on number of students)
District	:	200 (may be increased to 300 based on population)
Taluk	:	50 (may be increased to 100)
Primary Health Center	:	6 (may be increased to 10)

The Committee suggested also the staff who should be in position.

According to the Committee, the bed : population ratio which was 0.61 per thousand in 1967 was to be raised to 0.75 per thousand in 1971 and 1 per thousand in 1976.

Other policies and influences

The New Rural Health Policy, 1977, the Alma-Ata Conference (Primary Health Care) 1978, and New Health Policy, 1982 were the major influences which tried to make an impact on the Health Policy of the country.

The health policy of a country must assure equal access to health care for all. It would be ideal if the policy can ensure utilization and outcome of the use of health care services according to the need. This would be difficult but equity requires that there is equality of access to health care services for anyone in need of the services. Such access should not depend on the ability to pay, geographical location, sex of the individual or other non-medical issues. Health care services would improve quality of life.

Health policy should, in addition to ensuring access to health care, maximise the quality of care, minimise the cost and be acceptable. The available resources are limited; hence its allocation and distribution must be just and equitable.

Society has a duty to its members to:
- Allocate an adequate share of its total resources to health related needs, such as the provision of medical services; and
- Provide a just allocation of different types of health services, including primary, secondary and tertiary care.

Many questions arise:
- What share of total resources should be allocated for servicing health care needs?
- How should such allocation be divided among the different types of health needs?
- What is an individual's fair share of such healthcare services?
- How should the cost of such services be met?
- Who should pay for them?

Hospitals and other health care institutions have an important role to play in making sure that healthcare services are made available and accessible to those who need the services. In India, we have three sectors: the Public or Governmental, the Voluntary or not-for-profit and the Private, for-profit. The health policy has to take into consideration all these sectors.

Equity of Access to Health Care

Measures of equality of access:
1. Equality of public expenditure

2. Equality of cost of health care
3. Equality of physical accessibility
4. Equality of use (the need)
5. Equality of outcome.

Equality of Public Expenditure

Allocation of the available resources to the members of the society in equal proportion. Different individuals have different health care needs. Equality of public expenditure may in reality be inequality.

Equality of Cost of Health Care

The cost of obtaining a health service should be the same for all the individuals. What about the ability to pay? Not all members of the society belong to the same economic class and have the same purchasing power. Equality of cost will result in inequality of opportunity to access.

Equality of Physical Accessibility

The distance an individual has to travel to reach a health care facility has a direct bearing on the extent to which he/she will use it. The use of health services is often a direct consequence of proximity to those resources. There is a "distance decay in the number of patients registered with a particular doctor with distance from the doctor's surgery". Travelling a long distance to make use of a health care facility will affect the actual use of it, for it involves loss of time, effort and money.

Equality of Use

Individuals will have access to health care whenever there is a medical need. Health status should determine access to health care. Often other factors determine use : availability of physicians, hospital beds, patient-doctor ratio, distance, social and cultural background, income, insurance coverage, etc; differences in attitudes toward health care; perceived subjective needs;

Equality of Outcome

May be measured in terms of age-specific death rate and life expectancies. There is no real definition of health: Clinical, physiological and biomedical measures; functional status, emotional health, social interaction, degree of disability; indicators of mortality and morbidity.

When is access to health care equal? How do we measure it? Should we allow universal access to poorer sections to all forms of available and validated health care services or only to select health services?

Targeting public spending on poorer areas with high mortality rates can bring about greater equality of health outcome.

Basic Health Care Needs

Prevention of illness through health education
Caring for the patients

Health Education

It would generate more demand for health care and minimise the burden of care by preventing illness.

Caring for the Sick

It includes listening to the patient, identifying and relieving anxiety, recognising and managing pain and other symptoms, compassimately attending to the general and specific needs of the patient and the family.

"The crisis of humane medicine is the result of the failure of secular democratic societies to inculcate moral and ethical values into their educational systems" - - S.M. Glick, Humanistic Medicine in a Modern Age, N. Engl.J.Med, April 23, 1981, 304:1038.

"Health Care differs from other societal activities in the greater expectations of the public that in addition to technical competence, personnel should have an abiding spirit of social service and should bring concern and humanity to bear on their activities. Unfortunately, the current trends in this regard are far from happy. The impersonal callousness which is bred in large hospitals is spreading and the system is getting dehumanized and even mercenary and corrupt. The public dis-satisfaction against these trends is manifest and spreading..... the only way is to reverse these trends and reinfect the health services with a spirit of service. This is partly a responsibility of training process"- - - Health for All, An alternative strategy, Report of a study group set up jointly by ICSSR and ICMR, New Delhi, 1980.

Overuse of Technology

- Financial stake of the concerned physician in referring his patients to a particular facility;
- Pressures from patients or family, peers and supervisors;
- Convenience of the tests ordered;
- Desire to avoid malpractice claims;
- Physician's personal whims and practices;
- Physician's inordinate zeal for certainty.

CONCLUSION

India had a fairly well-defined health policy but it has failed in formulating an action plan and implementing it. Hospital Administrators can play a crucial role in implementing an effective action plan with people's participation, thus ensuring better health for all the people.

Section 15: Summing Up

CHAPTER

38

Summing Up

Effective administration is a skill. You need practice; you need experience. Apply the principles, above all, apply commonsense.

Always aim higher, you will come up better. Remember your power. Do not underestimate your capacity and your powers. At the same time, do not underestimate your problems. Have faith in yourself and in your hospital "He who shoots at the sun will shoot higher than he who shoots at a tree".

You must be sincerely convinced of the merit of your hospital and what it does. If you have that conviction, it will go a long way in helping you in any aspect of administration. If there are aspects of the hospital functioning which are not up to the mark, you will take steps to improve it. You will make the place better. You will make your coworkers perform better.

Commit yourself to your hospital, to the staff working there and to the service to the people. The more committed you are to the objectives of your hospital, the more you will achieve. Get others also committed to the objectives.

Give credit to your fellow workers. Consult your colleagues. Their experience can be helpful. Let all the work be done seemingly by others. Use your authority sparingly and when truly indicated. When needed, show it with strength and vigour for the good of the institution.

Do your homework carefully. Others will then realise that you know what you are saying and what you are doing. If you have done your homework, you will be prepared to take calculated risks. You will know how much risk can be taken.

Use knowledge. Know everything about your institution. Know about your neighbouring institutions. Know about other hospitals elsewhere. Know what is happening in the field of health care all over the country. Know the National Health Policy and priorities of the Government.

Information services are available. They send, for a small consideration, clippings from newspapers. Subscribe for one of them. These will keep you updated. Do not forget to read them at the first opportunity. If you keep them aside to be read when you have leisure, you may not read them at all.

Important

Distinguish between what is 'important' and what is 'urgent'. The urgent will anyway be got done. It is essential that the administrator devotes sufficient time and energy for what is important.

Setting Priorities

You must set your priorities. These would depend on the goals and objectives. How important is each one of them? How quickly should each be done? Is the way you have planned it, the best way of getting it accomplished?

Index

A

ABC analysis 261
Abortion 351
Activity based costing 293
Acts 356
Administrator 7
   Role profile 12
Advertisements, unethical 346
Agent of change 5
Appraisal 234
   by objectives 242
   conflicts in 245
   critical incident 240
   forced choice rating 241
   forced distribution 238
   format 237
   free written ratings 237
   graphic rating scale 239
   interview 243
   ranking methods 238
Appraiser 234
Assets 291

B

Balance sheet 291
   assets 291
   liabilities 292
Bhore committee 373
Biodata 224
Brain storming 62
Budget 274
   appropriation 243
   capital 277
   cash 277
   operating 275
Buzz group 62

C

Capital 277
Cash budget 277
Casualty 138
   management problems 146
   medical officer 147
   objectives 139
Central sterile suppy 334
Committees 93
   administrative 94
   blood utilization 100
   infection control 338
   quality assurance 96
   theatre users 99
Communication 31
Confidentiality 345
Confidential record 225
Consumer Protection Act 359
Cost, centres 298
   consciousness 294
   factors 297
Cross-infection 339
CSSD 334

D

Day care 163
Decision making 41
Delegation 37, 83
Demand forecasting 250
Depreciation 284
   accelerated 286
   straight line 285
Diagnostic services 180
   physical facilities 182
   problems 184
Diary 56
Disagreement 72
Disaster 150
Discussion leader 73
Drugs and pharmaceuticals 347
Drugs and therapeutics
      committee 205
   functions 205
Drugs information centre 213

E

Economic order quantity 20
Endowment fund 241
Equity 349, 377
Ethics 341
Euthanasia 352
Evaluation 49
Expenditure 278
   containment 280
   control 281, 286
   capital 278
   direct 279
   fixed 278
   indirect 279
   recurring 278
   variable 279

F

Failure 4
Fertility, control of, 350
Finances 271
   internal control 286
Financial information 286
Financial
   objectives 272
   planning 273
Foeticide, female 271
Formulary 207
FSN analysis 262

G

Governing body 86
Group behaviour 61

H

Health care statistics 197
Health policy 371
Health Survey and Development committee 373
Health Survey and Planning committee 374
Hospital acquired
   infection 329
   prevention 332

Hospital Committees 93
Hospital, Organisation 76
   matrix 81
   tall and flat 81
Hospital, types 77
Human resources 221

I

Income and expenditure 289
Incompetance 265
Infanticide 352
Infection control 329
   committee 338
Information 24
Informed consent 343
Information flow 27
Innovation 67
Interview 223
Inventory conrol 257
   physical 263
   turnover 263

L

Laws 355
Leading 15
Liabilities 292

M

Maintenance 265
Management audit 268
Managerial functions 15
Manuals
   nursing 124
Materials management 247
   budgeting and planning 249
   demand forecasting 250
   issue/distribution 138
   objectives 248
Medical records 185
Medical staff 107
Meetings 58
Microbiology 228
Minutes 62
Monitoring 46

N

National Health Policy 379
Negligence 359
Negotiations 64
Nosocomial infection 217
Nurses
 responsibilities 132
Nursing administration 126
Nursin audit 137
Nursing service 124

O

Objectives 75
Operating budget 244
Operating department 171
Organisation 75
Organ transplants 353
Outpatients 155
 facilities 156
 location 155
 objectives 155
 problems 159

P

People's problems 225
Performance appraisal 234
Personnel 221
 appointment 224
 interview 223
 recuritment 222
 selection 222
 training 225
Personnel Officer 232
Pharmacy 204
 committee 103, 205
 equipment 216
 functions 205
 objectives 204
 orders 209
 physical facilities 215
Pilferage 211, 267
Planning 19
 operational 20
 strategic 20

Problem people 226
Problem analysis 20
Procurement of materials 251
 committee 105

Q

Quality 305, 315
Quality management 315
 techniques 319
 tools 323
Quality care constraints 310

R

Rare setting 282, 294
Rational drug use 146
Recruitment 222
Retraining 230
Right to health 348
Right to life 350

S

Selection 222
Sex pre-selection 351
Storage 210, 256

T

Team 9
Terminally ill 353
Theatre design 172
Theatre materials 176
Theatre staffing 177
Time 52
Tumor Board 102

U

User fee 296

V

VED analysis 262

EU GSPR Authorised Reprsentative
Logos Europe, 9 rue Nicolas Poussin
1700, La Rochelle, France
Phone: +33 (0) 6 67 93 73 78
E-mail: contact@logoseurope.eu

www.ingramcontent.com/pod-product-compliance
Ingram Content Group UK Ltd.
Pitfield, Milton Keynes, MK11 3LW, UK
UKHW021837210426
5322IPUK00021B/339